Care of
the arthritic hand

ADRIAN E. FLATT, M.D., M.Chir., F.R.C.S., F.A.C.S.

Clinical Professor, Division of Orthopedic Surgery,
University of Texas Southwestern Medical School;
Hunterian Professor of Royal College of Surgeons of England; Chairman,
Department of Orthopaedics, Baylor University Medical Center, Dallas, Texas;
Civilian National Consultant to U.S. Air Force in Hand Surgery;
Past President, American Society for Surgery of the Hand; Past
President, Midwestern Association of Plastic Surgeons

FOURTH EDITION

with **314** illustrations

Foreword by
Russell L. Cecil, M.D.

The C. V. Mosby Company

ST. LOUIS • TORONTO • LONDON   1983

MOSBY

A TRADITION OF PUBLISHING EXCELLENCE

Editor: Eugenia A. Klein
Assistant editor: Jean F. Carey
Manuscript editor: Carol Claverie
Book design: Susan Trail
Cover design: Suzanne Oberholtzer
Production: Kathleen L. Teal

FOURTH EDITION

The C.V. Mosby Company
11830 Westline Industrial Drive, St. Louis, Missouri 63141

Library of Congress Cataloging in Publication Data

Flatt, Adrian E.
  Care of the arthritic hand.
  Rev. ed. of: The care of the rheumatoid hand.
3rd ed. 1974.
  Bibliography: p.
  Includes index.
  1. Hand—Surgery. 2. Rheumatoid arthritis—
Surgery. I. Title. [DNLM: 1. Arthritis—Surgery.
2. Hand—Surgery. WE 830 F586ca]
RD778.F53 1982   616.7′22   82-6428
ISBN 0-8016-1585-2   AACR2

TS/CB/B 9 8 7 6 5 4 3   01/A/001

Foreword to first edition

Rheumatoid arthritis presents a difficult therapeutic problem to the physician—so difficult that the combined skills of the rheumatologist, orthopaedist, and physiatrist may be essential to the achievement of best results. In this timely monograph Dr. Flatt, in discussing reconstructive surgery of the rheumatoid hand, points out that although the development of new drugs and the evolution of specialists in arthritis have tended to overshadow the surgeon's role in the care of this disease, both the medical and the surgical approach are needed in most cases. This is particularly true today when such rapid advances are being made in the field of surgical rehabilitation of the rheumatoid hand and foot.

This informative monograph includes a review of the general principles of surgery of the rheumatoid hand, with emphasis on the importance of early intervention.

The importance of both physical therapy and occupational therapy preoperatively and postoperatively is stressed. Since early recognition of disturbance of hand function is essential, it is more logical to perform early surgery and prevent deformity than to do a radical salvage procedure later on a disease-ravaged hand.

The author points out the frequency of tenosynovitis of the fingers in the incipient stages of rheumatoid arthritis and its relation to later deformities. He states that surgery can be of great benefit in treating disease of the tendons and their synovial sheaths if the diseased synovium is removed before secondary changes have occurred. An interesting chapter on prosthetic surgery of the joints and arthroplasty of digital joints is included.

I am much interested in Dr. Flatt's discussion of ulnar deviation and his statement that the majority of cases of ulnar drift could be easily corrected to the midline. (Internists take heed!) There is an entire chapter on the dysfunctions and deformities of the thumb.

The final chapter deals with the nonoperative treatment of the rheumatoid hand, mostly splinting and physical and occupational therapy.

Altogether this is a most readable and informative book, full of useful practical knowledge for both rheumatologist and surgeon. I would consider it a privilege to have Dr. Flatt at my elbow when planning therapeutic procedures for a rheumatoid patient!

Rheumatology needs more specialists in this field, in some respects a narrow one, but so important in the rehabilitation of the rheumatoid patient.

Russell L. Cecil, M.D.

Preface

Never ask me what I have said, or
what I have written. But if you
ask me what my present opinions are
. . . I will tell you.

John Hunter

On June 14, 1962, I was privileged to deliver before the Royal College of Surgeons of England a Hunterian Lecture entitled "The Surgical Rehabilitation of the Rheumatoid Hand." I chose the above quotation by John Hunter for my lecture and for the first edition of this book because I believed it very aptly described the situation at that time regarding the care of the rheumatoid hand. Twenty years later a fourth edition of the book is necessary, and the implication in John Hunter's words is still valid.

The scope of improvement that surgical care of the rheumatoid hand provides is at last well established and needs no excuses or apologies for its employment. It is sad that our colleagues in internal medicine and rheumatology have not yet generally accepted the concept of early surgical consultation. It is easier to provide prolonged improvement early in the disease than it is to attempt salvage surgery after the devastating effects of the biomechanical imbalances have been established.

I believe a major factor in the improved results that are now being obtained is the evolution of a strong cadre of hand therapists. The help of these dedicated professionals in the postoperative care of patients is essential to a good result, and I regard them as an integral part of the therapeutic team.

This edition has been changed both in content and in title. I have introduced in the appropriate chapters descriptions of other arthritic conditions of the hand. These new portions are not meant to be exhaustive, but I have tried to include sufficient material to aid in differential diagnosis and in the operative care of these allied conditions. To compensate for these added pages, I have ruthlessly pruned out-of-date illustrations and text; despite this the number of pages and of illustrations has slightly increased.

I have maintained the format and order of chapters of the previous edition and have once again placed ulnar drift as the last chapter because an understanding of this compound deformity is really a synthesis of the whole book. I trust my style of writing does not offend; I have tried to make this a reasonable book, and I humbly submit it is no sin to deliberately split an infinitive. I am aware that lay people read this book; one excellent hand therapist tells me that three copies of the previous edition have been worn out by her patients as they learn about their disease. This is excellent. I do not believe that this book should be a closed trade treatise; I would hope that all who are interested in these conditions would be able to understand the concepts behind the suggested treatment.

It is impossible to name all those who have worked with me and helped me over these twenty years to gather this material about these varied conditions. The questions and the criticisms of my fellows and therapists have increased my understanding of these problems, which has been distilled into this edition; but I am solely responsible for it.

Adrian E. Flatt

Contents

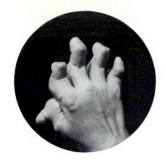

General principles of care

Arthritis is a symptom of over 100 diseases, and in a number of these diseases the hands are severely affected. In many patients the diagnosis is obvious from the characteristic patterns of involvement of the joints of the hand. The two major diseases to affect the hand are osteoarthritis and rheumatoid disease. Several other less common arthritides and collagen diseases also have a significant effect on the hand, amongst which are gout, systemic lupus erythematosus, psoriasis, scleroderma, mixed connective tissue disease, and hemochromatosis. These conditions are fully described in the appropriate specialized texts and are only discussed here in relation to their effect on the hand.

ROLE OF SURGERY

Many types of therapy, none of which is perfect, should be used to combat the symptoms of arthritis. Surgery is certainly not a cure. It must be regarded as only one of the available methods of treatment. Although surgery can alleviate symptoms, correct deformities, and restore function, it should not be advised hastily; the indications must be clearly established.

John Hunter has been aptly described as "the reluctant surgeon." He would never sanction surgery until he was sure that the failure of other methods of treatment had made surgery necessary. He used to tell his pupils, "If the disease is already formed, we ought to know the modes of action in the body and the parts, in their endeavor to relieve themselves; the powers they have of restoring themselves, and the means of assisting those powers. Or, if these prove insufficient, we judge, by all the attending circumstances, how far excision may be necessary, and what condition is most favorable for an operation. To determine on this last point is exceedingly difficult, and in some instances, exceeds our present knowledge."*

We have now gathered sufficient knowledge of the various forms of arthritis and its "modes of action in the body and the parts" to be able to define the role of surgery in the restoration of function. The actual operation is a small part of proper surgical care, which does not cease when the wound is sewn up. The operation can be successful only when combined with many other methods of treatment. Hand therapy may be a valuable part of the preoperative and postoperative care of an arthritic patient. Some believe it is possible to modify and reduce the extent of the operative plan because of successful therapy. Most of the late reconstructive procedures for the rheumatoid hand restore little more than basic functions and depend on postoperative therapy to achieve the maximum result.

An operative plan that does not consider recommendations for both preoperative and postoperative hand therapy is inadequate. For some patients it is wise to consult the social welfare agencies and the local counselor of the Vocational Rehabilitation Administration. One can then be certain that the results of the operation and therapy will be permanent improvement.

RECORDING OF FUNCTION

Probably the hardest task for surgeons working in the field of functional restoration is to produce an unbiased comparison of their patients' functional abilities before and after surgery. The surgeons' overconscientious desire to be objective produces harsh judgments that only too often clash with the somewhat rosy answers offered by loyal and anxious patients. Nurses and therapists are usually just as loyal, and their opinions of the surgical results are therefore equally suspect.

Despite all these problems, it is important that the results of treatment be expressed in terms of measurements that are generally acceptable and that avoid the ambiguity of words such as "good," "satisfactory," or "poor."

I make considerable use of photographic records and use a standard ordering sheet to obtain consistently comparable views (Fig. 1-1). In an attempt to be as objective as possible, I evolved a testing booklet that incorporated many of the more commonly used tests of hand function. The material finally selected for inclusion in the booklet was divided into the following four major sections:
1. Information about the patient and the therapeutic procedures used
2. Range of motion of various joints
3. Hand position and strength tests
4. Functional or "activities of daily living" tasks

The number of tests was large, and the booklet was designed as an experimental tool; it was not intended for use in everyday clinical practice. The format of the booklet was designed to allow a logical arrangement of data that could be readily transferred to punch cards and studied on a computer. More than 200 booklets were analyzed and subjected to various statistical studies.

---

*Kobler, J.: The reluctant surgeon, a biography of John Hunter, New York, 1960, Doubleday & Co., Inc., p. 165.

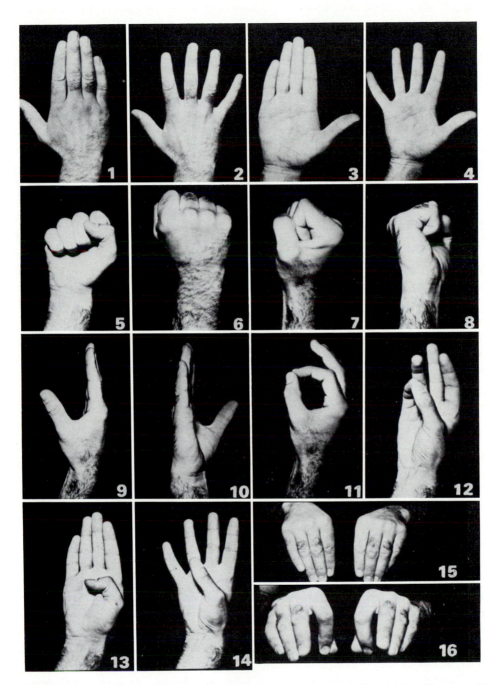

Fig. 1-1. Photographic records. Standardized positions for recording patients' hand deformities are useful for continuing comparative studies of the state of the hands.

The most important conclusion from this study was that the data in these 200 booklets do not show any direct correlation between the ranges of motion and the patient's ability to perform the functional assessment tasks. We had hoped that decreased anatomical range of motion might be significantly related to performance and that we would thus be able to derive some idea of disability from range-of-motion studies. In addition, we were unable to show that a limited selection of range-of-motion tests could be routinely used to predict a patient's ability to perform various functional tasks.

Despite these somewhat depressing results from our investigation, I believe that some form of standardized but simple testing must be developed for the periodical assessment of hand function. Many valiant attempts have been made to develop such a test but none has proved generally acceptable, and most hand surgeons have perforce developed record sheets for patient assessment of their own.

THE OSTEOARTHRITIC HAND

Osteoarthritis is not a systemic inflammatory disorder, but a strictly localized reactive reparative process occurring in one or several joints. Why it happens is not known, nor can its tendency to symmetrically involve the hands and to occur more commonly in postmenopausal women be fully explained. All men and women over the age of 60 show physical or radiological evidence of osteoarthritis, but only a quarter of the women and about 15% of the men are symptomatic. In some of the men the changes are occupational (Fig. 1-2). The degenerative changes in the hand most commonly affect the carpometacarpal joints of the thumb; the distal interphalangeal joints, causing Heberden's nodes; and the proximal interphalangeal joints (Bouchard's nodes).

Lewis Millender has pointed out that osteoarthritic patients tend to fall into one of three groups. The majority are in the first group, which includes involvement of the distal interphalangeal joints of the fingers and the presence of Heberden's nodes. Generalized osteoarthritis is the hallmark of the second group, with involvement of the distal interphalangeal joints and the carpometacarpal joint of the thumb; the proximal interphalangeal joints are only rarely involved. The third and least common group comprises those who develop erosive osteoarthritis of both rows of the interphalangeal joints.

The earlier stages of osteoarthritis are shown by a quarter to half an hour of morning stiffness of the interphalangeal joints; some reduction of joint space, which may be seen on x-ray films; and, often, soreness at the base of the thumb and weakness of pinch. Frequently, painful crepitation can be felt during both active and passive thumb motion. The osteoarthritic hand in the earlier stages responds well to conservative therapy consisting of education, medication, and splinting. Each patient must be taught that crippling is not inevitable, that osteoarthritis is different from rheumatoid disease, and that an arthritic joint must be moved to prevent stiffness. Movement must be judicious; some patients will aggressively overexercise while others will postpone activity as long as possible. Salicylates are still probably the best drug to use, but there are now a variety of nonsteroid antiinflammatory preparations that can be tried. Splinting is used to help patients through acute episodes of the

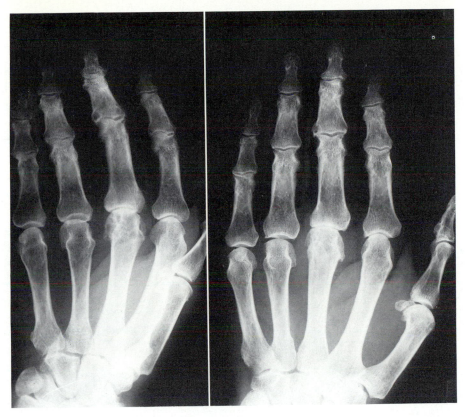

Fig. 1-2. Osteoarthritis of fingers. This professional wrestler's hand shows the results of repeated traumatic insults to the digital joints. (From Flatt, A.E.: Correction of arthritis deformities of the upper extremity. In McCarty, D.J., Jr.: Arthritic and allied conditions, ed. 9, Philadelphia, 1979, Lea & Febiger.)

disease—usually in the distal interphalangeal joints of the fingers and the basal joint of the thumb.

A small proportion of osteoarthritic hands require surgical treatment. The distal interphalangeal joints of the fingers often benefit from fusion and restoration of the digit contour. A few of these joints have been treated by implanting silicone substitutes, but the indications are not yet defined. I join with Dr. Millender in his reluctance to simply remove swellings and osteophytes; I have seen disasterous results from this type of surgery. The pain of degenerative changes in the proximal interphalangeal joints can be treated either by fusion or by prosthetic replacement. I tend to prefer fusion for the index finger because of the vital need for pinch stability. On occasion, however, I have inserted a prosthesis in this finger and in all the others. The basal joint of the thumb can and often should be replaced by a prosthesis when it is worn out and impairing hand function. Various methods are discussed in Chapter 9.

Erosive osteoarthritis

Erosive osteoarthritis is an inflammatory form of polyarthritis said to affect women in the postmenopausal age group, but it can also begin in the late 30's and early 40's.

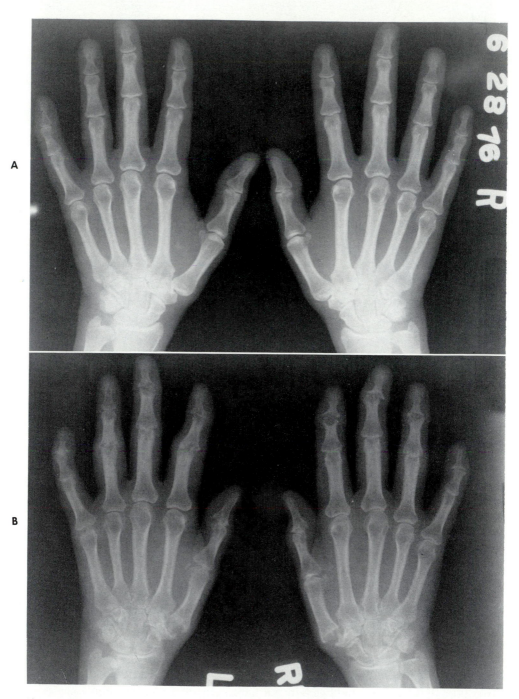

Fig. 1-3. Erosive osteoarthritis. **A,** In 1976 this woman's hands began to ache; these films were then taken. **B,** Three years later this devastating destruction had occurred.

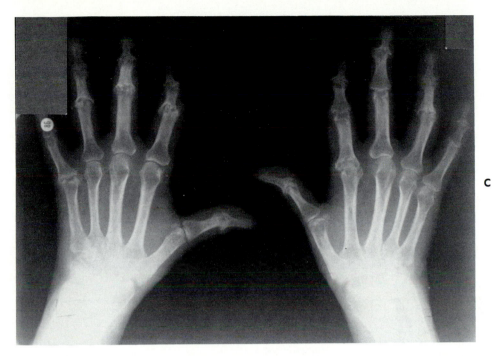

C

Fig. 1-3, cont'd. C, In 1981 the destroyed carpometacarpal joints of both thumbs were replaced with Neibauer prostheses; she continues to work as an executive secretary.

It is thought to be self-limiting over a period of about 10 years. Erosive osteoarthritis causes extensive destruction of articular cartilage and the subcondral bone, but in the early stages the characteristic marginal erosions seen in rheumatoid disease are not present. The metacarpophalangeal joints, which are commonly involved in rheumatoid disease, are rarely, if ever, affected by erosive changes. The principal changes occur in the proximal and distal interphalangeal joints, but the basal joint of the thumb is also commonly attacked (Fig. 1-3).

THE RHEUMATOID HAND

The late Dr. Philip Ellman, when teaching students "the rudiments of the art, science, and practice of rheumatology" always stressed the term *rheumatoid disease*, insisting that many tissues of the body were affected—not only the bones and joints. This is particularly true of the hand, in which every constituent tissue can be affected by the disease.

The long-term clinical course has been shown by Smyth to follow one of three basic patterns (Fig. 1-4). Unfortunately, we cannot accurately predict the incidence or duration of the remissions; nor can we predict the rate of progressive destruction of structures vital to the maintenance of hand function.

We have, however, accumulated sufficient knowledge to be able to forecast the final results of seemingly mild degrees of involvement of the hand. These results are so often crippling that there is no justification for a policy of "wait and see" such as was used for the patients shown in the opening illustration and in Fig. 1-5. Adequate

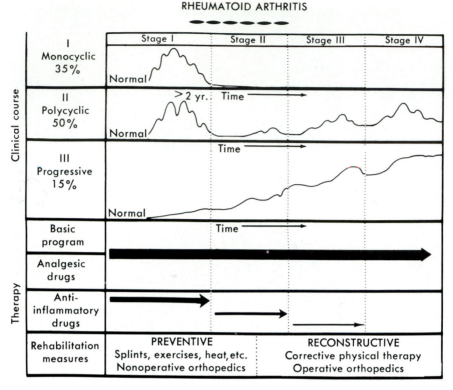

Fig. 1-4. Course of rheumatoid disease. The upper half shows three hypothetical clinical courses of rheumatoid disease, with early disease (Stage I) on the left and more advanced stages extending toward the right. Increases and decreases in disease activity are shown in the perpendicular axis, and time along the horizontal axis. The relationship of therapy to clinical course and stage is shown in the bottom half of the chart. Note that under Rehabilitation measures a dotted line in the area of Stage II separates nonoperative and operative orthopedics. The changing climate of medical opinion and Dr. Smyth's gracious permission have allowed me to shift this line to the left compared to its original position in the 1968 illustration. (From Smyth, C.J.: Med. Clin. North Am. **52**:687-698, 1968.)

surgical care of patients with rheumatoid disease is possible only if they are seen early in the development of their disease, are operated on as the indications become established, and are reviewed at regular intervals for long periods of time.

Sones has stressed that modern therapy of the disease requires a multidisciplinary approach. He correctly predicted that surgical treatment is destined to play an increasing part in the prevention and correction of the resultant deformities. The best interests of the patient are served when the particular skills of rheumatologist, surgeon, physiatrist, and therapist are used "in a flexible cooperative interplay of judgment and skills." Many centers have now achieved this liaison. Encouraging results are being obtained from the pooling of professional opinions regarding the suitability of different treatments.

The most urgent problem in the care of the rheumatoid hand is the early institution of various forms of preventive treatment. Correct treatment cannot be given

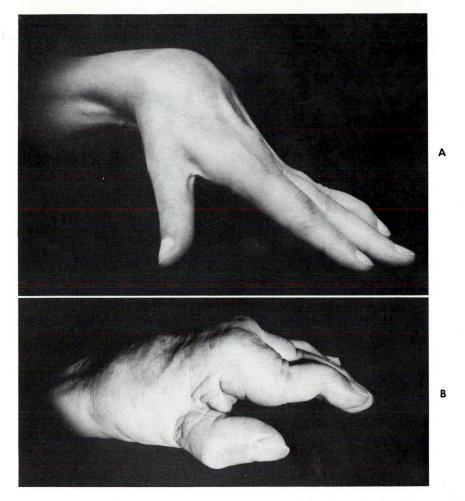

Fig. 1-5. "Wait and see." **A** and **B,** Ten years elapsed between these pictures. The diagnosis of rheumatoid disease was established at the time photograph **A** was taken. The patient was referred for "surgical treatment" at the time photograph **B** was taken.

unless the signs of early deterioration of function are recognized. It is impossible to treat diseases of the hand effectively without this basic knowledge. Early deterioration of hand function can be diagnosed only if normal patterns of use are understood. Because of the fundamental importance of understanding the anatomy of hand movement, the next chapter is devoted to its normal and abnormal kinesiology.

A deformity of the hand or an alteration of the kinesthetic balance must be fully understood before the correct treatment can be given. In his excellent discussion on dynamic factors in the deformity of the rheumatoid arthritic hand, Swezey has compared attempts to explain such deformities on the basis of single derangements to the 10 blind men describing an elephant by what each could feel. Deformities frequently can be corrected by surgery, but surgery must not be regarded as curative, however, since the dynamic state of the hand may be altered by the progression of the disease. The distressing fact is that this change in the dynamic state of the hand may so alter the surgical results in later years that occasionally the last state of the hand is worse than the first.

Within the hand, the basic tissue attacked is synovium; any joint changes that occur are the secondary result of a primary synovitis. Disease of the synovium affects the hand at two major sites, the extrinsic tendons and the digital joints. The synovial tissue expands from a membrane a few cells thick into a florid, villous mass many thousand times thicker. This swelling will occur wherever there is synovial tissue and is especially significant within the confined spaces beneath the extensor and flexor retinacula, within the flexor tendon sheaths, and within the capsules of the joints. The increase in tension caused by this swelling produces secondary effects on the structures in close contact with the swelling.

On the extensor surface of the hand the tendons beneath the retinaculum are directly invaded by disease or may undergo aseptic necrosis from obliteration of their blood supply. Similar changes occur in the flexor tendons, and, in addition, signs and symptoms of median nerve compression may be produced. Within the joints the swelling synovium distorts and destroys the supporting structures, causing subluxation and dislocation.

Prophylactic synovectomy would seem to be an admirable way of controlling this disease. Unfortunately, most patients are still seen far too late in the progression of their disease for prophylaxis to be truly possible, and most surgery is still performed on a catch-up basis.

In view of the episodic nature of the disease in most patients, proponents of prophylactic surgery are hard put to prove that an operation is entitled to full credit for any improvement in symptoms and signs. Some small collaborative controlled studies have been done in both the United Kingdom and the United States. Their results would seem to imply that there is little or no advantage to synovectomy. However, I strongly agree with Nalebuff who demonstrated the great difficulties encountered in attempting to maintain valid controls. He and I have been obligated to terminate prematurely a trial of unilateral operations because the hand not operated on—the control hand—had deteriorated rapidly while the synovectomized hand retained good function.

Both Lipscomb and Moberg deplore the use of the word *prophylactic*; the former advocates the phrase *arrestive synovectomy*, and the latter uses the term *preventive synovectomy*. Synovectomy done to prevent deformity from either occurring or increasing has merit, even though it is too late to be truly prophylactic. Fig. 1-6 from Moberg's paper is an illustration of the constant dilemma of the surgeon caring for the rheumatoid hand, the intermediate gray zone between preventive and reconstructive surgery. We are now seeing many more patients whose hands fall into this gray zone and for whom it is extremely difficult to select suitable therapeutic measures. I still confess to a general leaning toward conservatism in regard to these patients and advise surgery only when I believe it can restore a specifically requested absent function or when I can identify a significant threat of early functional deterioration.

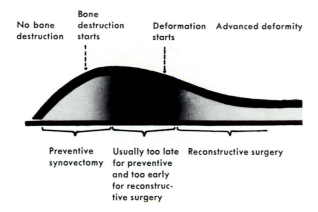

Fig. 1-6. The "gray zone." The intermediate phase of disease, in which it is hard to define the role of surgery since it is neither truly preventive or reconstructive. (From Moberg, E.: Early synovectomy in rheumatoid arthritis, Amsterdam, 1967, Excerpta Medica Foundation, p. 176.)

Many factors influence the decision to operate; some have virtue, others are part of the mythology that seems to surround this disease. It is clearly unwise to subject patients to elective surgery during an acute exacerbation of their general disease. On the other hand, I have never followed the theory that surgery should be delayed until the disease is quiescent and the sedimentation rate has fallen in order to decrease the risk of precipitating an acute exacerbation of the disease. High sedimentation rates and local signs of active inflammation have been ignored. In no instance has the disease been aggravated by surgery, and I believe that the sedimentation rate should not influence a decision to operate.

It is often said that patients with rheumatoid disease are poor subjects for surgery, but there is little to suggest that persons with early rheumatoid disease are psychologically different from normal persons. However, a surgeon must understand his patient's psychological response to the disease. I agree with Dr. Paul Brown, who maintains that many rheumatoid patients are unusual in their cheerful disposition and that their characterization as people who are depressed, complaining, and pessimistic is often a reflection of the physcian's attitude to the disease. Because of the capricious and unpredictable nature of the disease, one would expect rheumatoid patients to be "a dour, discouraged group and a depressing bunch to work with." He does not, and neither do I. The patient with osteoarthritis often fits this picture but only occasionally can the rheumatoid patient be characterized this way.

It is pointless to try to "sell" a patient an operation; the long-term results are far too uncertain to justify the exertion of any pressure. It has been my policy, whenever possible, to encourage potential candidates for surgery to meet others who have had the proposed operation. A demonstration of the results that can be achieved is often more helpful than any amount of theoretical discussion. Although the long-term results of surgery are often unfavorably influenced by progression of the disease, it is essential to avoid the "5-year cure" outlook of ablative surgery. Operations are completely justified if significant improvement is provided for even such short periods of time as 6 months or a year.

JUVENILE RHEUMATOID ARTHRITIS

Between 50% and 70% of children with juvenile rheumatoid arthritis will eventually go into remission. But the child with serious juvenile rheumatoid arthritis will have more stiffness, loss of motion, and ankylosis than an adult.

One of the earliest clinical signs of disease in the hand is a small loss of complete extension of the wrist, followed by ulnar deviation, and later by limited flexion of both the metacarpophalangeal and proximal interphalangeal joints. Granberry and Mangum believe that the main thrust of management should be to allow intercarpal and perhaps radiocarpal fusion to take place while splinting the wrist in a neutral functional position. A home program of therapy for the maintenance of digital motion is essential, and the patient's parents must be trained by the hand therapist.

In a growing child, many reconstructive procedures that are used in adults are not applicable because of the risk of producing epiphyseal arrest. The surgeon who treats a child with rheumatoid disease should do so conservatively, as surgery is rarely indicated. Digital joint synovectomy may have a place, but I believe that the risk of epiphyseal arrest is severe if joint clearance is done thoroughly. The nutrient artery to the growth plate runs subsynovially and can be easily damaged, either by surgery or by an expanding rheumatoid synovitis. I use thiotepa injections to reduce and control the synovitis more frequently than I do a synovectomy. When an expanding synovitis threatens to or has actually weakened the extensor mechanism, synovectomy can be reasonably combined with surgical repair of the tendons.

ARTHRITIS IN OTHER CONDITIONS
Gout

Gout is not a serious problem in the United States today; it is said to affect four people per 1000. It is 20 times more common in men, and the attacks are said to be more frequent in those who consume large quantities of beer. The wrist and fingers are one of the last sites to be involved. X-ray findings do not usually show positive indications until patients have had symptomatic gout for many years.

Both Riordan and Straub have reviewed gout as it affects the hand and find little indication for surgical intervention. Occasionally the tophi become so huge that the removal of these mechanical obstructions is justified. Draining sinuses and their causative tophi may also need to be excised. Considerable symptomatic relief can be achieved by aspiration of any tense joint effusions. Nowadays resorption of urate deposits can be accomplished with drugs, and remodeling and repair of damaged bones is often dramatic.

Occasionally I have had to fuse interphalangeal joints that have been destroyed and become unstable. I have never replaced such a joint with a prosthesis and do not know of any published reports of such an operation.

Systemic lupus erythematosus

Systemic lupus erythematosus commonly involves the hand but in a form different from that of rheumatoid disease. Raynaud's phenomenon is present in about half of the cases, and articular destruction and joint ankylosis do not occur. The skin of the hand is usually tight and the sensory examination normal. Aseptic necrosis of the carpal bones is not common. Deformities result from laxity of the supporting soft tissue structures; swan-neck deformities without tight intrinsics and hyperextension of the thumb interphalangeal joint are characteristic findings. The primary cause of disability in the hand is more frequently the result of Raynaud's phenomenon rather than of deformities caused by ligamentous laxity.

Psoriasis

There is no entirely satisfactory definition of psoriatic arthritis, and the true association of psoriasis and arthritis of the hand is hard to establish. It is known that 5% to 10% of patients with rheumatoid disease have psoriasis. It is also known that radiological changes typically seen in psoriatic arthritis precede the skin lesions in 10% of patients who eventually develop psoriasis.

The diagnosis of psoriatic arthritis rather than rheumatoid disease is usually considered when (1) the seronegative nodule-free patient has psoriasis, however mildly, and (2) the disease is patchy in distribution, less symmetrical, less aggressively progressive, and has attacked the distal interphalangeal joints of the hands in addition to other joints.

Clinically there is excessive fibrous tissue around the joints, and the metacarpophalangeal joints of the hand are stiff and flexed. There may be severe overriding of the bones, and the medullary canals of the metacarpals are small in diameter. There is much less synovial proliferation than in rheumatoid disease, but destruction of articular cartilage and subchondral bone does occur.

The excessive fibrous tissue around the digital joints can resemble the picture of Jaccoud's syndrome that is described by Bywaters as a postrheumatic chronic polyarthrosis. In this condition, there may be a history of recurrent attacks of rheumatic fever followed by the insidious development of symptomless ulnar deviation of the metacarpophalangeal joints without impairment of function. A characteristic "hook lesion," described by Bywaters in 1950, is seen in the sides of the metacarpal heads.

Radiologically, psoriatic arthritis is characteristically asymmetrical and often unilateral. It can also involve only the bones of a single digital ray. Malalignments of the digital joints is common, and subluxation occurs.

The results of surgery are not impressive. Fusion of individual joints may be helpful, but, in general, the results of soft tissue operations and joint replacements are less satisfactory than when done in rheumatoid disease.

Scleroderma

The soft tissue atrophy of the fingertips that occurs in scleroderma is usually associated with neurovascular disturbances such as Raynaud's phenomenon. Calcification of the fingertip pulp is common in scleroderma. When calcinosis occurs, about half the cases are associated with scleroderma or some other collagen disease and with Raynaud's phenomenon.

Absorption of the distal tufts of the terminal phalanges is the most common bony abnormality seen on x-ray examination. Articular bone or cartilage destruction is seen occasionally, the absorption of bone usually involving the middle and proximal phalanges.

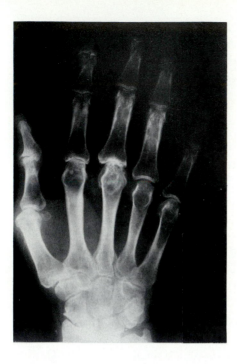

Fig. 1-7. Hemochromatosis. This surgeon's right hand has significant functional impairment because of multiple joint involvement, particularly of the metacarpophalangeal joints of the index and long fingers.

There appears to be a general drying out of the soft tissues of the hand in this condition. I have found that intrinsic muscle release may be of help as well as excision of symptomatic calcifications to improve hand function.

Mixed connective tissue disease

The hands of these patients differ from the hands of individuals with systemic lupus, rheumatoid disease, or scleroderma. The characteristic finding is a tightness in the flexors unassociated with skin or joint tightness. Occasionally tightness of the intrinsic muscles occurs. Steroid therapy is said to be helpful, and surgery may be needed to release adhesions, which occur in a high percentage of cases, between the superficialis and profundus tendons.

Hemochromatosis

A rare but important form of arthritis is that associated with hemochromatosis. Half of these patients will have arthralgia and arthritis with their hands characteristically affected. The proximal interphalangeal, metacarpophalangeal, and radiocarpal joints are all involved, and the triangular cartilage at the wrist may be calcified. Symptoms usually begin in the metacarpophalangeal joints, spread through the hand, and rapidly cause significant loss of function. I have seen few cases but, to my chagrin, have been sensitized to the diagnosis by missing it in the hands of a surgical colleague (Fig. 1-7).

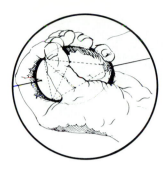

CHAPTER 2

Kinesiology

Bones of the hand
The wrist joint

Joints of the digits
Finger joints
Thumb joints

The hand in use
Anatomical patterns of prehension
Fingers in prehension
Functional patterns of prehension

Balance of muscle power within the hand

The posture of the normal hand is the result of the forces acting within it. Abnormal postures arising after the onset of rheumatoid disease have traditionally been described as bilaterally symmetrical. Such a generalization has little merit for a disease that is notorious for the variability of its intensity and of the sites it attacks. The patient's hands seen in Fig. 2-1 demonstrate different deformities in virtually all the fingers. Each deformity has developed in conformity with simple mechanical laws, but because selective and varying degrees of destruction by disease have produced different dynamic imbalances, the end results are asymmetrical.

The prime task in the assessment of deformity is the correlation of the anatomical and functional disturbances within the whole limb. The correction of hand deformities is pointless unless the proximal joints of the limb will allow the hand to be placed in a working area. In the normal limb the precise placing of the hand is largely controlled by the multiaxial wrist joint, after the grosser placement has been achieved by the shoulder and elbow.

A knowledge of the dynamic anatomy of the hand is fundamental in the recognition of factors that upset the normal muscle balance, produce the deformities, and thereby destroy function.

BONES OF THE HAND

Structurally, the hand consists of a linked system of longitudinal bony segments that are arranged in a series of integrated arches, the concavities of which face toward the palm, forming the hand into a cup (Fig. 2-2). The depth of the cup is varied by the controlled mobility of the fingers and the two borders of the hand. The thumb contributes the greater part of the border mobility because it can separate widely from

Chapter opening illustration from Littler, J.W.: On the adaptability of man's hand, The Hand **5**:187-191, 1973

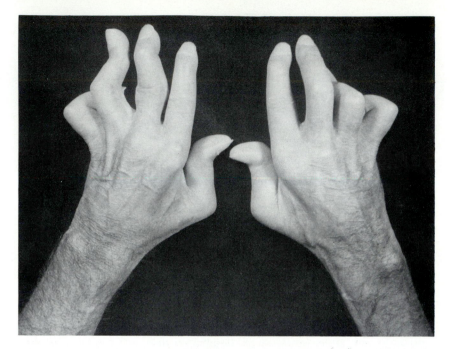

Fig. 2-1. Asymmetrical deformities. This patient's hands demonstrate different degrees of deformity in each of the fingers. Thus to say that rheumatoid disease is symmetrical is to make a generalization without merit.

the palm and swing around in front of, and oppose, any of the fingers. Mobility on the ulnar border is supplied by movement of the fourth and fifth metacarpals at their carpometacarpal joints. For control of the movement of the two borders, the metacarpals are slung from a centrally placed rigid pillar consisting of the metacarpals of the index and long fingers (Fig. 2-3). The thumb is connected to this rigid pillar by the intrinsic muscles, and the ulnar fingers are connected by the transverse intermetacarpal ligaments.

Although the extrinsic flexor and extensor muscles are largely responsible for altering the shape of the working hand, it is the intrinsic muscles that are responsible for maintaining the integrity of the arch system.

Movement of the borders of the hand passes through the mobile transverse arch at the level of the metacarpal heads. It is the mobility of this arch that allows the palm to adapt to objects of various sizes. A more proximal transverse arch is present in the carpus and is permanent in shape. The mobile longitudinal arches are made up of all the digital rays. The metacarpal forms one side of the arch with the apex or keystone at the level of the metacarpophalangeal joint, and the other side of the arch is made up of the phalanges. The longitudinal arches are more mobile than the transverse arches and can individually alter their shape in response to the demands of grasp.

The line traced by the sweep of the fingertips into flexion corresponds to a constantly recurring pattern in nature, the equiangular spiral. This logarithmic curve is determined by the ratios of the interarticular carpometacarpal and phalangeal bone

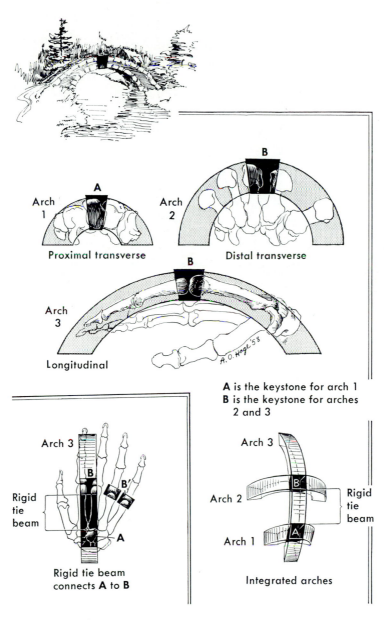

Arch 1
Proximal transverse

Arch 2
Distal transverse

Arch 3
Longitudinal

A is the keystone for arch 1
B is the keystone for arches 2 and 3

Arch 3

Rigid tie beam

Rigid tie beam connects **A** to **B**

Arch 3
Arch 2
Arch 1
Rigid tie beam

Integrated arches

B′ indicates keystones of mobile
longitudinal arches of ring and little fingers

Fig. 2-2. Arches of the hand. The bones of the hand are arranged in three arches: one longitudinal and two transverse. The rigid proximal transverse arch passes through the distal part of the carpus. The keystone of this arch lies in the capitate. The mobile distal transverse arch passes through the metacarpal heads. The two transverse arches are held together by the rigid central pillar of the hand acting as a tie beam. The four fingers make up the complex of the longitudinal arch. The longitudinal and distal transverse arches have a common keystone, the metacarpophalangeal joint. (From Flatt, A.E.: The care of minor hand injuries, ed. 4, St. Louis, 1979, The C.V. Mosby Co.)

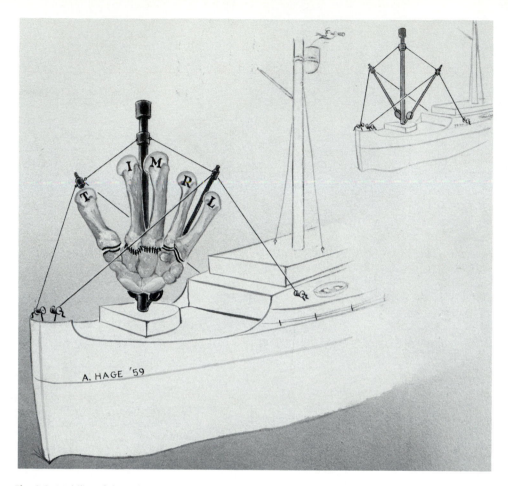

Fig. 2-3. Mobility of the palm. The shafts of the index and long finger metacarpals are firmly joined to the carpus and can be compared with the mast of a cargo ship. From the mast are slung two mobile borders, the thumb being on the radial side and the ring and small fingers on the ulnar side. The thumb is connected to the mast by intrinsic muscles, and the ulnar fingers by the transverse intermetacarpal ligaments. (From Flatt, A.E.: Hand deformities. In Traumatic medicine and surgery for the attorney, Washington, D.C., 1960, Butterworth, Inc.)

lengths that follow closely the Fibonacci sequence (1:1.618034). Littler has beautifully illustrated this concept by comparing the hand to the accretive shell of the chambered nautilus (Fig. 2-4). It can be seen in Fig. 2-4 that the sum of the interarticular lengths of the middle and distal phalanges is equal to the length of the proximal phalanx. The interarticular length of the middle and proximal phalanges is equal to the length between the metacarpal and the point in the capitate representing the axis of flexion of the wrist. It must be appreciated that the proportional lengths involved are not actual bone lengths but are measured between any two joint axes. This ratio is the mathematical basis for the shape of an egg, the nautilus shell, and even the spiral galaxies of outer space. The biomechanical efficiency of grasp is dependent on the

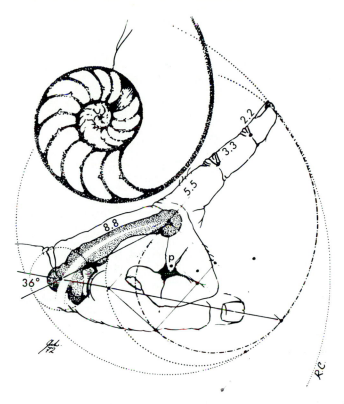

Fig. 2-4. The law of the logarithmic curve. This drawing compares the following circles of the digital joint arcs with the shell of the chambered nautilus. (From Littler, J.W.: The Hand **5**:187-191, 1973.)

retention of these proportional lengths. Rheumatoid disease destroys bone and dislocates digital joints, making efficient prehension no longer possible.

The wrist joint

The wrist includes eight carpal bones, the radiocarpal, the intercarpal, and the carpometacarpal articulations, ligaments, and soft-tissue structures. It transmits forces between the forearm and the hand, providing stability through the five primary extrinsic flexors and extensors passing over the carpus and inserting into the bases of the metacarpals. The wrist is the key joint in placing the hand in a working position, and, when its movement is considered in relation to finger movement, two independent actions are found to be possible. When the extrinsic wrist muscles stabilize the joint, the extrinsic and intrinsic finger muscles can alter the finger position. Conversely, when the finger posture is stabilized, the wrist can be moved in a variety of directions.

Anatomical deformity of any of the constituent parts of the wrist leads to instability and significant alteration of digital function. The key to understanding wrist instability and its influence on hand function lies in the "intercalated bone" concept of Landsmeer. Any multiarticulated mechanical system subjected to longitudinal stress will

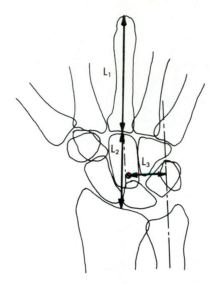

Fig. 2-5. Carpal height and carpal-ulnar distance. The carpal height ratio can be calculated as L_1/L_2 where L_1 is the length of the third metacarpal and L_2 is the carpal height. In the normal wrist this ratio is 0.54 ± 0.03. The carpal-ulnar distance and L_1 is the length of the third metacarpal. In the normal wrist this ratio is 0.3 ± 0.03. (Adapted from Youm, Y., McMurtry, R.Y., Flatt, A.E., and Gillespie, T.E.: Kinematics of the wrist, J. Bone Joint Surg. **60-A:**423-431, 1978.)

tend to collapse in a zigzag fashion. Thus a proximal deformity will tend to produce a reciprocal deviation down the line as the system attempts to balance its internal forces. In the subluxing wrist of rheumatoid disease, Linsheid and Dobyns have described two patterns of collapse. The more common palmar subluxation produces a zigzag collapse between the proximal and distal carpal rows in the flexion-extension plane, while the less common dorsal collapse is thought to be the result of compression stresses.

The various carpal collapse deformities caused by trauma or disease can be quantified by using the concept of carpal height (Fig. 2-5). By measuring the distance from the base of the third metacarpal to the distal articular surface of the radius on a posterior-anterior x-ray film, and dividing this length by the length of the third metacarpal, one gets a constant ratio of 0.54 ± 0.03 in the normal wrist. In diseased or deformed wrists, this ratio is decreased and may be quantified by subtracting the abnormal from the normal carpal height ratio.

Another clinically useful kinematic index is the carpal to ulnar distance (Fig. 2-5), which is measured from the center of rotation, for radial-ulnar deviation, to the distal projection of the longitudinal axis of the ulna. The carpal to ulnar distance, when divided by the length of the third metacarpal, results in a consistent ratio of 0.30 ± 0.03 in normal wrists. Any shifting of the carpus ulnarly by injury or by disease produces a decrease in this ratio and is termed *ulnar-carpal translation*. Once again, quantification is simply a matter of subtracting the abnormal value from the normal. Although these ratios have their limitations, they are particularly useful as a means of monitoring progressive deformity.

JOINTS OF THE DIGITS

The digital joints connecting the elements of the longitudinal arches all have the same basic anatomical form, which favors palmar flexion. The joint apparatus consists of a capsule and of a pair of strong collateral ligaments that pass around onto the palmar aspect to fuse with the sides of the accessory palmar plate. This plate consists of a tough fibrous portion in relation to the joint surfaces and a proximal membranous portion related to the metacarpal neck.

The palmar plate accounts for the different incidence of involvement of extensor and flexor tendons by diseased synovium of the digital joints. Expansion of the rheumatoid synovium can take place readily in the dorsal direction, leading to involvement of the extensor tendons, but the thick palmar plate effectively protects the flexor tendons from direct contact with the diseased synovium.

Finger joints

The type of movement in the digital joints differs in the interphalangeal and the metacarpophalangeal joints. The interphalangeal joints are simple hinge joints with congruous joint surfaces that travel on the same arc throughout their whole range of movement. The collateral ligaments, therefore, provide constant stability for the joints, since there is the same degree of tension on them in any position of the joint. The stability is greatly increased by the dynamic support of the flexor-extensor apparatus running over the joint. If the flexor and extensor muscles are completely relaxed, a little lateral movement of the joint can be passively produced.

The metacarpophalangeal joint has to provide mobility in two planes, and its mechanism is therefore correspondingly more complicated (Fig. 2-6). The collateral ligaments are slack when the joint is in extension, thereby allowing lateral movement to take place. Strength and stability of the extended joint are provided by the dynamic tone of the extrinsic muscles passing over the dorsal and flexor aspects of the joint. As the joint moves into flexion, the base of the proximal phalanx becomes firmly seated against the metacarpal head. This security is produced by a tightening of the collateral ligaments. The ligaments are fixed to the subcapitular portion of the metacarpal neck and become tight in two planes as the joint flexes. The joint is at its maximum tightness at approximately 70 degrees of flexion. The ligaments tighten in the longitudinal direction because they arise eccentrically in relation to the curve of the upper portion of the metacarpal head and because of the camlike action produced by the shape of the palmar portion of the metacarpal head. In the transverse direction the ligaments tighten over the bulging sides of the condyles (Fig. 2-6).

When rheumatoid disease attacks the metacarpophalangeal joint, the collateral ligaments are invariably weakened. The explanation is found in the mechanism of flexion of the joint. When an object is grasped and the fingers close around it, increasing tension is placed on the collateral ligaments. This tension, or stretching force, is increased until the object is securely grasped. If the integrity of the ligaments or their attachments has been weakened by the disease within the joint, disruption of the ligaments will occur. This stretching will produce an instability of grip, and correspondingly greater flexion power will be applied, leading to yet more stretching of the

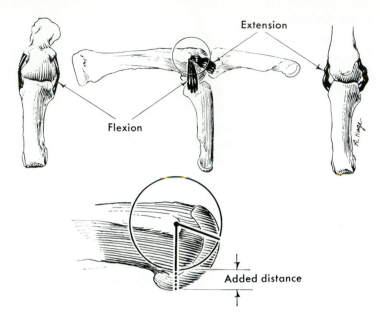

Fig 2-6. Metacarpophalangeal joint. When the joint is in extension, the collateral ligaments are slack, thereby allowing abduction and adduction to occur. The joint is stabilized when flexed because the ligaments are tightened in both the longitudinal and transverse planes. (From Flatt, A.E.: The care of minor hand injuries, ed. 4, St. Louis, 1979, The C.V. Mosby Co.)

ligaments. It is this vicious circle of stretching and lengthening that is primarily responsible for the dislocation of the metacarpophalangeal joint.

This dislocation results from progressive subluxation during which the base of the proximal phalanx moves in a palmar and proximal direction. Once the collateral ligaments have begun slackening, a major deforming force producing the dislocation is the pull of the intrinsic muscles via their insertion into the lateral bands and into the base of the phalanx (Fig. 5-5, p. 97). Progression of this deformity is inevitable, since there are no strong ligaments or muscles on the dorsum of the joint to counteract the deforming forces on the palmar aspect of the hand. The rate of progression of the dislocation will depend on the degree of activity of the disease.

Thumb joints

The three joints of the thumb are similar to the three joints of a finger in that the most proximal joint is the most mobile. Anatomically this joint is a carpometacarpal joint, which in the fingers would have very poor mobility. In the thumb, however, the range of movement is great, and the joint is almost universal in type. The joint surfaces are saddle shaped, and movement takes place through two main axes: (1) a radioulnar axis for flexion and extension and (2) a dorsopalmar axis for abduction and adduction.

When the proximal joint is in midposition, the capsular structures are slack and the articular surfaces are incongruous. In this state the important additional movement of longitudinal rotation can occur. When the thumb is fully abducted or

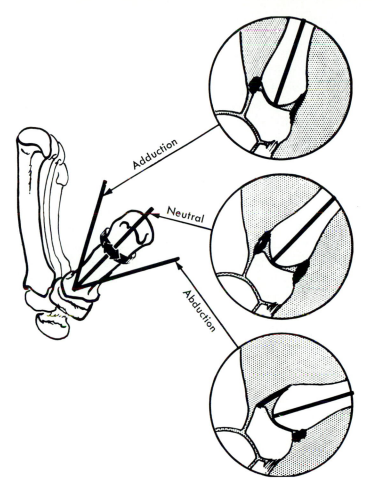

Fig. 2-7. Carpometacarpal joint of the thumb. This joint has two "positions of function": abduction and adduction. In these positions the joint surfaces are congruous and are held together by tense capsular and ligamentous structures. In the midposition the pericapsular structures are slack and rotation of the meta-carpal shaft is possible. Rotation of the first metacarpal at this saddle-shaped joint is possible only in the neutral position. (From Flatt, A.E.: Kinesiology of the hand, American Academy of Orthopaedic Surgeons Instructional Course Lectures, vol. 18, St. Louis, 1961, The C.V. Mosby Co.)

adducted, the joint's surfaces are congruous and are held close together by tense capsular and ligamentous structures. These two positions are regarded as the "positions of function" of the joint (Fig. 2-7).

Both the metacarpophalangeal and the interphalangeal joints resemble an interphalangeal joint of a finger and have strong lateral stability. However, the metcarpophalangeal joint does permit a few degrees of abduction and rotation that are of great functional importance in the finer movements of prehension.

Rheumatoid disease has a grossly adverse effect on the function of the thumb. The metacarpophalangeal joint dislocates in the same way as the similar joint in a finger and for the same basic reasons. To compensate for this dislocation and its resultant flexion contracture, a corresponding hyperextension deformity develops at the interphalangeal joint. Constant use of the thumb in grasp and pinch rapidly increases this dorsal dislocation of the distal joint (Fig. 9-4, p. 232). As the joint dislocates, a secure grip becomes increasingly difficult to achieve, and greater force is therefore applied in an attempt to restore efficiency. The dislocation continues, and eventually in many patients the joint literally falls apart. Disease of the carpometacarpal joint is frequent and often severely restricts the range of movement of the thumb. Disease in this joint and in the thenar intrinsic muscles commonly results in the typically stiff adducted thumb in which opposition is virtually impossible.

THE HAND IN USE

Proper grasp is impossible without adequate sensory information from the skin of the palm. The direction of mobility toward the palm of the hand is associated with a great concentration of sensory nerve endings in this area. Over a fourth of all the pacinian corpuscles in the body are present in the pulp and skin of the hands. Brand has shown that the power of grasp is controlled by the sensation of pressure on palmar skin and not, as formerly thought, by signals from nerve spindles buried in the muscles and tendons of the forearm. In patients with rheumatoid disease this vital sensory component of prehension is rarely affected. The most likely cause of impaired sensation is compression of the median nerve in the carpal tunnel, which in extreme instances produces a "blind" hand from median nerve paralysis.

The hand is used in two fundamentally different ways. The less common and completely unspecialized use is as a fixed end on a mobile arm. The hand acts as the passive transmitter of force, produced by the arm muscles, in such positions as the flattened hand or the clenched fist. The more common, skilled use of the hand is as a mobile organ at the end of a mobile limb. The movements used by the hand have been grouped by Stetson and McDill into three major types:

1. Slow to rapid movements, with control of direction, intensity, and rate
2. Ballistic or rapid repetitive motions
3. Fixations, including co-contractions yielding prehension

The slow to rapid movements consist of such actions as writing, sewing, and tying knots. Ballistic movements are usually repetitive rapid motions such as are used in typing or piano playing. Muscle power begins the movement and supplies momentum to the limb while the digits remain fixed in the required position. Fixations and prehensile movements are based on the so-called functional position. This is the position from which most prehensile actions of the normal hand develop, and it is this basic position that is modified when specialized activities are undertaken.

Anatomical patterns of prehension

In any prehensile activity the hand is considered to have two parts: the thumb and the rest of the hand. Most prehensile actions consist of an integration of the activities of the two parts, but occasionally pure finger prehension is used in a hook grasp. Thumb opposition is essential in all pinching or grasping movements. As the thumb opposes, it passes through a compound movement occurring at all three joints. The principal movements of abduction and rotation take place at both the carpometacarpal

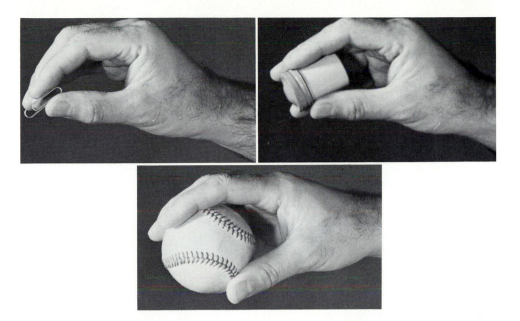

Fig. 2-8. Thumb in prehension. The fundamental position of abduction and rotation of the thumb relative to the palm is constant in all grasping actions. The basic position remains unchanged despite the variations in the size of objects held. (From Flatt, A.E.: Kinesiology of the hand, American Academy of Orthopaedic Surgeons Instructional Course Lectures, vol. 18, St. Louis, 1961, The C.V. Mosby Co.)

and metacarpophalangeal joints. This fundamental thumb position of abduction and rotation is constant in all grasping actions. This basic position will remain unchanged despite the size of the object held in the hand (Fig. 2-8).

Rheumatoid disease frequently affects the thumb and its intrinsic muscles, thereby interfering with the action of one half of the components of opposition. Involvement of the joints will affect the mobility of the bones, and involvement of the intrinsic muscles or pressure on the median nerve will destroy the subtle control necessary for skilled actions.

Fingers in prehension

Because of the large number of bones and joints within the fingers, it would certainly seem impossible to establish any form of coherent classification of finger movements. In fact, however, these finger movements fit into a relatively small number of patterns because of the overriding need for stability in the digital joints whenever prehension occurs.

Three patterns of prehensile movement can be recognized as most frequently occurring. These types of grip are derived from the basic functional position of the hand (Fig. 2-9) and are classified as tip, lateral, and palmar grips. The two most common prehensile movements are the picking up of an object and the holding of it for use. Keller and colleagues analyzed the type of grip used in these two forms of prehension and found that in both actions the palmar, or long-grip, pattern is the one

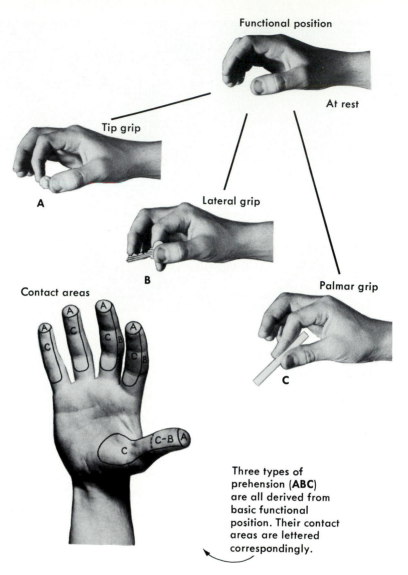

Functional position

Tip grip

A

At rest

Lateral grip

B

Palmar grip

Contact areas

C

Three types of
prehension (**ABC**)
are all derived from
basic functional
position. Their contact
areas are lettered
correspondingly.

Fig. 2-9. The functioning hand. In the functional position of the hand the wrist is stabilized in moderate extension and the thumb lies in line with the radius, with the metacarpal at right angles to the plane of the palm. The digital joints are held loosely in a semiflexed position. From this basic functional position are developed the fundamental prehensile grips **A, B,** and **C.** Their contact areas are lettered correspondingly. (From Flatt, A.E.: Hand deformities. In Traumatic medicine and surgery for the attorney, Washington, D.C., 1960, Butterworth, Inc.)

most commonly used. This predominance of palmar prehension was significant in both groups. The actual figures recorded are given in Table 1.

This overriding importance of palmar prehension must be appreciated in any attempt at splinting the hand or in reconstructive surgery. The dual importance of rotation and flexion of the thumb is unfortunately too often ignored in many splinting

Table 1. Comparative occurrence of the three types of grip used in prehensile movements*

Prehensile movement	Palmar	Lateral	Tip
Picking up	50%	33%	17%
Holding	88%	10%	2%

*Reported in Taylor, C., and Schwarz, R.: The anatomy and mechanics of the human hand, Artif. Limbs **2**:22-35, 1955; based on data from Keller, A.D., Taylor, C.L., and Zahm, V.: Studies to determine the functional requirements for hand and arm prosthesis, 1947, Department of Engineering, University of California at Los Angeles.

and operative procedures. A tip grip results from these inadequate forms of treatment because the pulp of the thumb cannot oppose the pulp of the fingers to produce palmar grip. Although tip grip presents only a relatively small surface contact area, it is still infinitely preferable to a lateral grip. In lateral prehension both the extrinsic and intrinsic thumb flexion power is brought to bear on the lateral side of the distal portion of the index finger. The only muscle available at the metacarpophalangeal joint to resist this power, which is being applied on a relatively long lever arm, is the first dorsal interosseous muscle. Unfortunately, this muscle is almost invariably weakened by rheumatoid disease, and the usual result of lateral grip pressure is to increase the tendency of the fingers to move into ulnar drift.

Functional patterns of prehension

Some have described the working hand with such terms as a hook, a ring, forceps, and pliers. Capener disapproved of such wholly mechanistic descriptions and stressed the dynamic quality of hand actions by pointing out that the thumb, the index finger, and the long finger form a dynamic tripod of prehension. The ring and small fingers are used largely for support and control.

Napier has also analyzed the use of the hand and has shown that two distinct patterns of function can be defined. He describes these patterns as power and precision (Fig. 2-10), using these terms in both dynamic and static senses. As a generalization, and therefore incorrectly, it can be said that in precision movements the fingers, although flexed, are abducted and held away from the palm. In the power grip the fingers are also flexed but are held clenched against the palmar buttress.

Landsmeer has carried this analysis a stage farther and has pointed out that there is a difference in quality between the power and precision grips. The power grip is characterized by a firm grasp that maintains constant pressure on the object despite movement that may occur in the wrist, elbow, or shoulder. In a precision "grip" the object is held relatively lightly between the tips of the digits and is manipulated by the fingers. Since the true use of the word *grip* is missing from this movement pattern, Landsmeer suggests that a more accurate description would be precision "handling." Although this may seem to be a semantic quibble, it is a description that I believe has practical value and one that should be generally adopted.

In precision handling the basic position of the fingers is one of flexion and abduc-

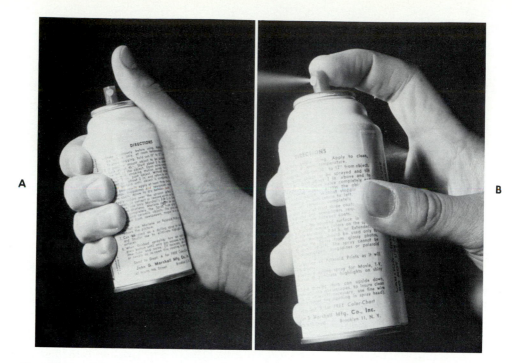

Fig. 2-10. Two types of grip. **A,** The cylinder is being held in a power grip between the flexed fingers and the palm. **B,** A precision grip pinches the cylinder between the flexor aspects of the fingers and the thumb. (From Flatt, A.E.: The care of minor hand injuries, ed. 4, St. Louis, 1979, The C.V. Mosby Co.)

tion at the metacarpophalangeal joints. In this position the span of the hand is increased, and a significant degree of opposition occurs in the fingers. The movement, which takes place at the metacarpophalangeal joint, is a combination of flexion, rotation, and ulnar deviation. By this action true pad-to-pad contact between thumb and finger occurs. Abduction of the thumb is necessary to provide the opposite pillar against which the fingers hold an object. When large objects are held, all the fingers are used; as the size of the object is reduced, however, the axis of grip moves to the radial side until finally only the index finger and thumb are used in the precise handling of small objects.

In power grips the thumb and thenar eminence provide the firm buttress against which the fingers press the object being held. Since the first metacarpal is not stable in the midposition, the thumb moves from its abducted precision position to the stable position of adduction. The fingers flex at both the interphalangeal joints and, by a combination of flexion, rotation, and ulnar deviation at the metacarpophalangeal joint, point toward the thenar eminence.

Backhouse has shown that in many hand activities the metacarpophalangeal joints are used, not in pure flexion, but with ulnar deviation and rotation. He believes that this is primarily caused by activity of the ulnar interossei of each finger and the flexor and abductor of the small finger, with the necessary flexor balance being supplied by the subordinate radial interossei.

This division of action of the digits, with the definition of two prehensile patterns,

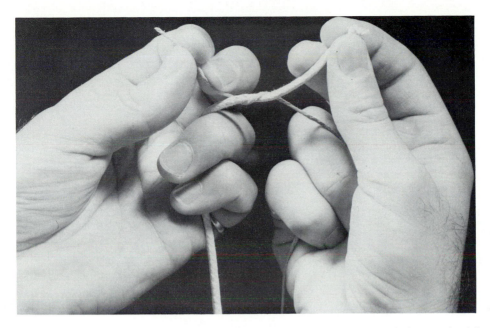

Fig. 2-11. Combined grip. When a knot is being tied, it is often necessary to grasp the loose ends of the string in a power grip with the ulnar border of the hands while the radial digits perform the precise work of forming the knot.

is not absolute. Each element depends on the other. The long finger can take part in either grip, and only rarely does a prehensile movement consist of pure precision or pure power elements. Many actions contain portions of each element, and it is the predominance of one or the other that will define the type of grasp. This mixing of action can be seen if a series of hammers of different weights are held, with a heavy hammer little precision is possible, and all energy is directed to grasping the handle against the palm of the hand. The thumb is used to reinforce the power grip by wrapping itself over the dorsum of the middle phalanges. When lightweight hammers are held, the grip moves to the radial side of the hand and the thumb provides a large element of precision. When medium-weight hammers are held, a mixture of these two extremes takes place. Occasionally the hand makes use of the two types of grip at the same time. If, for instance, a knot is being tied in two pieces of string, the power of grip needed to hold the ends is supplied by the ulnar fingers, while the precision work of tying the knot is performed by the radial digits (Fig. 2-11).

In summary it can be said that in both grip and movement the radial half of the hand provides precision, and the ulnar half provides power and stability.

BALANCE OF MUSCLE POWER WITHIN THE HAND

All these patterns of action of the normal hand are based on the mobility of the integrated group of skeletal arches. The individual longitudinal arch, or digit, alters its shape in response to the activity of both extrinsic and intrinsic hand muscles.

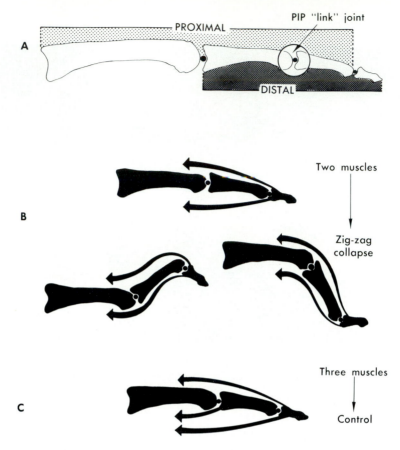

Fig. 2-12. Two biarticular bimuscular systems. **A,** The four bones of the longitudinal arch of a finger are shown as proximal and distal biarticular systems; the proximal interphalangeal joint is the "link" joint of the two systems. **B,** Three bones linked by two joints must collapse in a zigzag fashion if only two muscles are available as controls. **C,** The addition of a third force will add control and establish equilibrium.

Van der Meulen has stressed that in a mechanical sense a finger is a combination of two biarticular bimuscular systems (Fig. 2-12). The proximal system consists of the metacarpophalangeal and proximal interphalangeal joints, and the distal system is formed by the proximal interphalangeal and the distal interphalangeal joints. The proximal interphalangeal joint is thus the common, or link, joint between the two systems. A single biarticular system consisting of three bones and two joints, if controlled by only two long muscles, must collapse into a zigzag attitude, with one of the joints in a terminal position. Collapse could be prevented by providing a third muscle as additional control and thereby establishing an equilibrium of forces (Fig. 2-12). The intrinsic muscles are the third force that balances the more powerful but unequal forces in the extrinsic flexor and extensor muscles (Fig. 2-13).

At the metacarpophalangeal joint, the intrinsic muscles supplement the extrinsic flexor power and counterbalance the power of the extrinsic extensor digitorum com-

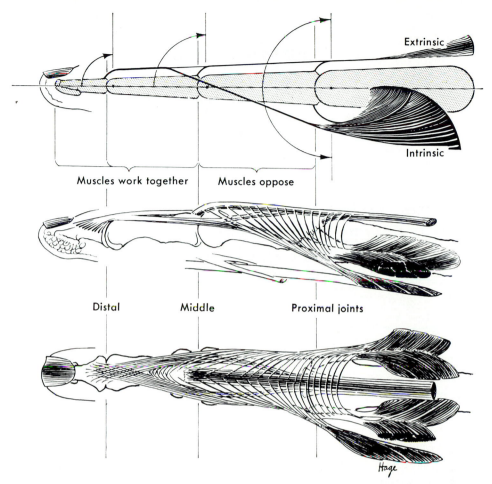

Extrinsic

Intrinsic

Muscles work together | Muscles oppose

Distal | Middle | Proximal joints

Hage

Fig. 2-13. Intrinsic muscles. These muscles approach the metacarpophalangeal joints from the depth of the palm and lie on the palmar aspect of the axis of the joints. The tendons then pass dorsal to the axis of the interphalangeal joints. The intrinsic muscles, therefore, flex the metacarpophalangeal joints and extend the interphalangeal joints. (From Flatt, A.E.: The care of minor hand injuries, ed. 4, St. Louis, 1979, The C.V. Mosby Co.)

munis (Fig. 2-13). Within the finger the tendons of the intrinsic muscles pass along the side of the proximal phalanx, cross dorsal to the axis of the proximal interphalangeal joint, and join the extensor mechanism. The intrinsic muscles thereby help the extrinsic extensor to balance the pull of the two extrinsic flexor muscles acting on the proximal interphalangeal joint. At the distal joint the intrinsic muscles provide a major part of the extensor power to balance the pull of the flexor profoundus tendon.

This balance of power is an extremely delicate mechanism and is totally dependent on the integrity of the joints and their supporting ligaments. Rupture of the extrinsic extensor or flexor tendons will produce a gross and obvious disturbance of function. Less obvious but equally important disturbances of function are produced

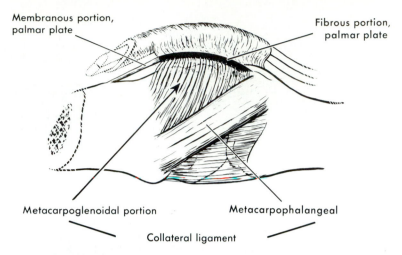

Membranous portion, palmar plate

Fibrous portion, palmar plate

Metacarpoglenoidal portion

Metacarpophalangeal

Collateral ligament

Fig. 2-14. Anatomy of the metacarpophalangeal joint. This drawing deliberately exaggerates the various structures to emphasize the differences in the anatomical constituents around the joint. Note that the collateral ligament has two distinct portions. (Modified from Flatt, A.E.: J. Bone Joint Surg. **48-A:**100-104, 1966.)

by synovitis of the digital joints or involvement of the intrinsic muscles. Swelling of the synovium alters the line of pull and the angle of attack of tendons passing over the joints and consequently alters their normal function. Rheumatoid involvement of the intrinsic muscles causes an exaggeration of their action, particularly at the proximal interphalangeal, or link, joint. In gross and neglected cases this exaggeration can result in extreme "swan-neck," or "intrinsic-plus," deformity. This link joint is also often affected in the opposite direction by a flexion, or boutonniere, deformity. In this instance collapse occurs because the expanding synovitis of the joint disrupts the extrinsic tendons and displaces the intrinsic tendons controlling the joint. Swanson and colleagues, in their excellent chapter discussing pathogenesis of rheumatoid deformities in the hand, have emphasized that once collapse has started, the axially applied forces of use further aggravate the deformation.

Zigzag collapse is the obvious external result of dynamic muscular imbalance of the hand, but equally significant disturbances can occur within the joints after destruction of the joint restraints or collateral ligaments. As this type of destruction increases within, a hand grasp weakens because it is basically dependent on the integrity of the longitudinal arch systems. A patient responds to the weakening grasp by exerting every effort to increase the power of the flexor tendons. It is this valiant but unwise effort that ultimately proves to destructive to the integrity of the arch system of the hand. The explanation lies in the route the flexor tendons take from their origin to insertion. Their line of pull is not straight, and wherever they change direction, restraints or pulleys are necessary. These restraints must therefore be subjected to large forces whenever the hand is used.

The anatomy of the metacarpophalangeal joint is not as simple as shown in Fig. 2-6. The collateral ligament is really two ligaments: a metacarpophalangeal ligament and a metacarpoglenoidal ligament (Fig. 2-14). The metacarpophalangeal portion is

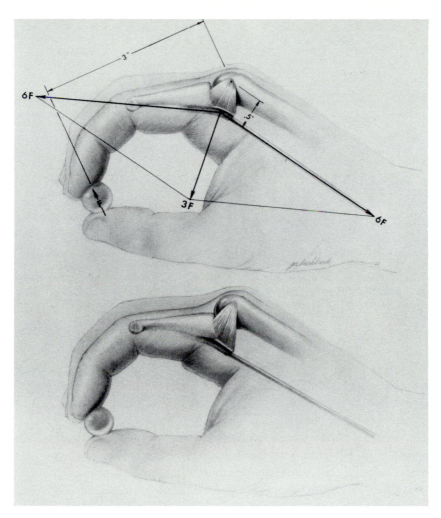

Fig. 2-15. Flexor tendon forces. The upper drawing shows the forces developed in the flexor tendons and the "sling" of the entrance to the tendon sheath when a pinch force acts on a moment arm six times that of the flexor tendons. The lower drawing shows the resultant palmar subluxation of the proximal phalanx when the diseased sling structures are elongated by the flexor forces. (From Smith, E.M., Juvinall, R.C., Bender, L.F., and Pearson, J.R.: J.A.M.A. **198:**130-134, 1966.)

the true bone-to-bone ligament holding the metacarpal and proximal phalanx together. The metacarpoglenoidal ligament is a U-shaped sling ligament coming from either side of the metacarpal neck, holding up the palmar plate and the flexor tendons just at the point where they change direction as they enter the finger.

Smith and colleagues were the first to emphasize the fundamental importance of this system on hand function. Because of the curved route the flexor tendons must follow, it can be shown that to obtain a 1F force output at the fingertip, a 6F pull on the profundus is needed, and that the dislocation tendency at the metacarpophalangeal joint is 3F (Fig. 2-15). Thus every time a patient with synovitis of the metacarpophalangeal joints pinches or grasps anything, a force three times greater is trying to

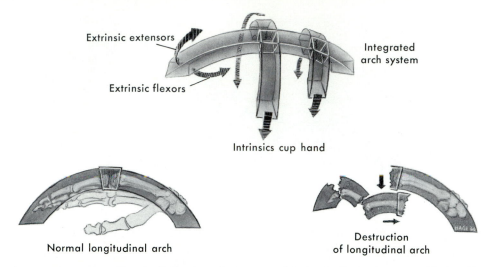

Extrinsic extensors

Integrated arch system

Extrinsic flexors

Intrinsics cup hand

Normal longitudinal arch

Destruction of longitudinal arch

Fig. 2-16. Destruction of longitudinal arches. The keystone of the longitudinal arch system of the hand lies at the metacarpophalangeal joint. Rheumatoid disease can destroy the arches by dislocation at the metacarpophalangeal joint and by hyperextension at the proximal interphalangeal joint. (From Flatt, A.E.: Lancet **1:**1136, 1961.)

dislocate the keystone joint of the hand. Once rheumatoid disease has weakened the collateral ligament or its bony attachment, subluxation followed by dislocation is the inevitable result (Fig. 2-15).

Dislocation of the metacarpophalangeal joint is usually into flexion, which breaks the curve of the longitudinal arch and sets the stage for more distal joint collapse. At the proximal interphalangeal joint the arch is more often broken by a hyperextension deformity (Fig. 2-16). This deformity is insidious in its onset and crippling in its fully developed state, since grip cannot be either initiated or sustained.

This discussion has considered the metacarpophalangeal joints only in the flexion-extension plane. Unfortunately, they are capable of motion in the ulnar-radial plane, and any deformity produced by the flexor tendons must therefore be a compound deformity affecting these two planes. The final result will be a distribution of the bearing forces on the articular surfaces of the joints proportional to the relative destruction in the collateral ligaments. Even in the normal hand the radial and ulnar metacarpophalangeal ligaments of each joint are not of equal size and strength. Hakstian and Tubiana have shown that in the normal hand the radial collateral ligament of the index and long finger metacarpophalangeal joints is thinner, longer, and attached more distally than the ulnar collateral ligament. This arrangement allows the small amount of ulnar drift normally present during firm grasp. If these radial ligaments become slackened by disease, the bearing forces on the articular surfaces will be unevenly distributed and wear will be concentrated in one area. A patient's hand at surgery is shown in Fig. 2-17. The palmar and ulnar worn spot on the head of the long finger metacarpal is associated with solitary destruction of the radial collateral ligament of this joint. It is the result of the complicated resolution of forces such as this

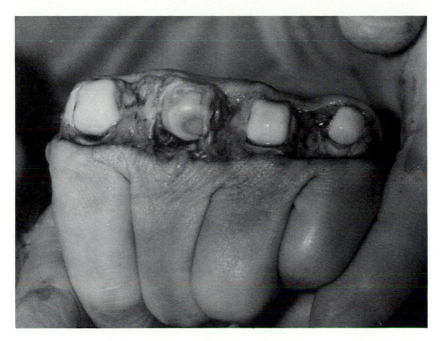

Fig. 2-17. Bearing forces on the joint. Unequal slackening of the metacarpophalangeal ligaments will allow uneven distribution of forces on the metacarpal head. The destruction of this patient's long finger meta-carpal head in the palmar and ulnar area was associated with solitary destruction of the radial collateral ligament of this joint.

example of early disease that have profound implications for those who prescribe physical or occupational therapy. The fundamental relationship of these forces to the cause of ulnar drift is developed in Chapter 10.

As the hand becomes more crippled by rheumatoid disease, it is the precision movements that first become increasingly affected. Patients rapidly develop trick movements in an attempt to compensate for these deficiencies, but these abnormal actions are not based on normal kinesthetic patterns, and function deteriorates. As precision movements are lost, the hand becomes steadily less agile, and the primitive prehensile movement of hook grip is often developed. The power for this grip is provided solely by the extrinsic muscles, and such a grip is rarely used in the normal hand. At the same time precision handling is deteriorating, the power of grasp is also failing because of the instability of the digital joints and the abnormal patterns of prehension that have developed.

Eventually the hands are reduced to such a state that a single-handed function such as holding a coffee cup becomes a two-handed action. Even at this stage many rheumatoid patients passively accept their lot, unaware that much could have been done and can still be done to restore function. Early recognition of disturbances of function is essential, since, as Marmor has pointed out, it is much more logical to elect to perform early surgery and prevent deformity than to be forced to do a radical salvage procedure on a disease-ravaged hand.

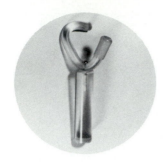

The arthritic hand often remains under medical supervision for many years and only infrequently during that time is surgery required. Nonoperative methods of treatment are certainly of use in the postoperative period, but they are also of great help at many other times. They must always be considered when undertaking long-term care of the arthritic hand.

This chapter is not a review of the various general and medicinal treatments available for the various forms of arthritis; such a discussion by a surgeon would be presumptuous. I have attempted to define, as I see it, the place of physical and occupational therapy and splinting and assistive devices in the care of the patient with an arthritic hand.

THERAPEUTIC ACTIVITIES

Physical and occupational therapies are of definite value in the treatment of arthritic hands. I believe that these forms of treatment are complementary to each other. They are not mutually exclusive, since they both have the same objective of restoring function to a disabled hand.

Recent years have seen the combination of the best of both physical and occupational therapies into the new discipline of *hand therapy*. Those who practice the highly skilled techniques of hand therapy need great patience and great empathy because so many of their patients are, or fear they are, severely handicapped. The good therapist is an expert psychologist and a dedicated teacher who can select the most suitable therapy for a patient at any given time in the treatment process.

When surgery is needed, development of the operative plan should include sessions with the hand therapist both before and after the actual surgical procedure. A good therapist may get more information about the patient from observation than by asking questions. Often considerable good comes from having patients work in small discussion groups made up of patients with the same or similar problems; apart from the therapeutic gains there are often psychological benefits for the patient from working with people with similar deformities. DeVore has made it a practice to encourage her rheumatoid patients to keep a "wish list" and a diary before surgery. A wish list may reveal totally unrealistic hopes that will have to be modified if the best possible results are to be obtained. Diaries often bring out problems that patients have deliberately forgotten. Many patients, however, resent the idea of keeping a diary and resist revealing their hidden frustrations. In an open discussion patients can often be encouraged to become active participants in the treatment plan. There is no common pattern of "good" therapy for all the various arthritic afflictions of the hand. The hand with rheumatoid disease may need varying types of supervision for months or years, while therapy for the other forms of arthritis usually has a finite time span. I believe that the key to therapeutic success is an understanding of the normal and abnormal forces present in the hand.

I have partially summarized the present state of our knowledge of the appropriate anatomy in Chapters 2 and 10. Landsmeer's work on tendon location analysis is directly applicable to the problem, since his mathematical theory helps to determine the effect of tendon location on interjoint coordination. It becomes possible to predict the relationship between muscle strength and the location of the tendon relative to the axis of rotation of the joint.

If this formulation is applied to the metacarpophalangeal joint, it can be shown that as the extensor tendon moves closer to the axis of joint rotation, it will become increasingly difficult to extend the joint. The converse is also true; if the flexor tendons should displace in a palmar direction, they will be further from the axis of rotation and will therefore increase their mechanical advantage.

There is a clear clinical application of this reasoning to a condition such as subluxation and ulnar deviation at the metacarpophalangeal joints, in which, despite full passive extension, active extension of the joints is often limited. The lack of extension can be directly related to the displacement of the extrinsic extensor tendons into the ulnar furrows of the metacarpophalangeal joints and the subluxation of the base of the proximal phalanx. These anatomical changes move the extensor tendon nearer to the joint axis and the flexor tendons away from the axis, thereby decreasing the effectiveness of the single extensor tendon and increasing the advantage of the two flexor tendons.

Smith has shown that the forces acting within the normal hand are potentially deforming but are restrained by healthy supporting tissues. Rheumatoid disease can and does disturb these normal anatomical restraints, and the forces can then act on this diseased tissue, increasing the potential for deformity. There are many sites in the wrist and hand where the anatomical restraints can be destroyed and aberrant forces allowed to develop. The tendon location theory can be applied to each of these sites, and it must be considered when it is proposed to strengthen muscle action on a joint that has a free passive range. The tendon location theory also carries the additional and very important implication that a patient's motivation cannot greatly improve joint range, regardless of the therapy employed, if the lines of tendon action have become aberrant.

I believe that the application of this knowledge disqualifies vigorous and resistive exercises. Resistive exercises apply additional forces to burden the diseased rheumatoid tissue. This cannot improve the weakened joint structures and may hasten the deforming process. If the tendons have already become displaced, muscle strengthening will not reposition the tendon nor will it strengthen the weakened soft tissues of the joint.

Others share our concern over the use of zealous exercise programs that are prescribed without a clear understanding of the deranged anatomy within the hand. Wozny and Long commented in their paper on electromyographic kinesiology of the rheumatoid hand that few, if any, gentle exercises can be devised that would do anything but hasten the process of deformity. They do suggest that passive stretching, applied to the side of the deformity opposite the side in which active forces may have a deforming effect, could be helpful. This stretching is better supplied by prolonged splinting rather than in short therapeutic sessions.

Despite the foregoing paragraphs, I am not entirely a therapeutic nihilist. Care-

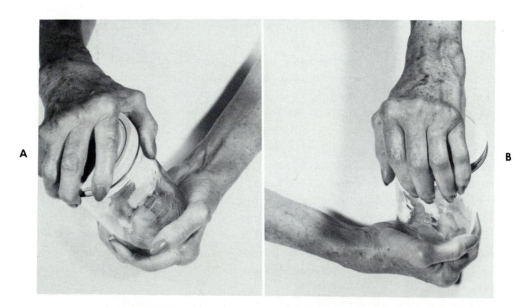

Fig. 3-1. Deforming forces of use. **A,** We live in a right-handed world, and most people use the right hand when unscrewing the lid of a jar. The fingers are forced into ulnar drift, which is devastating for the rheumatoid hand. **B,** Left-handed people gain a distinct advantage in this activity, and rheumatoid patients will also help their hands significantly if they will alter their habit patterns.

fully graduated exercise programs applied with intelligence can help gain limited objectives. But wholesale, unsupervised exercising of all the hand muscles can produce devastating results. Particular emphasis must be given to the protection of weakened joint supports during everyday use of the hand. Even seemingly innocent activities such as opening a screw-top jar can create enormous deforming forces (Fig. 3-1). Repetitive actions such as opening doors, using manual can openers, and turning keys can be devastating to a joint whose ligamentous structure has been compromised by disease.

JOINT PROTECTION MEASURES

A realistic therapeutic program that incorporates joint protection techniques can be designed for the rheumatoid patient, but to do this requires a great fund of knowledge. Hand therapists are trained to analyze how patients use their hands and to identify which activities are most likely to harm the hand. They can, therefore, devise programs that are both protective and helpful. Cordery and Melvin have both published useful guidelines in planning such protection. Their articles should be studied for a proper understanding of this vital concept, but the general principles on which this work is based are as follows:

1. Respect for pain
2. Balance between rest and work
3. Maintenance of muscle strength and joint range of motion (ROM)
4. Reduction of effort needed to do a job
5. Avoidance of positions of deformity
6. Use of the strongest or largest joints available for the job
7. Use of each joint in its most stable anatomical and functional plane
8. Avoidance of holding or staying in one position for prolonged periods of time
9. Avoidance of activities that cannot be stopped immediately if they become too stressful.
10. Use of assistive equipment and splinting to protect joints

Occasionally splinting can supplement this protection, providing it follows Bennett's principle that the ideal splint should "permit the normal planes of motion necessary for essential function, but block all faulty planes that might result in functionally significant deformity." A typical splint of this type is the "functional ulnar deviation cuff" designed by Quest and Cordery (Fig. 3-2). The splint is deliberately made to restrict full metacarpophalangeal flexion, thereby preventing the development of large subluxating torques, but it does provide a large working area of palmar skin. Detailed instructions for making this useful device are given in their article.

Patients must use their hands, and for many, provided they have been properly trained, this functional activity alone will be sufficient therapeutic exercise. I seriously question whether any additional exercises are necessarily beneficial. If therapists continue to be faced with patients in moderate or late stages of their disease who have not been treated surgically, the results of therapy will probably continue to be as unrewarding as in the past.

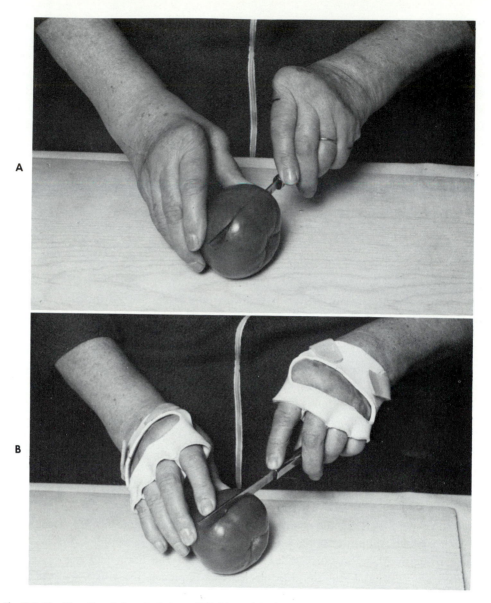

Fig. 3-2. The "functional ulnar deviation cuff." This useful splint, made of a thermoplastic material, restricts full metacarpophalangeal flexion by supporting the joint, but it does provide a large working area of palmar skin. **A,** Ulnar deviation while at work, **B,** Support provided by the splints. (From Quest, I.M., and Cordery, J.: Am. J. Occup. Ther. **25:**32-40, 1971.)

There is, however, a definite place for postoperative therapy. After surgery has realigned some of the aberrant forces, we can show that controlled exercises can double the strength of the hand. Therapy after synovectomy is also of definite value. I agree with Mongan and associates that there is a direct correlation between the end result and the extent of postsynovectomy therapy. Although some patients have the intelligence and drive to successfully carry out a home program, most need the incentive of regular outpatient vists to maintain their program.

In the first edition of this book, general hand exercise programs were included in the two sections entitled Physical Therapy and Occupational Therapy. All these exercises have been deleted because intelligent hand therapists with a knowledge of anatomy will be aware of any therapy that can be appropriately applied to the particular state of their patient's hands. If therapeutic activities are employed in the rehabilitation of patients with rheumatoid disease of the hands, one of the greatest problems that will be encountered is the varying pain tolerance of the patients. There is no doubt that activities that produce pain should be stopped and the hand rested. Unfortunately, rest is too often advised for discomfort rather than for true pain. Rose and Kendell have discussed this problem and pointed out that there is nothing therapeutic about rest but that its use may avoid flare-ups of the disease. Repeatedly cautioning the patient to avoid pain or soreness when using the hand does him a disservice. There is a distinction between pain and discomfort, and this fundamental difference must be fully explained to the patient. Discomfort during use of the hand must be expected and is no excuse for reduction in the program. Discomfort that rapidly recedes during a rest period is acceptable and allows the program to be gradually intensified. True pain that persists for several hours after activity is a warning that cannot be ignored; the program and the patient's daily activities must be modified. Short and frequent sessions of activity are of more value than a few protracted periods.

Flexion contractures of the digital joints are a frequent therapeutic problem. They occur more commonly at the proximal interphalangeal joint, but they are often associated with an apparent contracture at the metacarpophalangeal joint. This apparent contracture is usually a subluxation and, as such, cannot be improved by exercise. If it can be shown that the tendon mechanism passing over the proximal interphalangeal joint is intact, improvement can sometimes be obtained by exercising the muscles antagonistic to the direction of the contracture. Extension exercises should be done through the greatest available range. In the early phases the exercises may be almost isometric in nature because of the lack of range of the joint. Isometric exercises are useful in building muscle and should be used exclusively if the joints are too painful to move. In such cases the therapist must prevent joint motion during the exercise period. Isometric movements should be started as soon as possible to continue muscle development and to increase the range of joint motion. Passive exercises must be used to regain joint range and overcome contractures. These exercises must be used with great caution, since excessive stretching of contracted tissues produces pain and may produce hemorrhage, which in its turn will lead to further fibrosis. A series of passive resting splints is often useful to maintain the gains while providing support to the tissues. Increased range of motion produced by passive exercises is of no value unless there is sufficient muscle action to control the additional range of motion. Active exercises must follow passive exercises, but patients usually benefit more from assisted exercises in the early phase of treatment.

Even when flexion contractures are not a problem, it will usually be found that extension of the fingers is relatively weak when compared with flexion. Since it is vitally important to maintain extensor power, activities are often needed to build up the extensor muscles. Manual resistance by the therapist has been advocated as a method of developing strength in these muscles. Even though the degree of resistance can be varied easily according to the muscle being treated, I believe that the resistance used can often be harmful to the patient's joint structures.

MODALITIES OF TREATMENT

Treatments such as whirlpool, ultrasound, electrical stimulation, and massage are available only in the department. Others, such as local heat or cold applications, general functional activities, and exercises, can be used in the home. Close supervision is necessary in the early stages of treatment, but it should be directed toward helping the patient to understand the objectives behind the treatment so that he may become independent of supervision. To assist in this plan our patients are given illustrated exercise sheets and booklets containing the appropriate program of activities and treatments individually prescribed.

Local cold

We have carried out several experiments to assess the value of cryotherapy. At best our results are equivocal, and Rembe has shown that although postoperative edema appeared reduced, the difference was not significant at the 0.051 level. There is no doubt that in some patients the cooling has relieved postoperative discomfort and allowed an earlier onset of controlled exercising. Few, if any, patients will react adversely to the cold, but early complaints of increasing discomfort must be respected and the treatment abandoned.

In the immediate postoperative period the bandages are removed 5 days after surgery and the hand is placed in a disposable plastic glove or bag to protect the incision from the water. The hand is then immersed in water at 50° F for 4 minutes. Additional treatments of the same duration can be given on subsequent days. When the bandages should not be removed, cold treatments can still be given by applying cold packs outside the bandages. Studies have shown that if the cold is to penetrate the fluffed-up bandages effectively, the packs must be in place for a minimum of an hour.

Local heat

Heat treatment is usually given before exercise and is of definite help to some patients. Paraffin bath treatments are the usual method of providing local heat. We use paraffin because it supplies a uniform heat to the hand and is a method that can be easily learned by the patient. Our patients are given a booklet that describes how the treatment can be carried out at home, and they practice this method under supervision before they leave the department. When early movement is desirable in postoperative patients, paraffin bath treatments may be started as soon as the tenth postoperative day. However, I believe that this treatment is contraindicated for the edematous hand.

Whirlpool

Whirlpool treatments are useful for applying heat to the entire hand. Because the temperature of the water can be regulated according to the tolerance of the individual, these treatments are often preferred by patients who cannot tolerate the more intense heat of a paraffin bath. The water helps to support the hand and diminishes the effects of gravity. Often patients are more willing to start gentle isometric or isotonic exercises in the warm whirlpool bath at an earlier time than they will attempt similar exercises out of the water. Despite these apparent advantages, it is our impression that hands treated by whirlpool baths seem more edematous than those treated by other means, and we rarely use this modality.

Ultrasound

We have used ultrasonic treatments under water for some postoperative patients. The treatments have been prescribed principally for those few patients whose hands do not respond to whirlpool or paraffin bath treatments. These patients complain of a persistent mild ache in the hand, which may be relieved by ultrasonic treatment. The treatment is administered under water to ensure a good couple between the skin and the headpiece. The usual strength used is 1 watt per square centimeter, but it may be reduced to 0.5 watt per square centimeter. This treatment has been given even to patients whose hands contain metallic prostheses, and no ill effects have resulted from this order of strength.

ADAPTIVE AND ASSISTIVE DEVICES

Adaptive equipment is sometimes helpful even early in rheumatoid disease to prevent excessive strain on diseased tissues. However, patients with early disease are often still in the denial stage and cannot accept the concept of external aids and their implications of a crippling disease. This sense of defeatism is the greatest problem faced by the therapist. It is essential that patients actively participate in their therapy and assume responsibility for continuing their prescribed programs.

The opening illustration was deliberately chosen to emphasize the importance of assistive devices. This particular gadget had to be devised after the care of the arthritic hand was severely set back by the introduction of push-button openers for car doors. The force necessary to open these doors is far greater than should be put through the joints of even a normal thumb. Many such simple assistive devices are available to aid the handicapped hand in everyday activities, and proper nonoperative treatment should include the prescription of a suitable apparatus. Much useful information on many aspects of joint protection and assistive devices is now available from the Arthritis Information Clearinghouse.*

SPLINTING

Resting the hand in a splint is of great help during an acutely painful episode of any form of arthritis. Rigid splinting may also be necessary for immobilizing the hand after surgery.

---

*Arthritis Information Clearinghouse, P.O. Box 34427, Bethesda, Maryland 20034; 301-881-9411.

Some controversy still exists about the relative value of fixed, or traction, splints. This controversy stems from ignorance of the fundamental principles applying to the use of all types of splinting for the hand, whatever the primary indication. Certainly controversy exists regarding the value of splinting the rheumatoid hand. Its use has been well described by Souter as the Cinderella of our therapeutic armamentarium. It is a frequently neglected method of treatment, and I have drawn freely on Souter's excellent discussion of splinting to define the value of this method of treatment.

Splinting can be useful in three situations: (1) during acute exacerbations of disease; (2) instead of surgery; and (3) as an adjunct to surgery, either preoperatively or in postoperative therapy. A variety of splints, if properly prescribed, can be used for the relief of pain and maintenance of good position during acute flare-ups of disease, for correcting a deformity, for stabilizing some joints to allow movement of others, and for dynamic support of joints to counteract deforming forces.

Traditionally, splinting is applied at night and the hand is left free for use during the day. Swezey has stressed that since rheumatoid deformities are dynamically induced, nocturnal immobilization is an impractical protection against deforming forces that are operative only during the use of the hand.

Whatever type of splinting is prescribed, it must be acceptable to the patient. Rigid devices without soft covering or proper padding will not be tolerated. A loosely fitting splint is not mechanically efficient, and any mass-produced device must be modified so that each patient's limb may be individually fitted. A simple splint cheaply and easily produced is the ideal. Unfortunately, as the number of functions demanded of the splint increases, so does its bulk and complexity. Ingenuity of design frequently outstrips the patient's tolerance, and many apparently efficient but complex models are left neglected in closets.

Classification of splints for the hand is not easy because many of them serve several functions. A recently published book, *Hand Splinting*, by Fess, Gettle, and Strickland contains excellent discussions on the taxonomy, biomechanical effects, and therapeutic uses of splints. In the postoperative management of some patients several types of splints may be prescribed at different periods of time for use in one hand.

The splints generally used for the rheumatoid hand can be classified according to their function into three main types:

Rest splints—providing passive immobilization during active disease
Static splints—providing stabilization of joints and correction of deformity
Dynamic splints—used to counteract deforming forces

Splinting during acute disease

It has been repeatedly stressed that the wrist is the key joint for the position of hand function. This is because the joint influences, and is influenced by, the balance of the extrinsic muscles crossing the joint. In untreated acute rheumatoid synovitis of the wrist joint, flexion rapidly occurs and a compensatory nonfunctional position of partial extension of the fingers develops. The position used in splinting the wrist and hand is often a compromise between the most useful position of the hand and the position in which some joint stiffness would still allow a useful range of movement.

Every attempt should be made to prevent a lateral zigzag deformity leading to ulnar drift by correcting any radial deviation tendency of the carpus. A strong strut may be needed on the ulnar side of the small finger ray to control ulnar deviation. The thumb should be held in full abduction at the carpometacarpal joint, and care should be taken not to stretch the ulnar collateral ligament of the metacarpophalangeal joint.

During an acute flare-up of any arthritic condition and during temporary exacerbations, the wrist and finger joints should be protected until pain on motion has largely disappeared. Continuous immobilization is essential in the very active phase of rheumatoid disease, but as the symptoms improve, only intermittent immobilization is necessary. Rest alone is not adequate treatment. Rest is required during the very acute stage of disease, but it must be associated with properly controlled activity and the judicious use of local cold or heat applications.

As the acute inflammation and muscle spasm subside, pain decreases and joint movement becomes easier. Splinting must be continued until the pain has disappeared. Pain-killing drugs and steroids may give a false impression of rapid improvement. If early movement is started under the influence of such drugs, considerable damage can be done to the joints.

There is no danger that permanent stiffness will develop in finger and wrist joints from this type of splinting program. A correctly fitted, comfortable palmar splint puts the area at rest and allows the pain and the acute inflammatory process to subside rapidly. During the phase of intermittent immobilization, the splint should be left off for increasing periods during the day while the patient performs hand activities related to the skills of daily living. During this time strict attention to joint protection techniques may be necessary. The splint should be worn at night for several weeks after all acute symptoms and signs have subsided.

Materials such as plastics, epoxy resins, silicone rubbers, and plaster of paris are available for making temporary splints. I still believe that plaster of paris is the most efficient material from which to make these splints. However, its efficacy is destroyed if too much plaster is used, producing heavy splints. Rotstein's monograph gives a detailed description of the methods for making passive immobilization splints. When I make these splints, I first apply a stockinette sleeve over the forearm and hand. The wet plaster is applied directly to the stockinette on the flexor aspect of the forearm, across the wrist joint, and is carefully molded into the palm to maintain the position of function. If the finger joints need rest from acute inflammation, the plaster must be continued on the flexor aspect to a level distal to the involved joints.

About four to six thicknesses of quick-drying plaster bandage should supply sufficient strength for the splint. The wrist is placed in about 20 degrees of dorsiflexion, the fingers are flexed to a position of comfort, and the thumb is abducted at least 20 degrees. The plaster is carefully bandaged into place with a cotton bandage, and the forearm and hand are supported in the corrected position until the plaster has set.

When the plaster is dry, the bandage and the stockinette are cut through along the midline of the dorsum of the hand and forearm. The remains of the cotton bandage are removed, and any sharp projections are trimmed away from the edges of the cast. The stockinette is turned over the edges of the cast and held in place with either adhesive tape or some narrow strips of plaster bandage. The splint is now ready for use; it should be fixed to the arm by a self-adherent cotton bandage so that it can be removed during washing and exercising. Pressure is more evenly distributed on the forearm when the splint is held in place with a covering bandage rather than with individual straps.

Although rest splints are primarily used in acute disease, they have a definite place in postoperative care. Because they provide correct external skeletal support, they allow the dynamic supporting system to relax and also protect the joint-supporting structures against unwanted stresses. I use them both in the immediate postoperative phase and for rest periods during therapy in static or dynamic braces.

Static splints

Once instability and deformities have developed, a vicious circle of increasing malfunction is established. Deformities lead to lack of use of the hand, this lack of use leads to stiffness, stiffness leads to even less use of the hand, and contractures steadily increase. This vicious circle must be broken by encouraging constrained activity of the hand, by appropriate therapy, and by the use of static and/or remedial splints.

Static splinting is usually applied to the dorsum of the hand or forearm so as to free the working surface of the hand as much as possible. Palmar bars are essential for fixation, but their size must always be kept to a minimum. These splints can be used as a substitute for surgery and are also of value in postoperative care. Savill pioneered the use of this type of splinting, and Souter has illustrated the three standard splints (Fig. 3-3). Each has a dorsal plaster slab secured by Velcro bands and a palmar strut whose position determines the function of the brace. The No. 1 splint has the palmar strut in the palm and allows metacarpophalangeal flexion but immobilizes the wrist. The No. 2 splint allows flexion at the proximal interphalangeal joints and immobilizes the wrist and metacarpophalangeal joints. The third splint is difficult to construct because it only allows flexion of the distal interphalangeal joint. The distal edge of the palmar bar must be carefully molded to the different levels of the flexion creases of the individual fingers.

Dynamic splinting

In the past, manipulations have been used to break down contractures holding the hand in nonfunctional positions. The results were disastrous. Sudden violent manipulations of such contractures can only result in the tearing of scar tissue and adhesions; this trauma produces more bleeding, and the last state is worse than the first. Gradual application of dynamic traction provides a gentle, persistent force to which scar tissue will yield without excessive reaction. The principle of the application of gentle, persistent force in the stretching of scar tissue is whimsically illustrated in Fig. 3-4. Experience has shown that attempts to force contractures into new positions by applying unyielding splints are not as successful as the use of dynamic splints, which coax the joints into more functional positions. I do not believe that this type of splinting can be properly used on patients who live great distances away and who can see their physician only on an irregular outpatient basis.

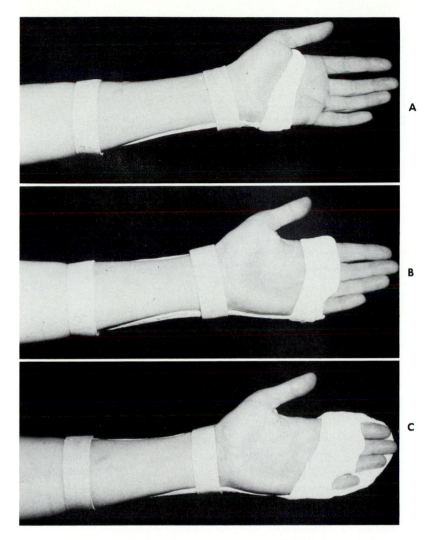

Fig. 3-3. Static splinting. These splints occasionally can be used as a substitute for surgery and are also of value in postoperative care. Three standard splints are illustrated. **A,** Allows metacarpophalangeal flexion but immobilizes the wrist. **B,** Immobilizes the wrist and metacarpophalangeal joints, allowing flexion at the proximal interphalangeal joints. **C,** Allows only flexion of the distal interphalangeal joints. (From Souter, W.A.: The Hand **3:**144-151, 1971.)

Dr. Sterling Bunnell pioneered in devising the principles on which these dynamic splints are built. He stressed that these splints must be lightweight and readily adjustable and must not interfere with the patients activities or therapy. The objective of dynamic remedial splinting is to gradually change the hand from a nonfunctional position into one of function. The tension for the splints is supplied by either elastic bands or springs, and frequent readjustment is needed to ensure that full benefit is being derived from the splint.

Few patients will tolerate indefinite use of splinting, particularly if it hampers

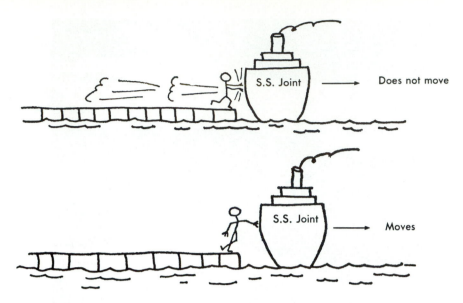

Fig. 3-4. Principle of dynamic traction. Sudden violent force applied to a stiff joint will not increase the range of movement in the joint. If, however, a gentle, persistent force is applied, the scar tissue will yield without excessive reaction. (From Howard, L.D.: Fractures of the small bones of the hand; booklet circulated privately.)

their existing functions. Some question whether they should even be asked to use these devices. Convery and co-workers reviewed 51 of their patients fitted with dynamic splinting and concluded that hand function was not increased while the splints were in use. Correction of preexisting deformity was not effectively achieved, and progression of deformity was not consistently prevented. They also believed that there was a greater limitation of motion than would have been expected if the hand had not been splinted.

However, others believe that this type of splinting can be of great value as part of either preoperative or postoperative care, but its design needs the most careful planning. The key to good design is placing the site of application of the dynamic forces in such a way that no adverse effect will be produced on the weakened rheumatoid hand. Souter has particularly warned against the possibility of increasing any subluxation tendency of the metacarpophalangeal joints with these splints.

Stiffness in varying degrees of extension in the proximal interphalangeal joints is common in some forms of rheumatoid disease of the hand. When this stiffness is particularly bad in the morning, it can be helped by the nighttime use of stretch gloves. Ehrlich and DiPiero have shown that gloves will control nocturnal pooling of tissue fluid and thereby decrease morning stiffness and increase the grip strength. A single finger can be treated by a miniature knuckle-bender splint (Fig. 3-5). A flexion deformity of a finger can be treated either by a miniature reversed knuckle-bender or the so-called safety-pin splint. It is difficult to apply the latter splint and more difficult to maintain an even pressure on the joint being treated. Because of these problems I prefer to use the reversed knuckle-bender splint (Fig. 3-5). Unfortunately, these

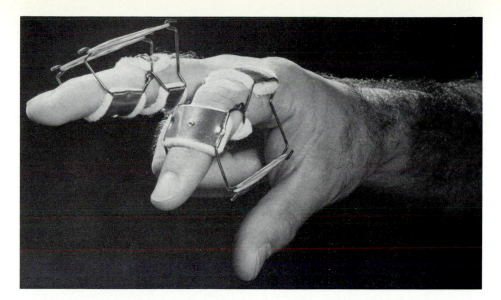

Fig. 3-5. Single finger splints. On the index finger is a knuckle-bender splint applied to the proximal interphalangeal joint. Pressure is applied to the dorsum of the proximal and middle phalanges by the elastic band, and the axis for movement is a small felt pad on the flexor aspect of the joint. On the long finger is a reversed knuckle-bender splint in which pressure is applied to the flexor aspects of proximal and middle phalanges against a pad on the dorsum of the joint, thereby straightening a flexion contracture.

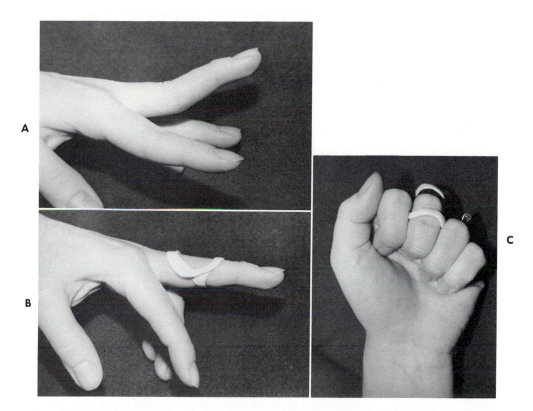

Fig. 3-6. Disposable finger splint. **A,** A swan-neck deformity before splinting. **B,** A small figure of 8, or donut splint, which is easily removable, prevents the hyperextension deformity. **C,** The splint does not inhibit full flexion of the joint.

commercially made splints are available in only a limited size range and frequently do not fit an arthritic finger.

The recent introduction of various thermoplastic materials has made it economically possible to provide splints fitted exactly to an individual digit. Since these materials can be easily altered to other shapes, it is possible to modify the splints as need arises. Because of their relatively small cost, a series of splints can be made and then discarded as gains are made through the therapeutic program. They are also of great use in demonstrating the possible gains that surgery has to offer (Fig. 3-6).

The most common use of the large or whole-hand dynamic splint is in the postoperative care of surgically treated finger joints. A dorsal splint is applied with a dorsal outrigger from which finger loops are suspended by rubber bands (Fig. 3-7). Few commercially available splints are of any use; the problems of custom-fitting these mass-produced devices to hands of all shapes and sizes are formidable. However, Swanson has introduced a mass-produced splint with sufficient potential for adjustment in the extensor assist overrider that has achieved general acceptance (Fig. 3-8). Whatever type of splint is used, I strongly agree with Souter's recommendation that a palmar strut is needed for stabilization of the finger joint to counter rotational forces (Fig. 3-7). Swanson also feels it is of value.

The recent surgical practice of balancing the wrist by transferring the extensor carpi radialis longus to the extensor carpi ulnaris during metacarpophalangeal joint reconstruction has created a great splinting problem. In these patients, wrist immobilization is essential and dorsal and palmar splint components are necessary. This makes independent donning of the splint extremely difficult and often requires the assistance of another. Since patients frequently substitute wrist flexion for metacarpophalangeal flexion, the immobilization of the wrist usually increases the active range of motion of the metacarpophalangeal joints despite the awkward splint.

It is widely believed that splinting has no place in the treatment of ulnar drift. I certainly believe it cannot be curative, since this is a dynamically induced deformity. However, an assistive dynamic splint that does not prevent prehension could be of use both preoperatively and postoperatively. Mannerfelt has recently introduced the DAHO splint illustrated in Fig. 3-9. I have no direct clinical experience with this device, but I have worn it for a number of hours and found it both comfortable and practical.

SPECIFIC POSTOPERATIVE TREATMENT

Postoperative therapy for the rheumatoid hand can be of definite use in certain specific instances when the therapy is properly supervised. We have found that the treatments suggested for patients who have had the following operations have been of value. The programs are, however, subject to variations according to the needs of each patient.

Intrinsic release

Therapy after intrinsic release must be concentrated on the restoration of flexion and the prevention of a hyperextension deformity of the proximal interphalangeal joint. However, it is important to remember that the operation removes the extensor

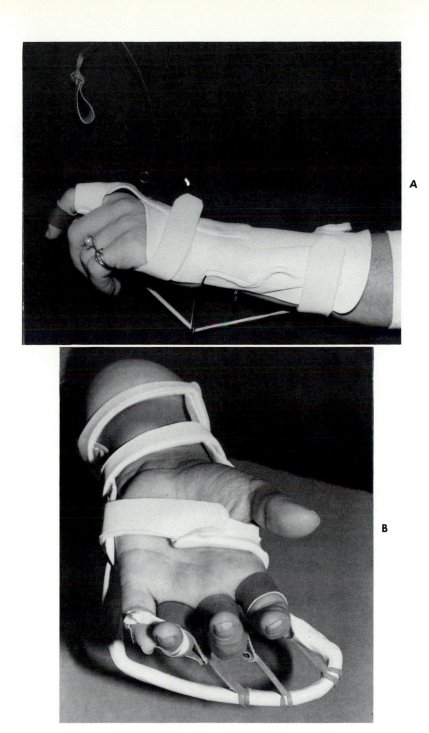

Fig. 3-7. Dorsal dynamic splint. **A,** This dorsal splint is used for exercising an arthroplasty of the index PIP joint. A cuff immobilizes the metacarpophalangeal joint, and the dorsal spring, steel wire and loop provide extension. Flexion is provided by the cuff around the finger attached to the rubber band stretched over the outrigger on the palmar side of the splint. **B,** This splint is used for exercising the metacarpophalangeal joints. A palmar strut has been added for stability, and the dorsal outrigger allows a radial placement of the rubber bands. Note that the small finger is ''buddy-taped'' and does not have a cuff and rubber band on its own.

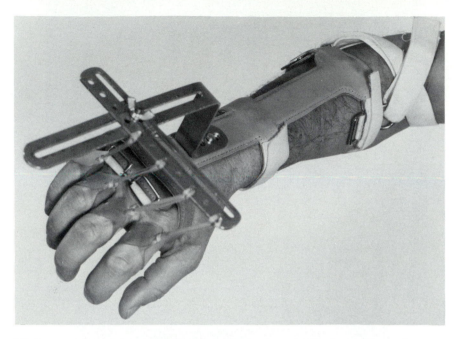

Fig. 3-8. Swanson dynamic brace. Stability is provided for the wrist. The finger slings assist metacarpo-phalangeal joint extension by lifting the proximal phalanx and prevent ulnar drift by pulling from the radial side. The rubber bands should be loose enough to permit 90 degrees of flexion, especially in the small finger. If flexion strength is weak, the slings must be periodically removed to allow a full range of joint flexion. Not shown is the palmar pad, which maintains the arch of the hand and helps prevent rotation of the device. (Illustration and legend courtesy Dr. Alfred B. Swanson, Grand Rapids, Mich.)

power of the intrinsic muscles from the finger. The fingers must therefore be exercised in both flexion and extension. The extrinsic extensor muscles will have to be reeducated and strengthened to take over the task of extending the interphalangeal joints. When exercising the extrinsic extensors, the fingers should be held in about 45 degrees of flexion at the metacarpophalangeal joint, since these muscles can extend the interphalangeal joints only when the metacarpophalangeal joints are held at less than 180 degrees.

Crossed intrinsic transfer

Technically it is difficult to sew in the transfer at the correct level, and 2 weeks should be allowed for healing before even gentle exercise is permitted. Even at this time the four fingers should be moved as a unit into flexion and extension and no attempt made to radially deviate the fingers. It is equally important to avoid firm grasping because of the natural tendency for ulnar deviation of the fingers. At 3 weeks specific radial deviation exercises with the hand flat on the table can be added to the program.

Tendon transfers

Most tendon transfers in the rheumatoid hand are done on the extensor surface to replace ruptured extensor tendons. On many occasions it is possible to defer sur-

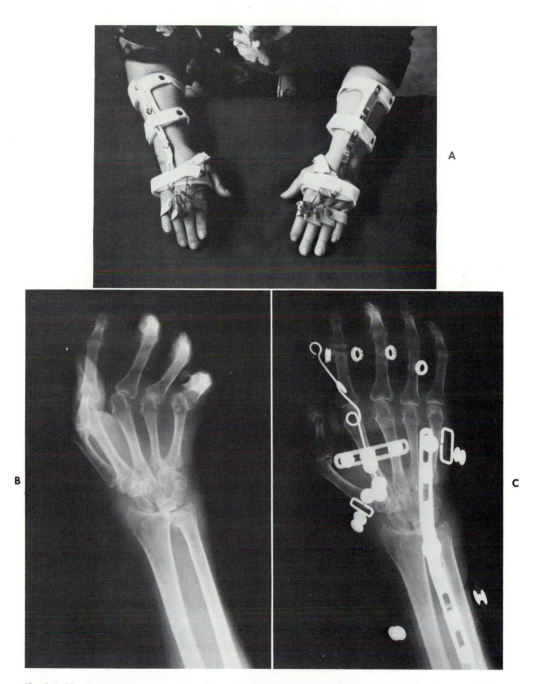

Fig. 3-9. The DAHO splint. An assistive dynamic splint that is comfortable to wear. **A,** The structure of the splint is kept dorsally away from the working surface. **B,** A hand before splinting. **C,** The hand with the splint in place showing the correction obtained. (Courtesy L. Mannerfelt, M.D.)

gery for some weeks while specific strengthening exercises are given to the muscle that will be transferred. After the operation a 3-week immobilization period is
necessary to allow healing of the transferred tendon at its new site. After this resting
period, therapy is aimed at teaching the patient the new function of the transferred muscle. Once this has been achieved, strength and endurance can be built
up.

Synovectomy and arthroplasty

Synovectomy and arthroplasty are designed to remove diseased tissue and to
restore joint alignment. They are performed at either the metacarpophalangeal or the
proximal interphalangeal joints. Therapy after these operations must be designed to
restore and increase the movements of flexion and extension. There is a risk of lateral
instability occurring in these joints; therefore exercises that require wide spreading of
the fingers or abduction/adduction movements must be avoided.

The bulk of surgery for the rheumatoid hand that requires postoperative therapy
is done at the metacarpophalangeal joints. Operations for synovectomy and joint
replacement both entail extensive dissection around the joint with a subsequent need
for tissue remodeling.

I have found that the best results are obtained in both procedures by using a
common postoperative program with a dynamic splint and finger traction bands. In
joint replacement procedures Madden and De Vore have shown conclusively that a
carefully followed management program will consistently yield good postoperative
motion.

The rationale of such therapy is that the capsular scar collagen remains metabolically active and changes configuration for months following surgery. For a synovectomy or an implant arthroplasty to succeed, the scar tissue on the dorsal and palmar
surfaces must be elongated sufficiently to allow flexion and extension. The collagen on
the sides of the joint must, however, be allowed to strengthen without lengthening,
thereby providing the necessary stability.

On the fifth postoperative day a dorsal splint is applied to hold the wrist in 15 to 20
degrees of extension. The metacarpophalangeal finger joints are held at zero degrees
of extension and 15 degrees of radial deviation by loops and rubber bands attached to
a dorsal outrigger. This splint, which is made out of thermolabile plastic, is reshaped
and adjusted as often as is necessary to maintain a perfect fit and is worn continuously
for 6 weeks. At the beginning of this time, active extension of the metacarpophalangeal joints is practiced; within a week active flexion of these joints is added. Passive
motion of these joints is done by the hand therapist daily with the objective of gaining
and maintaining at least 70 degrees of flexion. Usually 1 month after starting the
program a rubber-powered flexion band is applied with the fingers in radial deviation.
From the seventh to the fourteenth week the splint is removed during the day and
reapplied at night. Patients should be seen weekly from the fourth to the eighth week
after the operation and then monthly until 6 months have passed from the time of
surgery.

In spite of the complexity of this program, Madden, De Vore, and Arem found that patients' acceptance of the program was excellent. Using this program they obtained ranges of active and passive motion significantly greater than in other published reports. Their results certainly support their view that postoperative therapy is as important as operative technique and patient selection in determining the ultimate result.

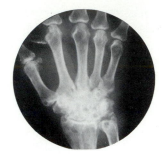

Both the elbow and wrist deserve greater consideration in terms of surgical care of the rheumatoid hand than they have been accorded in the past. Both joints frequently become weight-bearing joints for the patient with severe rheumatoid disease. Crutches can be used even with a fused shoulder joint but elbow and wrist disease may impose severe limitations on activity. A therapeutic plan for the rheumatoid hand that does not consider care of these joints must be regarded as inadequate. Surgical planning is frequently difficult because the question of priorities is hard to resolve. The elbow joint responds favorably to synovectomy even late in the disease, but the maximum benefit of synovectomy for the wrist is obtained early in the disease. Certainly if the integrity of the inferior radioulnar joint is to be maintained, surgery must be done before displacement of the extensor carpi ulnaris tendon and destruction of the triangular cartilage have occurred.

For a patient with significant disease in both joints, I usually operate on the wrist first, although on occasion it is suitable to clear both joints at the same time. When faced with severe disease in the hand and in the elbow, I generally choose to operate on the elbow as the second procedure. The combination of wrist and digital joint synovitis is best treated by giving priority to the wrist, provided gross mechanical disturbance of the tendon mechanism of the digits is not about to occur.

ELBOW

The elbow joint has a synovial cavity common to its three portions, the trochlea-ulnar, the capitellum-radial, and the radioulnar joints. The radioulnar joint is used in forearm motion, while the trochlea-ulnar portion transmits most of the forces crossing the elbow joint. Rheumatoid synovitis can therefore be expected to reduce both elbow motion and forearm rotation.

Limitation of elbow motion can be tolerated to a surprising degree if the retained motion is in an acceptable arc. Studies at the Mayo Clinic have shown that only 90 degrees of flexion/extension is required for 80% of the activities of daily living, provided the motion lies in the optimal functional range of 40 to 130 degrees. Only 50 degrees of pronation and 55 degrees of supination are required for the same activities. Even a small amount of elbow function, such as 30 degrees, will provide 50% of function if the motion lies between 80 and 110 degrees.

Souter has emphasized that the functional demands on the elbow may be threefold: as an important joint in positioning the hand, as the axis for the forearm lever, and as a weight-bearing joint in patients using crutches. The first two roles demand mobility but the second and third demand stability. The choice of operation—synovectomy (with or without excision of the radial head), arthroplasty, or arthrodesis—is therefore often extremely difficult.

Acute disease

During an episode of acute synovitis the joint needs rest, not surgery. Molded plaster splints in about 60 degrees of flexion provide excellent immobilization. These splints are for resting rather than for total immobilization. The splints should be removed several times a day, and active motions within the limits of discomfort should be insisted on. Pain is produced by too great a range of motion and is more commonly caused by ill-advised passive motion than by active contractions of the patient's muscles. Patients should be taught that the elbow is not normally a weight-bearing joint and that to use it as such via crutches or canes will greatly aggravate the condition of the joint.

Synovectomy

Physicians must remain alert to the presence of elbow synovitis because it is often relatively painless for a long while and the joint stiffens so slowly that the patient is unaware of it. Many elbows already show bony changes by the time symptoms attract attention, but Porter, Richardson, and Vainio have shown, in a review of 282 elbow synovectomies, that the severity of these changes does not significantly influence the outcome. They did show that synovectomy in joints with severe disease had few satisfactory results 3 years later. However, the study showed that in the usual case of moderately advanced disease, complete synovectomy provided pain relief in over two thirds of the elbows for up to at least 6 years.

Marked loss of pronation and supination can be caused by disease around the radial head or by concurrent disease at the wrist. A thorough examination of the distal radioulnar joint is mandatory in these patients. The rheumatoid patient needs pronation and supination but does not require the absolute mechanical stability of the normal elbow. Thus excision of the radial head can be readily considered as a means for improving forearm rotation. Excision of the distal end of the ulna may also need to

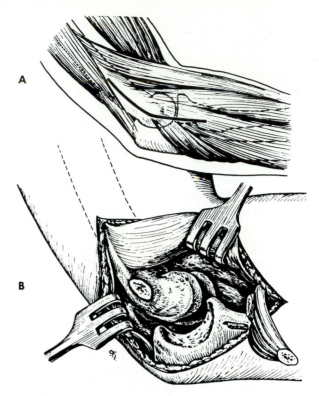

Fig. 4-1. Synovectomy of elbow joint. Surgical excision of the elbow joint synovium is a useful operation that relieves pain and restores movement. If it is done through a lateral approach, both anterior and posterior compartments can be cleared of disease. (From Edmondson, A.S. and Crenshaw, A.H., editors: Campbell's operative orthopaedics, ed. 6, St. Louis, 1980, The C.V. Mosby Co.)

be done to obtain a satisfactory increase in motion. If excisions are done at both ends of the forearm, artificial replacements should be considered to supply stability during forearm rotation. Excision of the head of the radius, with or without synovectomy, often gives marked relief of pain and increased flexion and extension. Forearm rotation is usually improved more in supination than pronation.

Synovectomy of the elbow can be successfully done through a lateral approach if the head of the radius is to be excised (Fig. 4-1). I agree with Wilson and associates that the single lateral incision carries a risk of subsequent recurrence because of inadequate clearance on the medial side of the joint. If excision of the radial head is not necessary, I do not hesitate to make a second, medial incision to ensure a thorough synovectomy. Inglis and co-workers enter the joint through a transolecranon approach, which, they state, gives a good exposure for complete synovectomy and permits early active motion, since the osteotomy is fixed both by a screw and a figure-of-eight stainless steel wire.

A voluminous soft compression dressing should be used around the joint, and early motion in both flexion/extension and pronation/supination should be started within the first two postoperative days.

It is rare for pain not to be relieved, but persistent discomfort with use is more common in those joints showing destructive changes. The postoperative range of motion varies; in Marmor's series of 25 elbows about half gained and half lost motion. Peterson and Janes showed a majority of "excellent" results in their series; and over half of the patients reported by Wilson and colleagues showed a gain in range. Inglis and associates observed an increased range of motion in 17 elbows, whereas 8 showed the same or a diminished arc of motion.

Arthroplasty

For grossly destroyed joints fusion can be considered, but it is rarely advisable because of the vital importance of retaining elbow motion. Rheumatoid disease affects many joints, and there are therefore great risks in fusing an elbow joint. Subsequent disease may so stiffen the opposite arm that the patient would be left helpless, with the two hands held away from the body. By contrast, excisional arthroplasty of the humeroulnar joint is an excellent operation and yields good long-term results. Good muscle control is essential for the success of any arthroplasty operation, and this is particularly important at the elbow because it is a hinge joint in the middle of a long lever arm. The operation necessarily destroys some of the stability of the joint, but this disadvantage is more than compensated for by the loss of pain and the increase in range of motion. The long-term rheumatoid patient often has greatly reduced muscle power, but when the joint is flexed after surgery the tightening of the muscles usually provides adequate stability for routine domestic tasks. Care must be taken in the selection of patients because the joint will not necessarily be sufficiently stable to support the extra demand of walking with a crutch or cane.

The operation is usually done through a posterior incision, with the humerus being approached through a slit made in the triceps muscle. Enough bone has to be removed from the lower end of the humerus and the trochlear notch of the ulna to produce a loose joint. No attempt is made to reproduce the exact bony contours, and only one condyle is made on the distal end of the humerus. The head of the radius is usually excised at the junction of the head and neck.

The traditional operation covers the raw bone ends with a large rectangular sheet of fascia lata cut from the thigh. Others have used cutis cut from the dense, elastic, deeper dermal layer obtained from the abdomen. A variety of flexible, synthetic, interpositional materials have also been employed.

Postoperatively, the arm is immobilized in a cast at 90 degrees of flexion and, in addition, is fixed in a shoulder abduction splint for the first 2 weeks to prevent rotational deformity. The skin sutures are then removed. During the next week the arm is held at rest in a gutter splint at 90 degrees of elbow flexion. Active movement of the finger muscles arising in the forearm is encouraged throughout the postoperative period. It is vital to maintain finger motion and to prevent circulatory stasis in the hand.

After 3 weeks a sling is used in the daytime, but the gutter splint is retained at night for about 2 months from the time of the operation. Active elbow exercises are started 3 weeks after the operation and must be continued for about 6 months. The

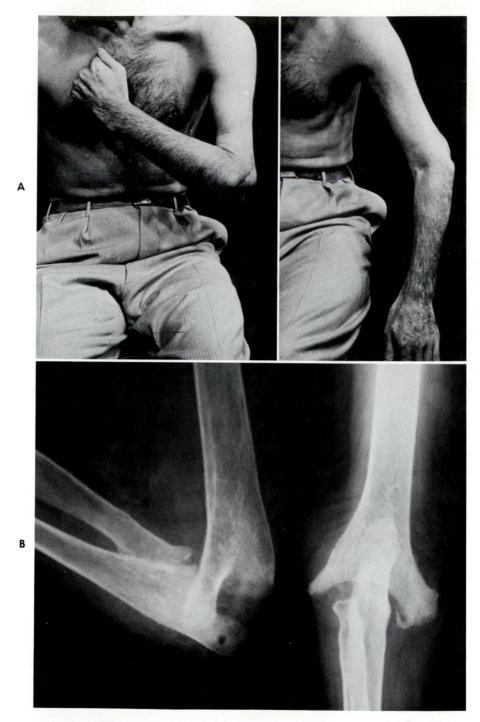

Fig. 4-2. Elbow arthroplasty. **A,** Restoration of a considerable range of motion can be achieved by elbow arthroplasty; this patient shows his range of motion 16 years after surgery. **B,** The x-ray film shows there has been a slow destruction of the lower end of the humerus, but it does not interfere with function. (From Flatt, A.E.: Phys. Ther. **44:**604-619, 1964. Reproduced by permission.)

long-term results of this operation can be excellent. The patient in Fig. 4-2 has now been followed for more than 16 years. Absorption of bone has occurred but has not adversely affected the functional result.

Dickson, Stein, and Bentley have reported improved results when the elbow is held flexed at 90 degress in neutral rotation by two Kirschner wires and protected for 6 weeks in a plaster backslab.

Prosthetic replacement

Because synovectomy of the elbow joint is not curative and excisional arthroplasty creates an unstable joint, the last 10 years have seen many attempts to produce an elbow prosthesis. The results are not impressive. The work has distilled into two approaches. The first replaces part or all of the articular surface on one or both sides of the joint and relies on the ligamentous structures for stability. The other separates the humerus and ulna by a mechanical hinge that provides angular and rotary stability.

Many varieties of both types have been tried, and several have already been withdrawn from the market. There are no detailed studies of long-term results available yet, but several short-term reviews imply that acceptable results are being obtained with the nonconstrained type of total joint replacement. Joint replacements with rigid internal restraints are subject to such severe shear and rotatory forces that loosening is inevitable.

It has become clear from this work that joint replacement of the elbow is technically extremely demanding. The short-term results being reported by those who have developed joint substitutes of either type are the best that can currently be obtained by experienced surgeons. These procedures should certainly not be performed by those who are unaware of the many biomechanical factors involved and who are inexperienced in the surgical techniques.

WRIST

It has been accepted clinical dogma for many years that positioning and integrity of the wrist joint have a profound influence on hand function.

The late Dr. Sterling Bunnell consistently taught that the wrist is the key joint in the placing of the hand and that the position of the joint has a significant influence on the function of the fingers. Dr. Arthur Steindler, in his book *Kinesiology of the Human Body*, stressed the interdependence of wrist and fingers: "Here is a chain of articulations, none of which operates in ordinary usage by itself; all depend for their mechanical effect upon intimate correlation."

Many others have echoed this view, but unfortunately only recently has the literature shown a more general appreciation of the fundamental effect wrist disease has on function of the whole hand.

Normal anatomy

In the normal limb the placing of the hand is largely controlled by the multiaxial wrist joint. The radiocarpal and radioulnar joints combine to provide a mobility

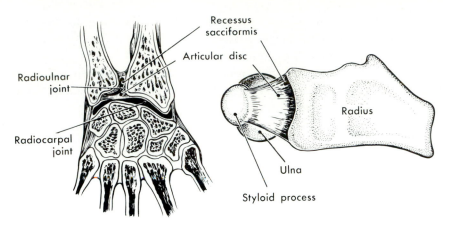

Fig. 4-3. Normal wrist joint. There is a considerable amount of synovial tissue in the radiocarpal joint and an extra amount in the recessus sacciformis more proximal to the radioulnar joint.

almost as great as a universal joint (Fig. 4-3). Cineradiography studies have shown that there is a considerable range of motion among the carpal bones. This movement is used in all directions of hand motion but is particularly utilized in palmar flexion.

All the muscles responsible for wrist movement pass over the carpal bones and insert into the bases of the metacarpals. Additional stability of the wrist is supplied by the extrinsic digital muscles as they pass over both the flexor and extensor surfaces. The stronger flexor muscles provide a more dynamic type of support than that provided by the extensors, which is of a more static quality. The tendon of the extensor carpi ulnaris has a profound influence on the balance of the wrist joint, since the line of pull of the tendon varies considerably according to the degree of rotation and flexion/extension at the wrist.

When movement of the wrist is considered in relation to finger movement, two independent actions are found to be possible. When the muscles controlling the wrist stabilize the joint, the extrinsic and intrinsic finger muscles can alter the position of the fingers. Conversely, if the posture of the fingers is stabilized, a variety of wrist joint movements is still possible. The effective length of the extrinsic finger muscles is the controlling factor in the range of combined wrist and finger movements. Neither the flexor nor the extensor muscles are sufficiently long to allow simultaneous maximum movement of wrist and fingers in the same direction at the same time. Thus it is impossible to completely extend the wrist and fingers at the same time because the flexor digitorum superficialis and flexor digitorum profundus do not have sufficient length to permit such a movement (Fig. 4-4). The extensor digitorum communis acts as a similar checkrein on the dorsum of the hand when attempts are made to flex the wrist and fingers simultaneously.

This checkrein action of antagonistic muscles creates a system in which strong wrist action is possible only if the fingers are neither fully extended nor fully flexed and in which a stabilized wrist is necessary for strong finger function. The range of

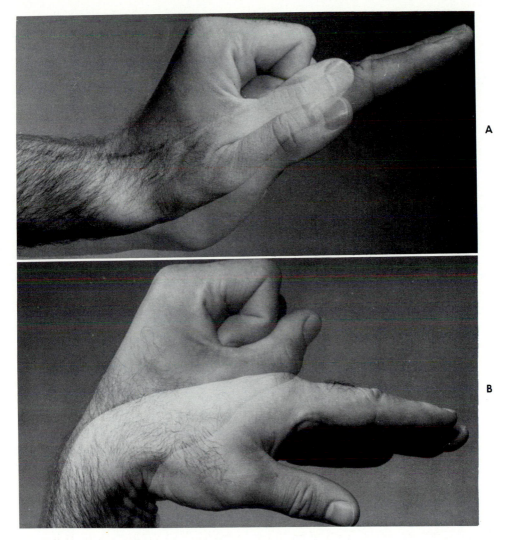

Fig. 4-4. Wrist and finger movements. **A,** The wrist and fingers cannot be fully extended at the same time because of the effective length of the extrinsic finger muscles. **B,** The wrist can be flexed further when the fingers are extended. (From Flatt, A.E.: Kinesiology of the hand, American Academy of Orthopaedic Surgeons Instructional Course Lectures, vol. 18, St. Louis, 1961, The C.V. Mosby Co.)

wrist movement needed to supply this stability is small. The most powerful extension of the fingers is achieved when the wrist is in a neutral or slightly flexed position. The most powerful finger flexion occurs with the wrist in slight extension.

The functional implications of this system for the rheumatoid patient are profound. In most patients the wrist is affected early in the disease and rapidly falls into a flexion contracture. This contracture immediately weakens the power of grasp, since grasp is more efficient with slight extension of the wrist. In the nonrheumatoid patient with a flexion contracture of the wrist, an attempt is made to compensate for the inefficient position by an increase in the intercarpal movements. In the rheumatoid patient, however, the disease almost always attacks the carpal region, thereby preventing the development of any compensatory movement in this area.

Abnormal anatomy

The key to understanding wrist instability and its influence on hand function is a grasp of Landsmeer's concept of the intercalated bone in a bimuscular, biarticular system. Zigzag collapse must occur in a three-link system with only two controls (see Fig. 2-12, p. 30). In the normal wrist the flexor and extensor muscles provide two controls, and the necessary additional third control is supplied not by a muscle but by the scaphoid bone acting as a rigid connecting rod. The studies of Fisk, Linscheid and colleagues, and others have clarified the maintenance of stability in this system, and Linscheid and Dobyns have further applied this knowledge to the rheumatoid wrist.

In the rheumatoid wrist two processes shatter the delicate mechanical balance of the carpus; both are directly attributable to the synovitis that occurs in at least 75% of all rheumatoid patients. Expanding synovium will weaken and destroy both the true wrist joint ligaments and the intercarpal ligaments. In addition, this disease leads secondarily to articular cartilage destruction and weakening of the carpal bones. They are then constantly subjected to crushing or compressive forces whenever the extrinsic tendons act over the wrist. Thus the strong extrinsic tendons responsible for accurately placing the hand are now forced to act over a "sloppy" mechanical system in which the constituent bones are smaller than normal and in which the ligamentous restraints are no longer intact. Deformity is inevitable.

Linscheid and Dobyns discuss in detail the more common patterns and combinations of deformity that are seen. Zigzag collapse can occur in the two basic planes of flexion/extension and radial/ulnar deviation. In the subluxating wrist the carpus and hand descent in a palmar direction and a concavity becomes apparent on the dorsum of the wrist (Fig. 4-5, A). This deformity is the result of a palmar flexion of the proximal carpal row on the radius. In effect there has been a zigzag collapse in the flexion-extension plane, and the intercarpal joint has buckled toward the palm. The opposite deformity, in which the collapse angles in a dorsal direction, is much less common, and the dorsal extension of the proximal carpal row on the radius is attributed by Linscheid and Dobyns to compression stress (Fig. 4-5, B).

A feature common to many of the zigzag collapse deformities in the plane of radial/ulnar deviation is the influence of the extensor carpi ulnaris muscle. Stack and Vaughan-Jackson have stressed the importance of its tendon in zigzag collapse of the wrist, and Bäckdahl devoted a considerable portion of his docent thesis, to the potentially deforming forces of the same muscle.

DeLeeuw has described the peculiar anatomical features of this muscle and its fibrous sheath. Its tendon crosses the dorsum of the distal radioulnar joint, but unlike all the other extrinsic extensor tendons, its position changes in pronation and supination (Fig. 4-6). During the movement from pronation to supination the tendon moves toward the radius and thereby tends to maintain a straight line from origin to insertion.

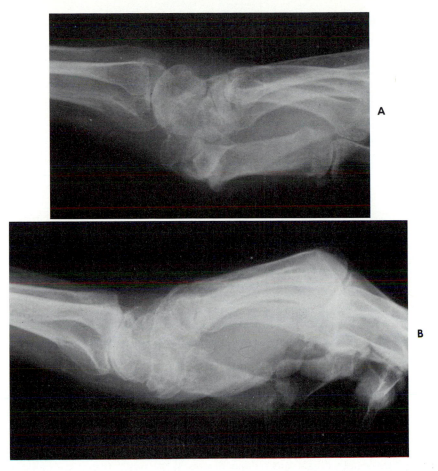

Fig. 4-5. Zigzag collapse of wrist. **A,** Rheumatoid wrist with loss of height of cartilaginous surfaces and attenuation of ligamentous structures. The normal balance of the intercarpal joint is diminished, and the position of stability becomes a zigzag collapse in which the proximal carpal row is in the palmar flexed position between the radius and capitate. This accounts for the frequently noted concavity, or spoonlike deformity, seen clinically and for the prominence of the extensor tendons at the wrist level. **B,** Lateral view of rheumatoid wrist, showing zigzag collapse of intercarpal joint under compression stress, with dorsal angulation of proximal carpal row in relation to distal forearm and carpometacarpal unit. This deformity occurs about one fifth as frequently as the palmar flexed position of the proximal carpal row. (From Linscheid, R.L., and Dobyns, J.H.: Orthop. Clin. North Am. **2:**649-655, 1971.)

Electromyographic studies have shown that this muscle always contracts in both wrist extension and flexion, but with the hand in pronation the tendon lies over the distal head of the ulna and the muscle acts more as a stabilizer than as an active extensor of the wrist. Thus constant activity of this tendon during wrist motion and stabilization subjects its fibrous sheath to constant stress. If the sheath is weakened by disease or underlying synovitis, it will yield and stretch, allowing the tendon to displace. This subluxation always occurs in an ulnar and palmar direction. Eventually the subluxation progresses to an irreducible dislocation, with the tendon lying on the

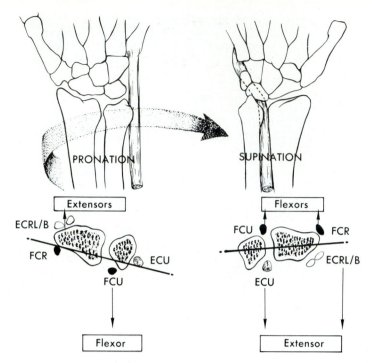

Fig. 4-6. Extensor carpi ulnaris tendon. The extensor carpi ulnaris tendon crosses the dorsum of the distal radioulnar joint, and unlike all other extrinsic extensor tendons its position changes in pronation and supination. During the movement from pronation to supination the tendon tends to maintain a straight line by moving toward the radius.

palmar side of the wrist axis, and the muscle's action becomes purely flexion. Since it is active during both dorsal and palmar flexion of the wrist, it becomes a constantly acting deforming force.

   This somewhat detailed discussion of a single muscle has been included to emphasize the importance of the torque of individual tendons as they cross the multiaxial wrist joint. Rheumatoid synovitis beneath the extensor retinaculum will expand the restraining tunnels through which the wrist tendons run, allowing alterations in their line of action. This destruction of normal equilibrium can produce profound disturbances in the placement of the hand, which, in turn, will profoundly influence the posture of the fingers and can in some instances be a major factor in the production of ulnar drift. On the radial side of the wrist the extensor carpi radialis longus produces a powerful radial torque and must be associated with the radial tilt of the bony carpometacarpal unit. By transferring this tendon to the extensor carpi ulnaris, the tilt is corrected and another factor in the production of ulnar drift is eliminated. This important concept is discussed more fully in Chapter 10.

Signs of disease

   To some the distinction will seem false, but I believe it is important to stress that disease of the extrinsic finger tendons as they cross the wrist is incidental to and independent from disease of the wrist and carpus, with which this chapter is concerned. Too frequently the word *wrist* is used in the literature as an all-inclusive term that fails to distinguish the enclosed joint systems from the more superficial synovium surrounding the extrinsic tendons (Fig. 4-7).

The active proliferative phase of rheumatoid disease almost invariably involves the synovium of the wrist and carpal joints. During the acute stage of the disease there is a strong tendency for the wrist to flex into a nonfunctional position. The optimum position for function of the normal hand is about 20 to 30 degrees of dorsiflexion. As the diseased wrist passes through neutral position and into flexion, the excursion and power of the digital flexor muscles are steadily diminished (Fig. 4-8).

The onset of rheumatoid disease of the wrist is hard to diagnose; late disease, however, is easily recognized. The articular surfaces of the normal radiocarpal and inferior radioulnar joints allow a considerable range of movement because there is little skeletal support. The integrity of these joints depends on their ligamentous support, which is much stronger on the palmar aspects. Synovitis of the joint, therefore, weakens the dorsal side of the joint earlier and more extensively than the palmar side.

The expanding synovium is restrained and concealed by the strong dorsal and palmar ligaments. It is only in the region of the ulnar and radial styloid processes that the wrist joint capsule is thinner, and it is here that early synovitis can be detected. Swelling in these areas should not be confused with the common wrist ganglion (Fig. 4-9).

Routine x-ray examinations will show alterations of the gross anatomy of the area, but only cineradiography will demonstrate the dynamic quality of the disturbance of wrist function. Arkless has reported a study of 110 wrists affected by rheumatoid disease. Among the major abnormalities found that were unsuspected from routine x-ray and physical examinations were various navicular-lunate subluxations, abnormal dynamics of the hamate-lunate interaction, diminished lunate and/or capitate rotation in dorsopalmar wrist movement, and abnormal contacts between the triquetrum and ulna.

The earliest radiological signs of wrist synovitis are seen at the ulnar styloid and head. There is involvement of the prestyloid recess and also of the distal radioulnar joint. On the radial side of the joint a notching is frequently seen on the radial aspect of the scaphoid. Marginal notchings at regions of synovial reflection are common in all joints affected by rheumatoid synovitis, but this radial notch in the scaphoid is common in other conditions as well. Although Swezey and Alexander found these notches to be present in 57% of a group of 14 patients with rheumatoid disease, they were also present in 33% of a group of 19 children and in 25% of adults' hand x-ray examinations of trauma.

Taleisnik considers that, in the rheumatoid wrist, this scaphoid notching is caused by synovitis between the radioscaphoid-capitate or "sling" ligament and the bone itself. Testut's ligament or the radioscaphoid-lunate ligament serves as a conduit for synovial invasion at its point of origin from the radius (Fig. 4-10, *A*). Gradual disso-

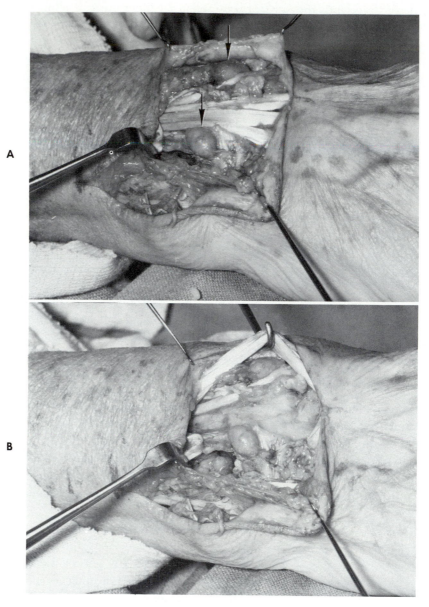

Fig. 4-7. Wrist joint synovitis. **A,** The arrows indicate two spherical projections on either side of the extrinsic extensor tendons. These projections were diagnosed as tendon synovial disease before surgery but are actually "blowouts," or herniations, of true wrist joint disease. **B,** With the tendons retracted it can be seen that the herniations have occurred not beneath the tendons but through the weak areas to the sides. **C,** The dorsal wrist capsule has been opened, and some of the extensive synovial disease of the wrist joint is shown.

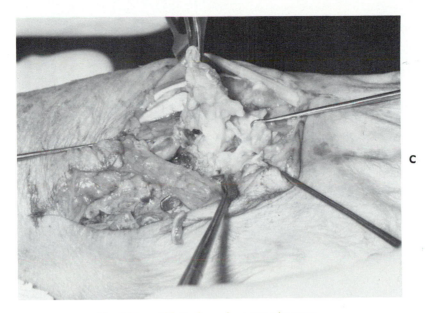

C

Fig. 4-7, cont'd. For legend see opposite page.

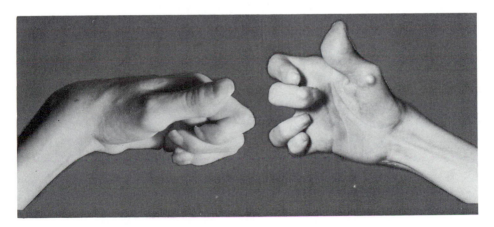

Fig. 4-8. Wrist joint disease. These two hands of a patient with juvenile rheumatoid disease show the gross wrist flexion contractures that had developed by the time he reached adult life. The flexion contractures of the fingers are largely caused by restriction of use because of the extreme wrist flexion.

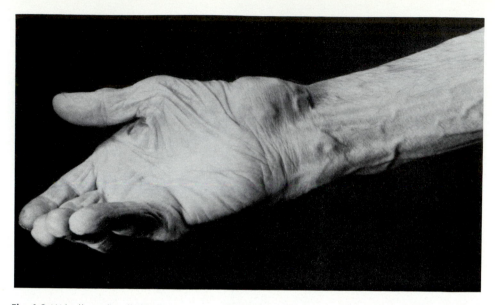

Fig. 4-9. Wrist "ganglion." This patient was referred for consultation with a diagnosis of "carpal tunnel and wrist ganglion." Removal of the rheumatoid synovium from the true wrist joint and around the flexor tendons relieved the symptoms.

lution of the carpal insertion of the ligament leads to the classic Terry Thomas sign* of scapholunate dissociation (Fig. 4-10, *B*), followed later by rotary subluxation of the scaphoid.

As the disease progresses the combination of synovitis and the forces inflicted on the carpus and wrist produces grave disturbances of function. The earliest restriction is usually in dorsiflexion. The onset of this flexion contracture is insidious and can be recognized only by repeated testing of the active and passive range of dorsiflexion of the wrist.

Disease of the radiocarpal and inferior radioulnar joints generally occurs together and produces a compound deformity. Bäckdahl's detailed description of the changes occurring in the distal radioulnar joint shows that the patient first complains of increasing weakness in the wrist, particularly during rotation, which is usually reduced in range. Later the head of the ulna projects prominently onto the dorsum of the wrist and shows an abnormal degree of dorsopalmar displacement. The ultimate complication of the caput ulnae syndrome is rupture of extrinsic extensor tendons so that there is a dropping of one or more of the ulnar fingers.

Treatment

Although the wrist is a vitally important joint, it may not be treated without regard to the patient's total disease.

Systemic treatment is essential, as are rest and the avoidance of undue stress on

---

*Mr. Terry-Thomas, a British comedian with an upper central dental diastema. See Clin. Orthop. **129:**321-322, 1977.

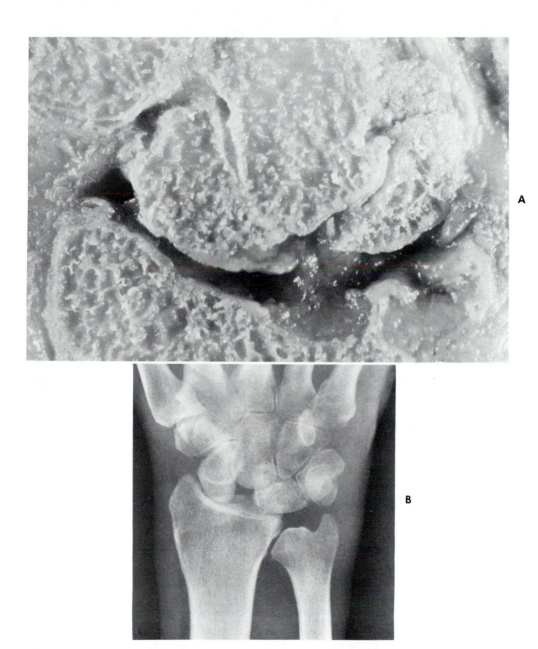

Fig. 4-10. Testuts' ligament and the Terry Thomas sign. **A,** Coronal section of a rheumatoid wrist. The radius shows cavitation of its articular surface at the site of origin of Testuts' ligament. There is separation of the scaphoid and lunate bones. **B,** The Terry Thomas sign of scapholunate dissociation. Because the lunate is dorsiflexed it is superimposed on the capitate (From Medical radiography and photography, 52, Rochester, New York, 1976, Health Sciences Markets Division, Eastman Kodak Company. Courtesy Dr. Donald Resnick.)

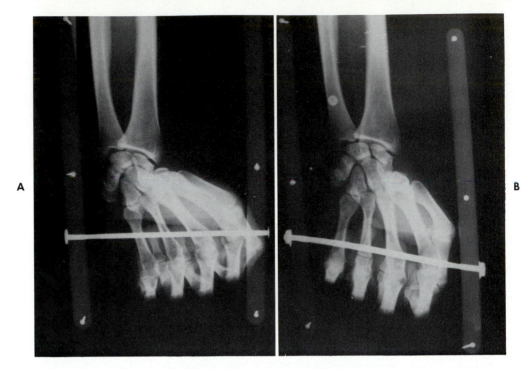

Fig. 4-11. Crutch handle. **A,** Conventional horizontal handle showing the radially deviated hand and poor anatomical alignment of the articulating structures in general. **B,** An obliquely positioned handle aligns the hand better and produces a more equal distribution of the bearing forces. (From Powers, W.R., and Flatt, A.E.: Arch. Phys. Med. Rehabil. **43:**570-573, 1962.)

the wrist. A frequent source of grossly abnormal forces on the wrist is the common crutch. The horizontal handle of the standard appliance forces the hand and wrist into an absurd caricature of wrist position. The design of this medieval support should be changed so that its handle slopes to accommodate to the normal inclination of grasp and thereby distributes the bearing forces in a more normal direction (Fig. 4-11).

Splinting the wrist is of definite value. It does not need to be forced up into the 30 or more degrees of dorsiflexion associated with the so-called functional position. A simple plaster splint can be made for use at night; the wrist should be in neutral position or in a few degrees of dorsiflexion and in neutral radial/ulnar deviation. A similar splint is of use during acute flare-ups of disease, and repeated changes of this type of splinting can gradually reduce significant flexion contractures.

Injection of various substances into the cavities of the wrist joint has not been shown to give anything other than symptomatic relief. It may therefore be useful in acute flare-ups of the disease when combined with proper rest, but it has not been my practice to use corticosteroids or the alkylating agents in this relatively large joint.

Surgical treatment for wrist disease includes synovectomy, tendon transfers, arthroplasty, and arthrodesis. Only one hand should be operated on at one time. To immobilize both hands simultaneously cripples a patient and can be so distressing as to even cause transient mental disturbances. In addition, Peacock and Holbrook have pointed out that simultaneous marked postoperative elevation of both hands increases the risk of respiratory accident.

SYNOVECTOMY

Pain around the wrist joint can be caused by a variety of conditions, and careful diagnosis is needed to ensure that synovectomy of the wrist joint would be the most appropriate procedure. Disease involving the flexor or extensor tendons or the inferior radioulnar joint can produce considerable disturbance of function and would not be improved by synovectomy of the radiocarpal or intercarpal joints.

Whether or not the long-term result of synovectomy will be good must depend on the aggressiveness of the patient's general systemic disease. One can, however, be reasonably certain that the short-term results will include relief of the pain and usually an increase in the stability of the joint and sometimes in the range of motion. Synovectomy will also have a profound effect on the more distal finger function. We have studied 10 patients in whom we performed early synovectomy at the true wrist joint. The early results, which are shown in Table 2, are satisfactory; there was no decrease in range of motion of the joint, and there was a significant increase in postoperative pinch strength.

Synovectomy of the true wrist joint is carried out through a lazy S-shaped dorsal incision, illustrated in Fig. 6-1, p. 112. The venous drainage system must be preserved wherever possible and the dorsal branches of both radial and ulnar nerves sought and protected in the borders of the incision. The extensor retinaculum is hinged on one side, and the extrinsic tendons are retracted. A transverse incision across the dorsum of the joint should be placed to leave sufficient material attached to the radius so that the dorsal capsule can be reconstituted after clearance of the radiocarpal joint. Distraction of the hand and forearm usually opens the wrist joint cavity sufficiently for the synovectomy to be performed, but it is often very difficult to adequately clear the areas adjacent to both the radial and ulnar styloid processes. Every attempt should be made to retain the triangular cartilage and even to repair its radioulnar attachments. Occasionally a longitudinal incision may be necessary over the inferior radioulnar joint to do a complete synovectomy of the joint and the saccus recessifomis. Linscheid and Dobyns recommend correction of any tendency toward ulnar translation of the carpus or angulation of the proximal carpal row by manipulation and temporary fixation with Kirschner wire pinning. The dorsal capsule is tightly sewn together and then reinforced by passing the extensor retinaculum between it and the extensor tendons.

Taleisnik has stressed that synovitis of the wrist also affects its palmar aspect. The synovitis shows as a bulge through thin portions of the palmar capsule or it can protrude between fibers of the intact deep radiocarpal ligaments. These herniations cannot be properly seen until the superficial capsule is retracted. The approach to the palmar aspect of the wrist is the same as the longitudinal approach for a carpal tunnel decompression. The only occasions on which I have done a palmar synovectomy of the wrist have been in association with median nerve decompression and flexor ten-

Table 2. Wrist joint synovectomies

A. RANGE OF WRIST MOTION

	Hand	Patient	Deviation, radioulnar		Dorsiflexion–palmar flexion	
			Preoperative	Postoperative	Preoperative	Postoperative
Wrist	R	J.A.	83-105	90-105	45-110	48-105
Wrist	R	L.I.	65-113	66-108	67-135	45-142
Wrist	R	W.L.	78-110	90-112	47-122	45-120
Wrist	R	Y.J.	98-110	90-125	80-120	90-105
Wrist	R	R.W.	78-112	75-105	45-115	32-142
Wrist	L	S.J.	75-115	75-108	38-120	45-148
Wrist, extensors*	R	W.G.	75-120	80-112	45-142	48-135
Wrist, extensors*	R	P.K.	78-122	75-130	37-135	35-148
Wrist, extensors*	L	Y.J.	80-113	105-127	100-120	85-115
Wrist, extensors, ulna*	R	M.C.	115-115	90-120	125-135	103-135
AVERAGES			83-114	84-115	63-125	58-130

NOTE: By this method of recording, the "neutral" position of the wrist is at 90 degrees in both ranges of motion.
*Additional adjacent procedure also.

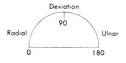

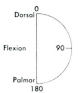

B. STRENGTH OF PINCH GRIP IN POUNDS

Patient	Preoperative			Postoperative			Postoperative test time (months)
	Tip	Lateral	Palmar	Tip	Lateral	Palmar	
J.A.	UA	4.5	4.5	6.5	8.5	6.5	4
L.I.	2.0	2.0	2.0	2.0	3.0	4.5	2
W.L.	8.5	10.0	10.0	10.0	10.0	10.0	4
Y.J.	UA	UA	4.5	UA	UA	4.5	5
R.W.	UA	UA	8.5	4.5	4.5	6.5	2
S.J.	2.0	1.0	3.0	4.5	6.5	4.5	3
W.G.	4.5	4.5	4.5	4.5	8.5	6.5	3
P.K.	1.0	4.5	3.0	4.5	6.5	6.5	7
Y.J.	2.0	4.5	2.0	2.0	1.0	2.0	4
M.C.	1.0	4.5	2.0	1.0	1.0	2.0	2
AVERAGES	2.1	3.6	4.4	4.0	5.0	5.4	

UA = Unable to perform test adequately.

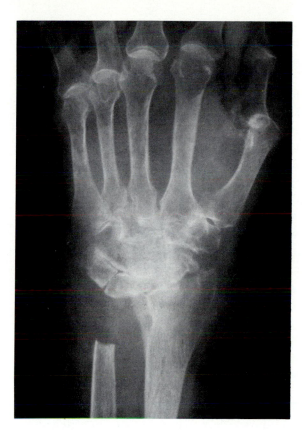

Fig. 4-12. Excision of distal ulna. Radical resection of the distal end of the ulna in a patient whose carpus has already shifted in an ulnar direction may lead to gross instability of the carpus on the radius.

don synovectomy. I have also done the traditional dorsal synovectomy at the same time and have not encountered any problems with postoperative healing.

The wrist must be protected by splinting in a midpronated position for 3 to 4 weeks to allow adequate healing of the capsular tissues, but finger and thumb motion should be encouraged throughout the recovery period.

It has been uncommon for me to perform an isolated synovectomy of the wrist joint; more commonly I combine this procedure with a synovectomy of the extensor tendons or a resection of the distal ulna, or even with both these procedures. Excision of the distal ulna provides a wide corridor to the joint, and synovectomy is not difficult (Fig. 4-12). Unfortunately this attractive entrance carries potentially severe liabilities, which are discussed in the section on arthroplasty.

Synovectomy and the necessary postoperative immobilization may lead to temporary, and in some cases permanent, small limitations of motion. Some believe that this limitation of motion in a wrist joint is of such fundamental importance that synovectomy should not be performed. I respect such views but personally believe that the operation is of value both in the relief of pain and in the prevention of further destruction within the joint. Such small limitations of motion that I have seen have not bothered the patient and more often than not have been helpful in stabilizing what would otherwise have been a somewhat floppy wrist.

Savill recorded that, in his patients, disabling symptoms in the wrist are more often related to the tendons and to the inferior radioulnar joint. He performed synovectomy at this joint, usually combined with resection of the distal ulna, but was reluctant to do synovectomy of the radiocarpal joint in early stages of the disease because of the risk of limitation of joint range. Backhouse and Kay recognize the value of resection of the distal end of the ulna but comment that the reduced range of motion may be an advantage for patients in whom there was formerly some degree of wrist instability. Bäckdahl stated that the results of radiocarpal synovectomy are not very good and remarked on the difficulty of the operation.

I agree that technically it is difficult to do an adequate clearance of the radiocarpal joint and that it often has to be combined with an excision of the distal ulna. When synovectomy of the extensor tendons is added to a wrist joint synovectomy, with or without excision of the distal ulna, we have also found little, if any, disturbance of wrist motion.

Table 3 shows the preoperative and postoperative ranges of motion of 13 hands in which the combined operation was performed. The range of motion in the thumb and the fingers is also recorded, and no significant disturbance of motion can be detected.

The intercarpal joints are frequently attacked by synovitis, but early disease may cause little or no change in the radiological findings, and the swelling synovium in these joints is often hard to detect because it is usually masked by a tenosynovitis of the extensor tendons. Synovectomy of this area was first reported by Fernandez-Palazzi and Vainio in 1965. They combined a dorsal tenosynovectomy with an intercarpal synovectomy on several occasions during their trial of this operation on a total of 47 wrists. The great majority of their patients showed diminution of pain (85%) and of swelling (71%), and the power of grip was generally increased by 63%. The range of both dorsiflexion and palmar flexion was significantly decreased.

The approach to these joints is through the lazy S-shaped dorsal incision illustrated in Fig. 6-1, p. 112. After retraction of the extensor tendons the individual intercarpal joints are opened through a dorsal incision and a piecemeal clearance of the diseased synovium is carried out. The capsule of each joint that has been opened must be individually sutured. Postoperatively the wrist is immobilized in neutral position, and active finger motion is started immediately.

I have been unable to find any other published results for this operation, but I would now agree with authors' opinion that it is a useful procedure that should be retained and that it is most suitable for patients in whom the articular cartilage is still fairly well preserved.

ULNAR HEAD RESECTION

A frequent symptom in the rheumatoid wrist is pain caused by a dorsal dislocation of the ulnar head. Firm depression of the ulnar head usually increases the pain, increases the synovial bulge on the ulnar side of the wrist, and may increase the radial deviation of the wrist. The displacement of the ulnar head occurs after the rheumatoid synovitis has destroyed the integrity of the triangular radio-ulnar articular disk (Fig.

Table 3. Synovectomy of wrist and extensor tendons

	Preoperative		Postoperative	
	AVERAGE OF 13 PATIENTS' RANGES OF MOTION			
	Preoperative		**Postoperative**	
Wrist				
Radial deviation	7		7	
Ulnar deviation	25		25	
Palmar flexion	38		39	
Dorsiflexion	26		32	
	Extension	**Flexion**	**Extension**	**Flexion**
Thumb				
MP	17	55	18	52
Carpometacarpal				
Abduction	54		49	
Adduction	9		0	
IP	22	51	24	50
Fingers				
MP Index	17	80	23	74
Long	22	85	17	79
Ring	18	81	12	72
Small	10	76	8	69
PIP Index	8	78	6	74
Long	5	80	8	79
Ring	3	84	6	82
Small	6	84	9	83
DIP Index	7	50	5	52
Long	8	60	8	61
Ring	5	56	9	58
Small	4	60	4	59

MP = Metacarpophalangeal.   PIP = Proximal interphalangeal.
IP = Interphalangeal.   DIP = Distal interphalangeal.

4-3). Attempts to repair or to replace this vital ligament have proved useless, and resection of the ulnar head is the operation of choice.

Riordan has stressed that the amount of bone removed must be small and that the resection should be carried out subperiosteally to preserve the ligamentous structures as much as possible. The length removed need not be greater than 1.5 cm, and most of the bone should be nibbled away from the articular and dorsal surfaces. The stump of the ulna must be stabilized by a flap of local tissue from either the palmar or dorsal capsule. The extensor carpi ulnaris tendon must be returned to, and retained in, its proper dorsal relationship. With this limited resection of the ulna, stability will be maintained by the pronator quadratus and the interosseous membrane. A good clearance of the radioulnar joint will also be accomplished.

The excised bone can be replaced by a Silastic ulnar head implant to maintain the length of the ulna and the balance of the wrist. The implant also provides a smooth articular surface for the radius, the carpal bones, and the overlying extensor tendons. Elimination of potential dead space by the implant allows better reconstitution of the

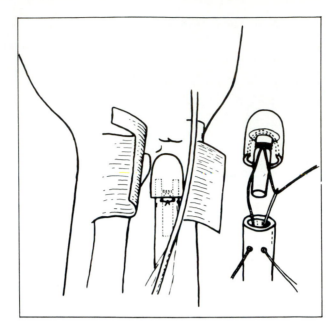

Fig. 4-13. Ulnar head implant. The implant should be secured to the ulnar shaft by passing a 2.0 Dacron suture around or through the stem and then through the two holes in the ulna. The roof of the sixth dorsal compartment should be incised so as to preserve a narrow, radially based distal flap and a wide, ulnarly based proximal flap. The narrow, radially based flap is used as a check ligament for the extensor carpi ulnaris. (Courtesy Dr. Alfred B. Swanson.)

ligaments in the area, although the remnants of the triangular ligament usually have to be removed.

The implant should fit loosely in the bone, and care must be taken not to strip back the periosteum excessively. A 2.0 Dacron suture should be passed through the implant and two holes drilled in the ulnar shaft to hold the implant in the proper position during the early weeks of healing. The distal ulna must be pressed closely against the radius before a dorsal retinacular retaining flap is sutured in place. An additional small flap must always be used to retain the extensor carpi ulnaris tendon in a dorsal position (Fig. 4-13).

Four to 6 weeks of postoperative immobilization with a dorsal plaster slab is needed, but if implants have been placed at the metacarpophalangeal level during the same operation, the dynamic splint is a satisfactory substitute for the dorsal plaster splint.

ARTHRODESIS

External support of a painful radiocarpal joint by rigid splinting is a useful, temporary expedient but is not a practical, permanent solution for the destroyed wrist. Surgical fusion of the wrist supplies the same painless immobilization and a single permanent solution to the three basic problems of pain, instability, and weakened hand function. It must be explained to the patient that while forearm rotation will be retained, wrist flexion and extension will be lost but can be substituted for by elbow and shoulder motion.

The advisability of wrist fusion is often hotly contested and is certainly under scrutiny in these days of man-made joint substitutes. However, the literature consistently contains reports of large series of good results particularly in rheumatoid patients. No doubt the pendulum will continue to swing between retaining motion and fusion, but I am impressed by how most patients gladly tolerate wrist stiffness as long as the position is proper and forearm rotation is good.

The usual indications for fusion are varying combinations of malposition, pain, and weakness, but Nalebuff and Millender regard pain as the prime indication. They will consider patients for fusion relatively early in the progression of their disease. These candidates have persistent wrist joint pain and have derived no relief from splints or occasional steriod injections. Their x-ray films show loss of joint cartilage or early carpal destruction.

Usually when many procedures are advocated for a single purpose, the implication is that no procedure is wholly satisfactory. This is not true in the case of the rheumatoid wrist; fusion can be readily obtained by a variety of techniques. The fundamental problem is not so much technique as it is the selection of the correct position for the fused wrist. The rheumatoid patient's limb is usually far from normal, and the flexion deformity of the wrist occurs because flexion is the functional position for many of the most vital uses of the hand. During feeding or dressing, the wrists are almost always flexed, and perineal toilet is impossible with the wrists held in the so-called functional position. Straub and Ranawat point out that although traditionally some dorsiflexion has been suggested, the prime consideration is to relate position to the desired function. They recommend that the dominant hand should be fused in the straight position and the minor hand should be fixed in some degree of palmar flexion (Fig. 4-14).

The radial/ulnar deviation plane is equally important. The follow-up studies of Pahle and Raunio show that a position of 5 to 10 degrees of ulnar deviation is the most desirable. This position will counterbalance the zigzag collapse and ulnar drift of the fingers that are associated with radial deviation of the metacarpals.

OPERATIVE TECHNIQUE

Carpectomy is an essential part of wrist fusion in the rheumatoid patient. Removal of bone will allow the flexion contracture to be adequately corrected and will expose good raw surfaces of bone across which fusion will occur. Partial or complete carpectomy will relatively lengthen both the flexor and extensor tendons, since the effective length of the forearm and palm has been shortened. The lengthening of the flexor tendons is helpful because it provides a greater range for the fingers, but the lengthening of the extensor tendons decreases the ability to open the hand. The total effect is often helpful, since the extensor power may be built up by appropriate exercises.

I do not use one operative technique to the exclusion of all others, but I confess to a preference for the addition of autogenous bone assisted by some means of internal

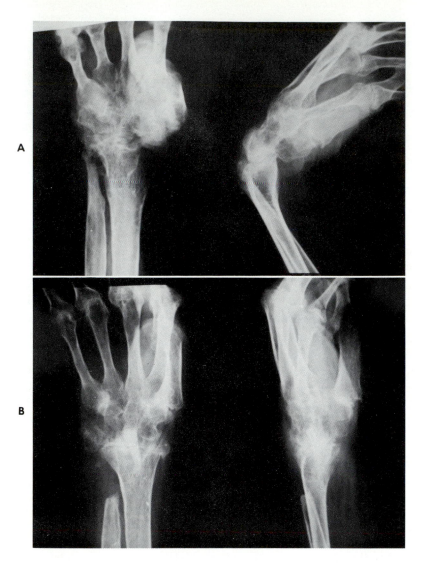

Fig. 4-14. Wrist fusion. Stabilization of the wrist is a valuable procedure, but the angle of fusion should be chosen with great care. It is not advisable to fuse the wrist in dorsiflexion because of the limitation in function imposed by such a position. **A,** Preoperative malposition in palmar flexion. **B,** Postoperative fusion in neutral position, allowing improved function of the hand. (From Flatt, A.E.: Correction of arthritis deformities of the upper extremity. In McCarty, D.J., Jr.: Arthritic and allied conditions, ed. 9, Philadelphia, 1979, Lea & Febiger.)

fixation. I always supplement this fixation with a cast in the early postoperative period.

Mannerfelt and Malmsten advocate a technique using internal fixation that does not require additional external fixation. Nalebuff and Millender report a comparable technique of internal fixation that they supplement with a removable palmar splint during the early postoperative period if soft bone prevents firm fixation. Mikkelsen has slightly modified the original method of Mannerfelt and Malmsten by inserting a Rush pin in the second metacarpal. Mannerfelt has for some years used the third or second metacarpal, depending on which gave the best position of the hand. Others have suggested the use of more than one Rush or Steinman pin for intramedullary fixation, but virtually all agree that cancellous bone should be packed between the raw surfaces of the carpus and radius. I believe that the distal end of the ulna should always be resected. I therefore obtain the necessary spongy bone from the ulnar head.

Some physicians question whether the carpometacarpal joints should be included in the fusion. Those who do not include these joints imply that the motion that develops at these joints may be useful. I agree with this assessment for fusions other than in rheumatoid joints, but it seems illogical to me to exclude the second and third carpometacarpal joints in a condition that primarily involves synovial joints and in an operation that is designed to give painless stability.

At the terminal stage of whatever technique I have chosen, the extensor tendons are laid back in their normal position, but superficial to the extensor retinaculum. The skin is closed with interrupted nylon sutures. A drain may be necessary. A complete plaster cast over a minimum of padding is then put on the limb in the operating room. Many surgeons protect their wrist fusion operations by a long arm cast for the first few weeks. I believe that for a rheumatoid patient it is wrong to immobilize more than the minimum number of joints. In most of these patients the degree of supination and pronation of the forearm is considerably reduced, and I therefore prefer to use a below-the-elbow cast. The cast should extend from below the elbow to the level of, but excluding, the metacarpophalangeal joints. The cast must be incised throughout its length while it is still wet. It is considerably easier to do it at this time than in the small hours of the first postoperative night when the question of adequate circulation in the hand may arise. The sutures are removed between 10 to 14 days after the operation, and a dorsal plaster slab is applied at the appropriate time to protect the healing tissues around the distal ulna.

ARTHROPLASTY

For those who are adamantly opposed to wrist fusion, the operative choice lies between excisional arthroplasty and total wrist arthroplasty. Both have their proponents, and neither consistently yields good results. True excisional arthroplasty of the wrist joint has had little place in the care of the rheumatoid wrist because of the technical difficulty of supplying stability as well as motion. An arthroplasty operation is, in effect, a failed fusion. Sufficient stability is desired to hold the bony surfaces together, and yet the stability must be loose enough to allow motion. Such a state of affairs is hard to achieve in the wrist. The palmar shelf arthroplasty described by Albright and Chase has provided a technique that offers stability while preserving a significant range of motion.

Arthroplasty is a salvage procedure and is a combination of synovectomy of the radiocarpal and intercarpal joints, excision of the distal ulna; and sufficient shortening of the radius to eliminate tension in the soft tissues when the wrist is reduced to

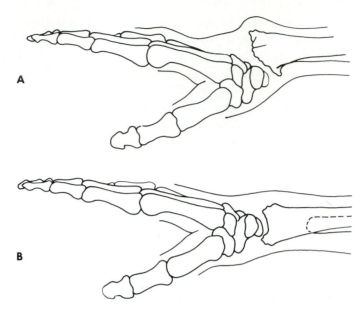

Fig. 4-15. Wrist arthroplasty. **A,** In the preoperative deformity the distal end of the radius is distorted by erosion and palmar radial spurs, which block satisfactory reduction of the subluxation. **B,** The spurs have been removed, and a shelf has been made on the palmar aspect to accommodate the carpal bones. This shelf extends the full width of the radius but does not project more than 2 or 3 mm, so that it does not block wrist flexion. (From Albright, A., and Chase, R.A.: J. Bone Joint Surg. **52-A:**896-906, 1970.)

neutral or slight extension. A small palmar cortical shelf is made on the distal end of the radius (Fig. 4-15). Fusion is avoided by not disturbing the articular surfaces of the carpal bones and, where possible, by suturing the capsule of the wrist joint to the dorsal radial cortex. Stellbrink and Tillman have modified this part of the operation by using the dorsal retinacular ligament for both interposition and the prevention of palmar displacement. Its midportion is sutured to the palmar joint capsule, the proximal edge to the dorsal radius, and the distal edge to the dorsal capsule of the carpus. If there is sufficient length, this distal edge can also be brought proximally and sutured to the dorsal radius.

The joint is transfixed for 4 to 6 weeks with Kirschner wires and splinted part-time until healing is complete some months later. Finger motions are encouraged throughout the postoperative period. I have used this procedure and I like it, but I cannot go so far as to say that I have abandoned proper fusion of the wrist, which I still regard as a useful alternative to a deliberately induced failed fusion of the joint.

TOTAL WRIST ARTHROPLASTY

Several mechanical substitutes for the wrist have been produced in recent years but none has found general acceptance. A Silastic spacer is also available but it is not a true joint substitute. There are significant design problems in replacing this complex joint with a simple mechanical device.

The wrist is a biaxial joint with two degrees of freedom, radial and ulnar deviation

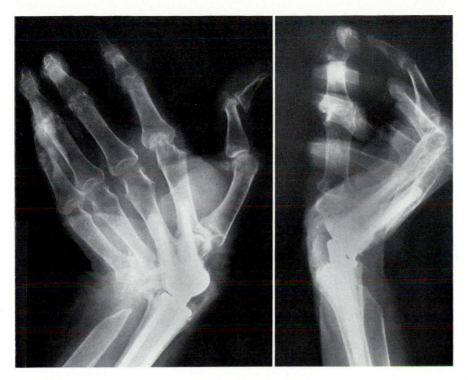

Fig. 4-16. Total wrist arthroplasty. Any unconstrained total wrist substitute must have its axes correctly placed to obtain a proper balance among the 22 extrinsic tendons crossing the wrist. This patient's wrist is locked in an end position.

and flexion/extension. The latter motion does not take place in a true sagittal plane since there is a radial deviation on extension, while flexion occurs in an ulnar direction. The centers of rotation for motion in these planes are located in the head of the capitate and are therefore on the line of the third metacarpal. Any satisfactory prosthesis must place its center of rotation directly on this line or run the risk of imbalance between the moments of force of the 22 major extrinsic tendons crossing the wrist. That this is a major design problem is shown by the ease with which the hand may fall into an end position following prosthetic insertion (Fig. 4-16). Considerable force, which may not be available to the rheumatoid patient, is needed to initiate motion from an end position.

A competent total wrist prosthesis must provide at least two degrees of freedom, with an intersection of the axes at the proper site in the head of the capitate; the mobile radial and ulnar borders of the hand must remain free to move; and the rigidity of the fixed unit of second and third metacarpals must be maintained. In addition, the moments of the 22 extrinsic tendons must be balanced. Such a complex demand could be simplified by producing a constrained cone within which the hand could operate without reaching the limiting end positions. This constraint would then impose significant forces on the stems of the device and threaten the biological interface between human tissue and the implant.

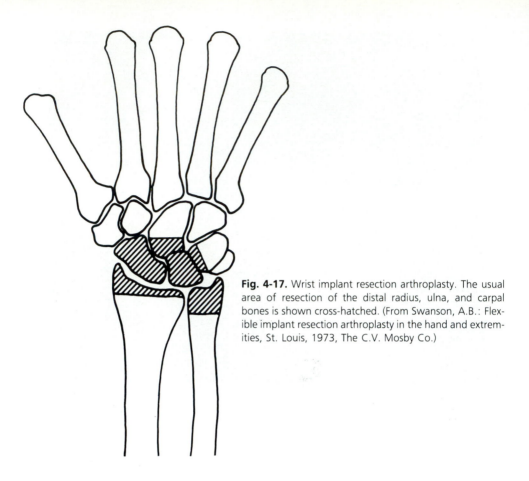

Fig. 4-17. Wrist implant resection arthroplasty. The usual area of resection of the distal radius, ulna, and carpal bones is shown cross-hatched. (From Swanson, A.B.: Flexible implant resection arthroplasty in the hand and extremities, St. Louis, 1973, The C.V. Mosby Co.)

It is for these major reasons that the currently available total wrist devices are "unforgiving" and the better results are reported from the experiences of the original designers. I have examined the biomechanical characteristics of many of these total joints and have used several clinically. However, I have used more Silastic spacers because I have found that they relieve pain and that the limited motion they provide is adequate for most rheumatoid patients.

As in all excisional arthroplasties, successful results are only obtained when the excision of bone is sufficient for proper decompression of the joint.

No matter what device is used, most of the proximal carpal row is removed together with the distal end of the radius. Frequently, but not always, the distal end of the ulna must also be removed. The amount of bone removed when the Silastic spacer is used is shown in Fig. 4-17. Note that the distal end of the ulna is cut off about 1 cm proximal to the distally cut end of the radius. A Silastic ulnar head is recommended (Fig. 4-18). Excision of the distal ulna is not always necessary. I make the decision to excise after removal of the requisite amount of carpus and distal radius and after test fitting the implant. Fig. 4-19 shows a 3-year follow-up of a Silastic wrist implant. Fifty degrees of painless motion is possible despite an apparent impaction on the distal end of the ulna.

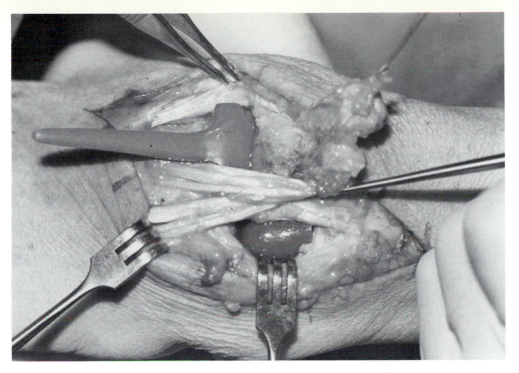

Fig. 4-18. Wrist implant resection arthroplasty. In this patient, an ulnar head replacement was judged necessary. Note the relative level of the end of the ulna implant and the crossbar of the radial component.

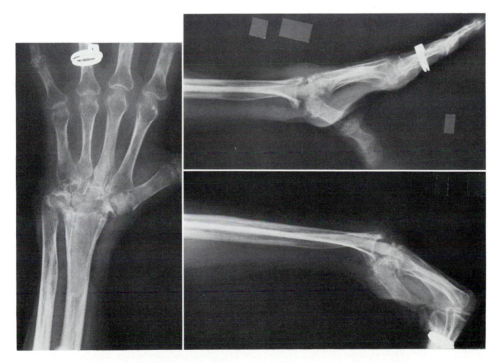

Fig. 4-19. Wrist implant follow-up. These x-rays were taken 3 years after a wrist implant; an ulnar head replacement was not judged necessary. Fifty degrees of painless motion is possible. A trapezial implant has also been used.

In the postoperative management of this operation, I use a well-padded dressing and a palmar plaster slab. The hand is elevated for about 48 hours, and the drain removed after 24 hours. A short arm cast is then applied in the neutral position. Finger movement is encouraged.

There is often an extensor lag at the finger metacarpophalangeal joints that can be helped by loops and elastic bands. This elastic traction should be suspended from an outrigger incorporated into the dorsum of the plaster cast. Sutures are removed after about 10 days, and a definitive cast is applied for about another month. Continued support for finger extension may still be needed throughout most of this time.

Carpal arthritis

Primary osteoarthritis of the intercarpal joints is uncommon and tends to be concentrated in the pantrapezial area. Secondary or postarthritic degenerative changes are much more common. The major causes of these secondary changes are scaphoid and lunate fractures, Keinboch's disease, scapholunate dissociations, persistent perilunar dislocations, and collapse deformities secondary to ligamentous disruptions.

The literature contains a large number of case reports concerning a variety of isolated involvements of various carpal bones. Some of the secondary changes are helpful in retrospective diagnosis; other changes are so characteristic that they point to a primary diagnosis. A progressive narrowing of the intercarpal articular spaces is frequently seen in juvenile rheumatoid disease. In many patients this leads to complete ankylosis by adulthood. Aseptic necrosis of the capitate is rarely seen but for some unknown reason, when it does occur, it is often associated with systemic lupus erythematosus. Degenerative arthritis of the pisotriquetral joint can occur either primarily or secondarily to old fractures or dislocations. The diagnosis, once thought of, is easily made by point tenderness over the pisiform and by crepitation caused by passive lateral movement of the pisiform on the triquetrum. Routine x-ray views will not profile the joint cavity, which can be shown by a lateral view with the forearm in 30 degrees of supination. If conservative treatment methods fail, the pisiform should be shelled out of the tendon of the flexor carpi ulnaris.

REPLACEMENT OF CARPAL BONES

Localized disease in a carpal bone with secondary peripheral arthritic changes was treated in the past by excision. Nowadays the cavity can be filled with an "anchovy" made from rolled up tendon, or silicone rubber implants can be used as spacers after resection of the trapezium, and the scaphoid and lunate bones. Careful technique is needed to reinforce the capsuloligamentous system around the implants to minimize the risk of dislocation. The scaphoid and lunate bones should be temporarily fixed in place by absorbable sutures or removable pins. An important point when excising the discarded bone is to leave a thin cortical wafer of bone behind in the depths of the wound, thereby leaving the important palmar carpal ligaments intact. I believe that the wrist should be immobilized in a short arm cast for at least 6 weeks to allow proper healing to occur. After the cast is removed, the patient should be cautioned to mobilize the wrist slowly and to only gradually increase the demands made on it.

INTERCARPAL FUSIONS

Localized intercarpal arthrodeses have recently become popular in the treatment of degenerative change following long-standing carpal instability. The infrequent occurrence of various congenital synostoses between carpal bones is cited as a justification for fusion, since these fusions do not appear to cause pain or significant limitation of motion. I believe this to be fallacious reasoning because those with congenital synostoses have never had normal intercarpal motion and should not be compared to those who are deprived of earlier motion by deliberate fusion. However, there is no doubt that successful fusions do relieve pain by restricting intercarpal motion. After fusion of the triscaphoid joint, approximately 80% of flexion/extension and 66% of radial/ulnar deviation remain in the wrist. These fusions are certainly an attractive short-term solution to a currently unsolved problem; but I am concerned that later there may be adverse results for wrist motion. Radial deviation of the wrist takes place at the radiocarpal joint with little or no intercarpal motion, but the greater range of ulnar deviation demands motion between virtually all the carpal bones. To restrict this motion by selective fusions must throw a heavy load on the remaining intercarpal joints. I believe the risk of later degenerative changes in these joints is real and could produce a serious long-term problem, perhaps necessitating wrist fusion.

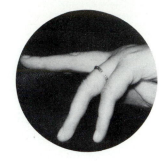

THE SKIN

Involvement of the skin of the hand is not common in rheumatoid disease. Iatrogenic thinning of the dermis by steroid medications is common and sometimes reduces the skin to tissue-paper thickness. Postoperative healing is usually normal, even in these patients, unless there is a concomitant arteritis. Arteritis usually is found only in those patients with a high titer of rheumatoid factor; some believe it is more common in patients treated with steroids. Minor lesions of the digital skin, usually adjacent to the nails and consisting of minute punctate hemorrhages or infarctions of similar size, are not uncommon in patients with more severe rheumatoid disease, but frank ulceration of clinical importance is rarely found. The few patients whom I have seen with the fully developed picture of vascular disease have usually been so ill that reconstructive surgery of their hands has not been justified.

Small tender nodules in the terminal pulps of the fingers or thumbs often precede the full-blown picture of arteritis. They should not be confused with the larger nodules that arise in response to pressures of use and are found on the working surfaces of the palmar aspect of the fingers and thumb. The grossest examples of these nodules are found along the subcutaneous border of the ulna. I have not found any constant association between these nodules and those occurring in the tendons.

Subcutaneous and intracutaneous nodules of the digits or elbow that arise in response to pressure wax and wane with no predictable pattern. Excision is the only useful treatment, but the patient must be warned that recurrence is likely if similar pressures are applied in the future. Above all, the physician must remember that these multiple nodules are often a signal of marked rheumatoid involvement and merit a cautious prognosis for the general disease.

NEUROPATHY

Impairment of peripheral nerve function is common in rheumatoid disease. Unfortunately, the discomfort of the paresthesias is frequently dismissed as "rheumatic pains," and the condition is not recognized until frank signs of palsy, such as sensory disturbances or muscle weakness and atrophy, become obvious. Chamberlain and Bruckner have studied the three distinct types of peripheral neuropathy seen in rheumatoid disease and categorized them as follows:
1. A distal sensory neuropathy with a good prognosis
2. A severe fulminating sensorimotor neuropathy
3. Entrapment neuropathies often found in early disease

Patients in the first group usually have a mild form of general disease and a patchy glove-and-stocking type of hypesthesia and hypalgesia. The electrophysiological findings are frequently normal. Patients in the severe group have a malignant form of disease with a high titer of rheumatoid factor. Nerve conduction studies show severe denervation of the nerves supplying the involved muscles. Mortality and morbidity in this group are high.

The neuropathy is probably associated with an occlusion of the vasa nervorum by arteritis. Some believe this arteritis can be associated with corticosteroid therapy, but Chamberlain and Bruckner could not detect any convincing association, and Pallis and Scott were also unable to show any direct cause-and-effect relationship.

Entrapment syndromes

Peripheral nerves passing through relatively confined and anatomically rigid areas are subject to compression by expanding adjacent synovium. In the upper limb of the rheumatoid patient this compression affects the median, ulnar, and radial nerves. The classic example is the carpal tunnel syndrome, in which the median nerve is compressed by the thickening of the synovium around the flexor tendons.

MEDIAN NERVE

There is a close association between rheumatoid disease and carpal tunnel syndrome. Polley and Lipscomb, reporting on more than 1,200 patients with carpal tunnel syndrome, noted that 29% of these patients has shown additional signs of rheumatoid disease. One hundred of these patients had rheumatoid disease and symptoms of median nerve compression simultaneously.

It is not uncommon to have the diagnosis of rheumatoid disease clearly established by the pathological study of the synovium removed from a patient operated on for idiopathic carpal tunnel syndrome. It is probable that nearly one quarter of all rheumatoid patients suffer from median nerve compression in the carpal tunnel.

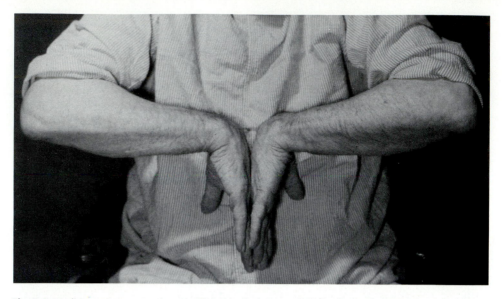

Fig. 5-1. Median nerve compression test. The wrist flexion test of Phalen for median nerve compression will usually quickly reproduce the patient's symptoms. Pressure must be applied along the forearm to press the wrist into flexion. (From Flatt, A.E.: Geriatrics **15**:733, 1960.)

The pain is characteristically troublesome at night, waking the patient, and can be relieved only by vigorous movement of the hands for a considerable time. During the day it is brought on by any activity that involves persistent grasping, particularly of small objects. Tingling and numbness occur in the thumb and in the index and long fingers, with frequent involvement of the radial side of the ring finger. The symptoms can be reproduced by asking the patient to flex the wrist by pressing the backs of the two hands against each other for about 1 minute (Fig. 5-1). The paresthesias, which are particularly troublesome at night, are caused by anoxia of the nerve produced by venous stasis. Nighttime inactivity does not provide the necessary muscle pump activity to promote adequate venous return. It is significant that the nighttime symptoms can be relieved by moving or shaking the hands, thereby increasing the activity of the muscle pump. Some have believed that the anoxia of the nerve is produced by obstruction of the arterial flow rather than by stasis of the venous return. In 1957 Vainio published a "stasis test" that clearly showed that the paresthesias were caused by venous congestion rather than arterial insufficiency. I have used this test on several occasions, both before and after surgical decompression of the carpal tunnel, and am convinced that venous congestion is the underlying cause for the symptoms in median nerve compression.

Rheumatoid patients do not often volunteer complaints referrable to the median nerve, and it is important that they be directly questioned about these symptoms. Although the classic case of carpal tunnel syndrome can be diagnosed on clinical evidence, electrodiagnostic techniques will also be positive in many cases. Barnes and Currey, in a study of 45 rheumatoid patients, found that electrodiagnostic tests for carpal tunnel syndrome were abnormal in 49% and that the condition occurred at all stages of the disease. The tests should include electromyography of the abductor pollicis brevis muscle, measurement of the motor latency between this muscle and the median nerve at the wrist, and determination of the sensory conduction time between the index finger and the wrist.

I do not believe that every rheumatoid patient should be subjected to these diagnostic tests, but I do believe that the sensory conduction times are particularly helpful in doubtful cases.

Patients with doubtful or mild signs of median nerve compression are entitled to conservative treatment with rest splints and possibly injection of hydrocortisone into the swollen synovial tissue within the carpal tunnel. Such treatment cannot be curative but it may temporarily produce sufficient shrinkage of the synovium to give some relief from the pressure symptoms. Splinting the wrist incurs the risk of increasing venous congestion by restricting use of the hand. The hydrocortisone cannot penetrate throughout all the diseased synovium, and many patients do not obtain adequate relief from such injections. Long-term follow-up of those who did receive relief shows that in most cases the improvement is only temporary.

By far the most satisfactory treatment for the established condition and the relapsed mild case is surgical decompression of the carpal tunnel by incision of the transverse carpal ligament. This is a relatively minor operation that usually gives immediate and dramatic relief of symptoms (Fig. 6-3, p. 116). In fact, most patients will voluntarily state that they had their first good night's sleep in months the night after their operation.

A surgeon undertaking carpal tunnel release in a rheumatoid patient must be prepared to proceed to a complete flexor compartment synovectomy, a much more formidable operation (p. 115).

Carpal tunnel syndrome in children is said to be rare, but when it does occur, there is a high rate of association with juvenile rheumatoid disease. Ishikawa and his colleagues at the Heinola Rheumatism Foundation Hospital have shown that the occurrence of symptoms can help in establishing the diagnosis of juvenile rheumatoid arthritis. The symptoms are produced by a proliferative flexor tenosynovitis. Thenar atrophy is common. Unlike the adult case of carpal tunnel syndrome, in children unilateral disease is frequent, sensory disturbances are rare, and thenar atrophy often improves after release of the carpal tunnel.

ULNAR NERVE

Entrapment of the ulnar nerve at the wrist is much less common than median nerve involvement because there are no tendons and therefore no expanding diseased synovium in Guyon's canal. There can, however, be a spillover effect from severe synovitis of the carpal canal. A significant number of patients may benefit from decompression of Guyon's canal. Some surgeons routinely explore around the ulnar nerve in all cases of median nerve decompression. In doubtful cases I frequently measure the conduction times of both ulnar and median nerves. Conservative treatment is of little use, and relief is best obtained by surgical decompression of Guyon's canal.

RADIAL NERVE

An inability to extend the fingers at the metacarpophalangeal joints is not necessarily caused by the rupture or dislocation of the extensor tendons; it can be caused by a radial nerve lesion. The differential diagnosis for drooped fingers is between posterior interosseous nerve compression and tendon rupture. Rupture of the extensors of all fingers does not usually occur at one time, and concomitant rupture of the extensor carpi ulnaris virtually does not occur at all. Therefore the patient who has a sudden inability to extend the fingers, which is associated with a radial deviation of the wrist, is probably suffering from paralysis of the extrinsic communis extensors and the extensor carpi ulnaris as a result of posterior interosseous nerve palsy. Often the extensor indicis proprius tendon is not immediately involved, because its nerve supply comes from the deepest and most protected fibers that are only involved in severe compression.

Additional helpful tests and signs in examining these hands are as follows: (1) Passively push the wrist into flexion; if the fingers extend slightly, then their tendons are intact because of the tenodesis effect. (2) Passive full extension of the fingers that can then be maintained by the patient shows that the muscles are not paralyzed but that the extrinsic extensor tendons had been dislocated below the axis of flexion of the metacarpophalangeal joints. (3) If direct electrical stimulation to the muscle produces extension of the fingers then their tendons are intact and the nerve supply to the muscle is at fault.

In all cases the nerve is compressed between an expanding synovitis of the elbow joint and the deep surface of the supinator muscle. Rapid recovery of function may follow a steroid injection in the elbow joint cavity, but if it does not, then synovectomy of the elbow and proximal radioulnar joints must be done.

MUSCLES

Involvement of skeletal muscles is usually early and widespread in rheumatoid disease. The weakness and wasting commonly occurs without neurological involvement. Both the extrinsic and intrinsic muscles can be involved, but the degree of involvement varies from time to time. In general, the trend is toward increasing weakness.

Some of the corticosteroids have been regarded as responsible for increasing the incidence of muscle fatigue, muscle wasting, and atrophy. Paul has pointed out, however, that many of the side effects attributed to the use of steroids are probably histopathological changes normally present in rheumatoid disease but possibly accentuated by the use of steroids. Strandberg agrees with this point of view in a study of the fluorine-substituted steroid, triamcinolone, and raises the question as to whether this drug simply exaggerates a common action of all steroids.

Intrinsic muscle disease

Changes in the state of the intrinsic muscles produce a gross disturbance in the delicate balance so necessary for normal finger function. This disturbance of balance is first shown by an exaggeration of the action of these muscles that can be detected very early in the disease by use of the appropriate test. Neither myositis nor spasm can be

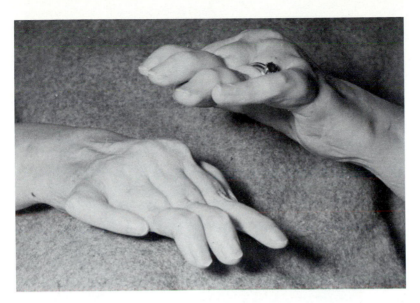

Fig. 5-2. Swan-neck deformity. The classic, fully developed deformity in patients with rheumatoid disease can be caused by permanent contracture in the intrinsic muscles. (From Flatt, A.E.: Geriatrics **15**:733, 1960.)

blamed for this aberrant action. Myositis of the intrinsic musculature is not a consistent finding in rheumatoid disease. The myositis that does occur is mild and not associated with serum enzyme elevations typical of true polymyositis. Wozny and Long have shown that spasm—in the sense of contracture of intrinsic muscles accompanied by action potentials—does not exist in rheumatoid hands, and "intrinsic plus" deformity does not subside in patients receiving either general or axillary block anesthesia.

Swezey and Fiegenberg have put forward a unifying concept that explains intrinsic muscle weakness and atrophy and the increased intrinsic tension without invoking either myositis or spasm. They suggest that painful stimuli originating during stretch of the inflamed capsule of the metacarpophalangeal joint induce a "protective" flexion contracture in the interosseous muscles. Since the muscles cannot fully stretch, they are subject to secondary fibrosis, scar in the shortened length, and thus create a mechanical restraint to extension of the metacarpophalangeal joint. Vainio has demonstrated at surgery on these cases the presence of nodules in and adhesions of the intrinsic tendon to the capsule of the joint. Although he suggested these changes as a primary mechanism, it now seems more likely that they occur secondary to the initial dynamic phase of the deformity.

SWAN-NECK DEFORMITY

Shortening of the intrinsic muscles eventually collapses the beam system of the fingers by pulling the metacarpophalangeal joint into flexion and hyperextending the proximal interphalangeal joint. The head and beak of the swan are formed by secondary flexion of the distal interphalangeal joint (Fig. 5-2).

All degrees of this exaggerated action of the intrinsic muscles are shown by an

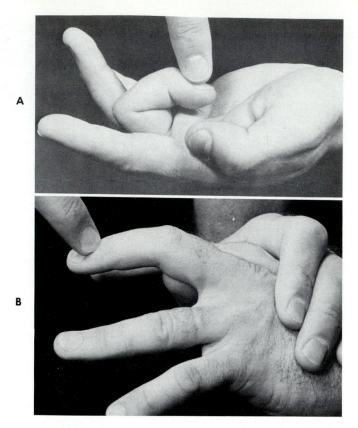

Fig. 5-3. Test for swan-neck deformity. **A,** First stage of the test applies passive flexion to all three digital joints to exclude pathological conditions of the extrinsic extensor tendon or the digital joints. **B,** Second stage of the test tenses the intrinsic muscles by holding the metacarpophalangeal joint in full extension and applying dorsal pressure to the tip of the finger. In patients with rheumatoid disease the degree of resistance to passive flexion is directly proportional to the severity of the disease.

inability to flex the interphalangeal joints when the metacarpophalangeal joints are held extended. The test for this condition is carried out in two stages (Fig. 5-3). The first stage applies passive flexion to all three digital joints. If flexion is possible, it establishes that there is no restriction to motion caused by pathological conditions of the extrinsic extensor tendon or the digital joints. In the second stage of the test the intrinsic muscles are tensed by pushing the metacarpophalangeal joint into full extension and then applying dorsal pressure to the tip of the finger in an attempt to produce passive flexion. In the normal hand passive flexion is still possible in this position. If rheumatoid disease is affecting the intrinsic muscles, the degree of resistance to passive flexion is directly proportional to the severity of the disease.

This test is extremely simple to do, yields valuable information, and should be routinely employed in the examination of all rheumatoid patients.

In the early stages of rheumatoid involvement of the intrinsic muscles, the average patient is not likely to notice any functional disturbance. Patients with skilled occupations may notice some loss of dexterity, but the changes are so insidious that even this loss may not be noticed. As the condition progresses, the exaggeration of the action of the muscles eventually produces the fully developed swan-neck deformity, which shows a flexion of the distal interphalangeal joint as well as hyperextension of the proximal interphalangeal joint. Tightening of the intrinsic muscles extends both interphalangeal joints; it cannot flex the distal interphalangeal joint. This flexion is a secondary development. It can be produced by the continuous pull of the flexor profundus muscle, gradually overcoming the resistance of the oblique ligament of Landsmeer and the extensor expansion over the dorsum of the joint. In addition it is possible that relative tightening of the profundus and its lumbrical may play some part in production of flexion of the distal joint. If the profundus is made taut because of an anterior carpal dislocation, the lumbrical would be likely to extend the proximal interphalangeal joint, and the profundus would flex the distal joint. Whatever the cause of the fully developed deformity, the resulting effects on function are disastrous (Fig. 5-4).

METACARPOPHALANGEAL JOINT DISLOCATION

For the purposes of anatomical description the interosseous muscles are divided into palmar and dorsal interossei. Boyes has pointed out that this division is of no value when considering the function of these muscles. It is better to group them into two types according to their insertion: (1) those with an attachment to the extensor mechanism and (2) those attached solely to bone.

The interosseous attachments to the extensor tendons are those responsible for the swan-neck deformity. The skeletal attachments are inserted into the bases of the proximal phalanges and normally produce flexion of the metacarpophalangeal joint and adduction/abduction movments. As the shortening of muscles becomes permanent, the abnormal flexion power becomes a deforming force. In long-standing disease of the metacarpophalangeal joints, it is common to see a palmar and proximal dislocation of the base of the proximal phalanx in relation to the head of the metacarpal. This dislocation can take place only after destruction or lengthening of the collateral ligaments. Once the dislocation has started, the pull of the bony insertion of the diseased intrinsic muscles, coupled with the pull of the superficialis and profundus flexor tendons, overcomes any remaining dorsal resistance and steadily increases the dislocation.

The resultant of the pull of these forces lies at an angle to the long line of the finger (Fig. 5-5). In long-standing, slowly progressive disease the palmar half of the metacarpal head and the dorsal half of the base of the proximal phalanx disappear, and the two joint surfaces articulate in a plane between 30 and 60 degrees to the long line of the digit. This plane is inherently unstable, and the displacement will continue until the dislocation is complete. In such cases the base of the proximal phalanx will eventually lie within the palm, with the dorsal surface of the phalanx resting against the palmar aspect of the neck of the metacarpal (Fig. 5-6).

The onset of this dislocation is insidious. If it can be diagnosed in the very early stages, it is theoretically possible that splinting may be of value. The use of splints does not retard the progression of the disease within the joints or muscles, and splints

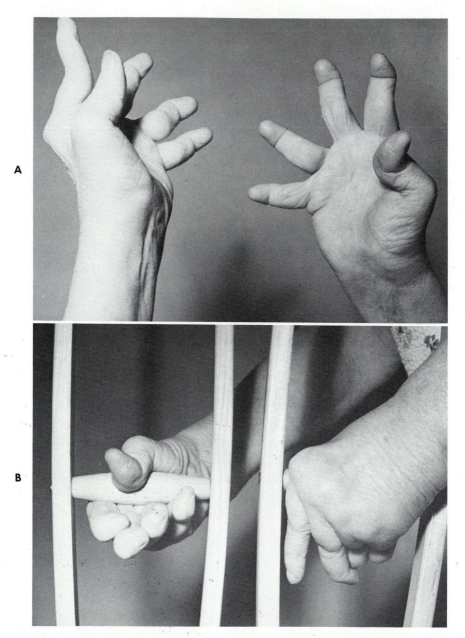

Fig. 5-4. Function and swan-neck deformity. **A,** In patients with fully developed rheumatoid disease grotesque deformities of the hand occur, and function is grossly disturbed. **B,** Principal disability is inability to curve the hands around any object, making proper grasp almost impossible.

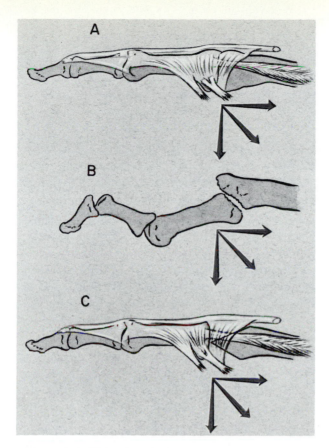

Fig. 5-5. Metacarpophalangeal joint dislocation. The forces pulling on the base of the proximal phalanx are principally the extrinsic flexor tendons and the intrinsic muscles. **A,** These two forces pull at an angle of 90 degrees to each other, and the resultant is at a 45-degree angle to the long line of the digit. **B,** Distortion of the adjoining surfaces of the two bones forming the joint is frequently at a 45-degree angle. **C,** Arthroplasty operations designed to correct this deformity must take into account these deforming factors. If they are left intact, the deformity is liable to recur. (From Flatt, A.E.: Ann. R. Coll. Surg. Engl. **31:**283, 1962.)

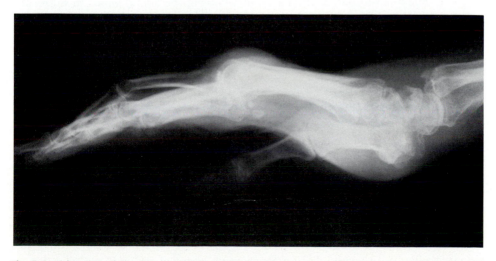

Fig. 5-6. Dislocation of the metacarpophalangeal joint. This lateral x-ray film of the hand of a patient with long-standing disease shows the classic palmar and proximal dislocation of the base of the proximal phalanges in relation to the metacarpal heads.

cannot be of lasting value. Surgery can produce such excellent results that it is more logical to treat the condition at its primary site by appropriate surgery to the metacarpophalangeal joints and the intrinsic musculature.

SWAN-NECK DEFORMITY—DIFFERENTIAL DIAGNOSIS

Unfortunately, this posture is frequently considered to be solely caused by intrinsic muscle disease. Although it is true that involvement of the intrinsic muscles is the commonest cause, many other conditions are capable of producing the deformity. The swan-neck position represents an imbalance between the muscle power on the flexor and extensor aspects of the finger. Thus the imbalance that follows a mallet finger injury or the quite common congenital swan-neck predisposition, can also be responsible. Snapping swan-neck deformity can occur in the absence of rheumatoid disease and is basically caused by the initial failure of the long flexors to overcome the hyperextension of the proximal interphalangeal joint. Eventually flexion of the joint occurs with a distinct snap as the lateral bands move from their dorsal position to the side of the joint. It is often helpful to reinforce the power of the long flexors by stabilizing the metacarpophalangeal joint in extension. Even dislocation or disturbance of wrist mechanics can produce this disturbance of balance in the fingers.

Shapiro has suggested that instead of being caused by an "intrinsic plus" state the posture can also be produced by an "extrinsic minus" situation in which the length between origin and insertion of the extrinsic muscles has been shortened by carpal collapse. This is a reasonable explanation for the established observation that in some swan-neck hands initiation of finger flexion is greatly helped by distraction of palm and forearm.

Welsh and Hastings have pointed out that swan-neck deformity may follow primary synovitis of either the proximal interphalangeal or the metacarpophalangeal joint.

With proximal interphalangeal synovitis, the palmar plate support is weakened, allowing hyperextension to occur while the capsular distention stretches out the transverse fibers of the retinacular ligament, allowing the lateral bands to subluxate dorsally. The imbalance of force over the dorsal aspect of the joint produces the characteristic hyperextension of the middle phalanx while the distal joint is decompressed by the relative lengthening of the lateral bands and thus drops into flexion.

When the metacarpophalangeal joint is primarily involved the expanding synovitis allows a more direct pull on the base of the middle phalanx. The action of the long flexors joins the bony insertion of the intrinsic muscles in producing palmar subluxation of the metacarpophalangeal joints. The resultant tightness in the intrinsic mechanism pulls the lateral bands dorsally causing the characteristic deformity.

EXTRINSIC TENDONS

Disease of the extrinsic tendons is common in rheumatoid disease. It has been said that over half of all patients have tendon disease, but the true figure must be much higher. The extensor tendons are frequently involved, but disease of the flexor tendons is often not diagnosed. In a consecutive series of 300 patients attending a medical rheumatic clinic, Savill was able to demonstrate disease of the flexor tendons in 50% of those attending. Brewerton found abnormalities of the hand tendons in 64% of an identical-sized series. He pointed out that tenosynovitis among the flexor tendons at the wrist is common and is clinically very important, since it can cause generalized pain throughout the hand. Scandinavian workers have been prominent in publishing descriptions of typical rheumatoid tendon lesions, and papers reporting large series of tendon lesions still tend to come from Scandinavia. The most commonly reported lesions are rupture of tendons from various causes, snapping fingers, tendinitis, peritendinitis, and nodule formation within tendons. Inability to extend the fingers does not justify a diagnosis of extensor tendon rupture; posterior interosseous nerve paralysis must always be excluded.

Histological study of the ruptured tendon ends has proved to be particularly unrewarding. No constant cellular patterns have been reported.

Ehrlich and colleagues found no evidence of ischemic infarction in their specimens, and Vaughan-Jackson described the tendons in his patients as "remarkable for their macroscopic and microscopic normality." Kellgren and Ball considered the primary pathological change was fibrinoid degeneration of the collagen fibrils within the tendons, whereas Laine and associates believed that rheumatoid granulomas were an important etiological factor in rupture of the extensor pollicis longus tendon.

The integrity of a tendon and its tensile strength can be weakened by direct invasion of the rheumatoid process, by chronic chafing, by involvement of its normal synovial tissues, by interference with its blood supply via the mesotendon, or by formation of intratendinous rheumatoid nodules. I believe that most tendon ruptures occur because of a combination of factors and that few are caused by a "pure" etiological factor such as ischemia or attrition.

Synovial disease

Disease of the synovium is a primary precipitating factor in subsequent disease of the tendons. It is significant that disease or rupture of the tendons occurs only in that part of the tendon that is surrounded by the synovial sheath. Disease and spontaneous ruptures do not occur in that part of the tendon that is covered by paratenon.

Experience shows that it is impossible to predict the future rupture of either extensor or flexor tendons from examination of the associated mass or from the length of time the mass has been present. It is, however, true that patients who do not respond to proper medical treatment or who have rapidly progressive disease are prone to tendon rupture. On the dorsum of the hand the ruptures commonly occur at the level of the distal edge of the extensor retinaculum. In the extensor pollicis longus tendon the site of rupture is associated with the change in angle of the tendon at Lister's tubercle.

Rheumatoid disease may first appear as isolated attacks of tenosynovitis. These swellings usually are not large and have slight symptoms (Fig. 5-7). Unfortunately these signs and symptoms frequently respond to a variety of medications and give the false impression that the disease is being controlled. More often than not, only the acute edema has been reduced, and the synovial granulation tissue continues to invade the tendons, with gradual dissolution of normal tendon fibers. This dissolution

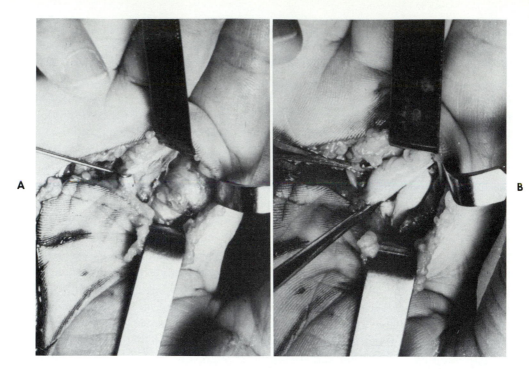

Fig. 5-7. Tenosynovitis of tendons. In the palm, swelling around the flexor tendons may be obscured by the dense palmar fascia. **A,** Tenosynovitis at the level of the metacarpal head of the index finger. **B,** After the sheath has been opened and the diseased synovium removed, involvement of the tendons can be seen.

allows gradual lengthening of the tendon, leading to a decrease of strength, and eventually may cause rupture with loss of function (Fig. 6-8, p. 122).

Backhouse and colleagues have published an extensive review of tendon involvement in the rheumatoid hand and as a result of this study have proposed a tendon damage mechanism that is related to the tendons and sites subject to the greatest movement and stress. They reason as follows:

> *At the termination of a synovial sheath the synovium normally rolls around from parietal to visceral layer as the tendon moves. Normal synovium has little bulk, and efficient lubrication results in easy movement. In rheumatoid disease synovial bulk may be enormously increased and lubrication less efficient. Easy movement of the synovium is thus no longer possible; it will neither slip easily under the retinaculum nor will it move readily round the corner from parietal to visceral layer. Furthermore there is often a great deal of fluid and debris within the synovium. When a tendon is pulled beneath a retinaculum under load, the passage of the diseased, thickened synovial sheath is difficult because of mechanical blocking. Thus, synovium and contents tend to be forced distalwards to the blind synovial end, which is thus subjected to a pumplike action with increased pressure on itself and the underlying tendon (Fig. 5-8).*
>
> *As the end of the synovial sheath is the site of greatest damage, no matter what the tendon, it would appear that such an effect distal to the nearby direct tendon-loading zone could be the cause of so much tendon damage.**

---

*From Backhouse, K.M., Kay, A.G.L., Coomes, E.N., and Kates, A.: Tendon involvement in the rheumatoid hand, Ann. Rheum. Dis. **30:**236-242, 1971.

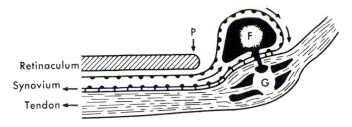

Fig. 5-8. Tenosynovitis of tendons; mechanism of damage. This illustration from the paper by Backhouse and colleagues summarizes their proposed mechanism of tendon damage within the hand. *P,* Point of maximal pressure; *F,* collected synovial fluid and debris; *G,* granuloma or other tendon damage. (From Backhouse, K.M., Kay, A.G.L., Coomes, E.N., and Kates, A.: Ann. Rheum. Dis. **30:**236-242, 1971.)

This theory certainly fits the observed facts that certain sites and tendons are found to be more vulnerable to disease than others. The main sites in all tendons are distal to the wrist retinacula or proximal to the digital fibrous flexor sheaths. The highest incidence of involvement is in the profundus tendons and the least is in the wrist joint flexor tendons.

Tenosynovitis of the wrist flexors occurs as frequently as in the extensors, usually concurrent with carpal tunnel syndrome. When the symptoms of median nerve compression are associated with limited active flexion of the fingers, flexor tenosynovitis can be diagnosed with confidence. In the palm the dense palmar fascia will prevent gross swelling, but it can usually be seen and felt near the metacarpal heads (Fig. 5-7). When the patient flexes and extends the fingers, a creaking and even crunching sensation can be felt over the line of the flexor tendons.

After the tendons have entered the fibrous flexor sheaths they are tightly enclosed, and relatively slight synovitis can have a profound effect on finger function. Stiffness, locking, or snapping of the fingers may be found, and flexion often occurs in a cogwheel fashion. Savill has described a useful lateral pinch test for nodular disease within the finger.

Another, but less common, result of tenosynovitis of the flexor compartment is the development of adhesions between the superficialis and profundus tendons. These adhesions restrict the full travel of the profundus tendon and hamper finger flexion. Surgical clearance can be satisfactory if the adhesions are slight. Unfortunately they are usually strong and extensive, and the most satisfactory treatment is excision of the superficialis tendon, which restores unrestricted profundus action.

Avascular necrosis

Pressure from edematous diseased tissue is particularly noticeable beneath the tendon retinacula because of the narrow tunnels through which the tendons pass. Although any extrinsic tendon can be affected by this process, it is the extensor pollicis longus that is most frequently affected. This tendon comes from the deep muscle group on the extensor surface of the forearm, passes around Lister's tubercle, beneath the extensor retinaculum, and inserts into the distal phalanx of the thumb. Rupture of this tendon is common in the elderly patient after Colles' fracture and is usually attributed to attrition rupture on spurs of bone left after imperfect reduction of the fracture. This mechanistic explanation has traditionally been used to explain the rupture of this tendon in patients with rheumatoid disease, but such a rupture frequently occurs early in the disease and certainly long before bony changes are demonstrable.

The explanation of the rupture is to be found in pressure obliteration of the blood supply to the tendon. Smith and Trevor both stressed the importance of inadequate blood supply as an etiological factor. The anatomist D.V. Davies pointed out that there is a critical point in the tendon at which the proximal and distal blood supplies meet. The muscle belly and proximal part of the tendon obtain their arterial supply from vessels that enter their deep surface after piercing the interosseous membrane from its anterior surface. Beyond the wrist, branches derived from the radial artery provide a relatively good blood supply to the distal portion of the tendon. The watershed between these two supply systems is in the area of Lister's tubercle. It is in just this area that the tendon usually ruptures (Figs. 5-9 and 6-9, p. 125).

Obliteration of the blood supply and subsequent avascular necrosis are significant factors in tendon rupture and occur as frequently in the flexor compartment as in the area of the extensor tendons. Rupture of the flexor tendons in the carpal tunnel is more common than is usually believed (Fig. 5-10). Both the superficialis and profundus may be affected, but it appears that the deeper profundus tendons more commonly rupture. The flexor pollicis longus tendon is also frequently affected, but this rupture is readily diagnosed because of the significant loss of function in the thumb.

BOUTONNIERE DEFORMITY

Dissolution of a length of tendon can also be caused by an associated interference with its blood supply. The edematous diseased tissue presses on, and obliterates the lumen of, the blood vessels supplying the tendon.

The proximal interphalangeal joint is a common site for such slow insidious destruction of tendon tissue. The fully developed result of this condition is the boutonniere deformity, which is the exact opposite of the swan-neck, or intrinsic-plus deformity. Like the swan-neck deformity it is not specific to rheumatoid disease and is caused by a tendon imbalance over the proximal interphalangeal joint. The fully developed deformity has three components: flexion of the proximal interphalangeal joint, hyperextension of the distal interphalangeal joint, and hyperextension of the metacarpophalangeal joint. The deformity begins at the proximal interphalangeal joint, and the changes in the joints on either side are secondary (Fig. 5-11) This distortion of the normal functional arch of the finger is caused by the expanding synovium weakening the terminal portion of the central slip of the extrinsic extensor tendon and of the lateral fibers that normally retain the lateral bands in place. The weakening and consequent lengthening of the fibers allow the lateral bands of the intrinsic apparatus to dislocate in a palmar direction. During this dislocation the lateral bands cross the axis of the joint and, instead of being extensors, become flexors of the joint. This change in function of the lateral bands has two results. One effect is that it allows the lateral bands to act more strongly at their insertion and thereby

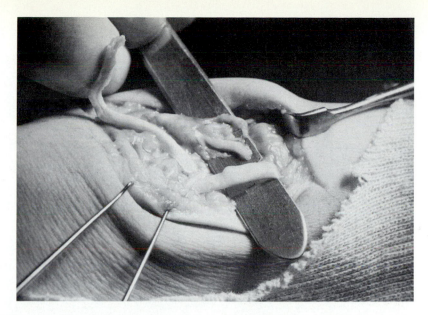

Fig. 5-9. Rupture of extensor tendons. This illustration shows the disease on the dorsum of the wrist of a 21-year-old man with rheumatoid disease of 6 months' duration. The ruptured extensor pollicis longus tendon can be seen in the top left-hand corner. In the center of the picture, on the knife blace, is the ragged ruptured end of the extensor carpi radialis longus tendon surrounded by edematous diseased synovium. Toward the bottom of the picture, lying across the knife handle, can be seen an early rheumatoid nodule developing within the tendon of a common extensor to the fingers. (From Flatt, A.E.: Ann. R. Coll. Surg. Engl. **31:**283, 1962.)

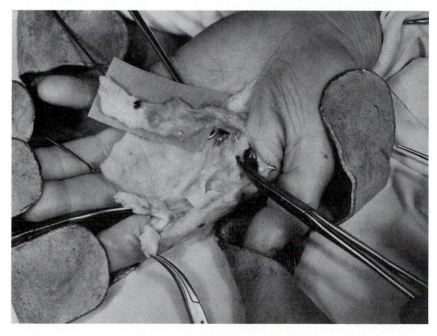

Fig. 5-10. Rupture of the flexor tendons. This patient presented with a fusiform swelling of the palm at the base of the index finger. He was unable to flex the index finger. Exploration showed extensive rheumatoid tenosynovitis and spontaneous rupture of both the superficialis and profundus tendons to the index finger. The ragged distal ends are held in hemostats. The thickened diseased synovium lies toward the upper portion of the picture on the rectangular piece of paper.

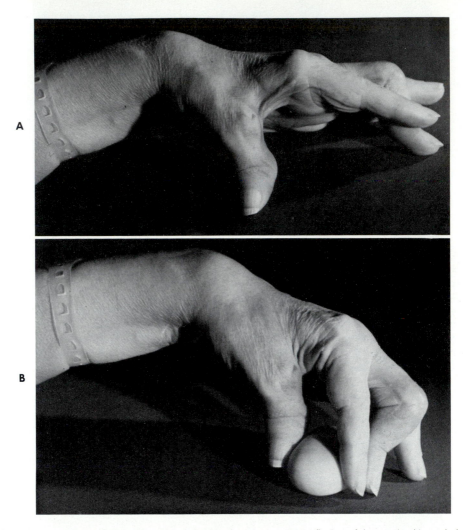

Fig. 5-11. Boutonniere deformity. In this deformity there is a persistent flexion of the proximal interphalangeal joint and a compensatory hyperextension of the distal interphalangeal joint. This patient's long finger shows the classical position of the deformity in extension, **A,** and in flexion, **B.**

produce a hyperextension deformity of the distal interphalangeal joint. The other effect is to produce a constant flexion pull on the proximal interphalangeal joint. This pull tends to push the two bone ends forming the joint up between the two dislocating lateral bands and through the thinning central slip of the extrinsic extensor tendon (Fig. 5-12). Because this deforming mechanism exactly resembles a knuckle being pushed through a buttonhole, it is known among English-speaking physicians as the boutonniere deformity. To the French it is known as "le buttonhole." Unfortunately the deformity is self-perpetuating once the lateral bands have dislocated to the flexor side of the axis of the joint.

When the flexion deformity of the proximal interphalangeal joint becomes signif-

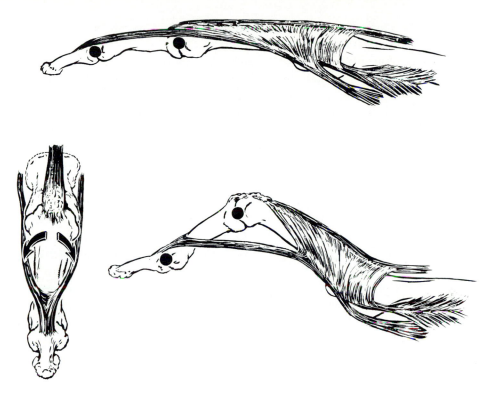

Fig. 5-12. Boutonniere deformity. The anatomical basis of the boutonniere deformity is shown in this drawing. There is a thinning of the central slip of the extrinsic extensor tendon and a dislocation of the lateral bands to the flexor side of the axis of the joint.

icant, a compensatory hyperextension of the metacarpophalangeal joint occurs. In the early stages these deformities are flexible and passively correctible. Later, after the shortening of the particular tissues, the deformity becomes fixed.

Boutonniere deformities are difficult to treat by surgery. In rheumatoid disease they seem to be particularly resistant to the usual methods of treatment. Fortunately, the functional loss is usually minimal until the late stages of the deformity. Several operative procedures that are of use are described in Chapter 6.

Attrition rupture

Rupture of the extrinsic extensor and flexor tendons can occur from attrition against a bony spur produced by reaction to the disease. This form of rupture is quite common, and both Vaughan-Jackson and Straub have analyzed the significance of attrition rupture in the loss of tendon function. Attrition rupture usually occurs in the extensor tendons at the place where they pass over the inferior radioulnar joint.

Vaughan-Jackson graphically described his findings in a series of patients with attrition ruptures. He likened the central area of rheumatoid tissue to a sea anemone because there is a mass of fibrils, tendrils, and edematous granulation tissue surrounding a central pore. Nestling deep in this pore can be found a sharp spicule of abnormal bone derived from the distal end of the ulna. The extensor tendons rub against this spike of bone and eventually rupture.

Chronic chafing of the extensor tendons against an isolated bony spike is not the only etiological factor of tendon rupture in this area. As the disease affects the distal radioulnar joint, it disrupts the structures responsible for the integrity of the joint. The triangular cartilage between the radius and ulna is destroyed, and the distal end of the ulna becomes loose and displaced. This laxity is often associated with a scalloping of the ulnar side of the distal radius as if from a pressure erosion; this defect can be clearly seen on a posteroanterior x-ray film of the wrist. As the displacement increases, the ulna moves dorsally and radially. Since the extensor tendons to the ring and small fingers cross over the distal radioulnar joint, the radial encroachment of the diseased distal end of the ulna will restrict free movement of these extensor tendons and present a large bony surface against which they can rub. Other sites for attrition rupture are recorded, but the tendons most commonly affected are the extensors of the ring and small fingers and the extensor carpi ulnaris.

Attrition rupture of the flexor tendons tends to occur more on the radial side of the hand. Mannerfelt has shown that the cause is bony spurs on the palmar aspect of the scaphoid or trapezium. The flexor pollicis longus is most commonly affected, but both the profundus and superficialis tendons of the index finger can also be involved. Only very rarely is the profundus of the long finger affected. Involvement of the thumb and index finger could be misdiagnosed as an anterior interosseous nerve palsy, and electromyographic tests may be needed to establish the diagnosis.

Nodular disease

Rheumatoid involvement of the tendons can be confined to the formation of a nodular thickening within the length of the tendon, but more commonly there is an accompanying synovitis. Nodules are formed by infiltration of the expanding synovium between the tendon fibrils. When found at this stage they can be reduced by meticulous removal of the invasive synovium from between the intact fibrils. If left untouched, these nodules enlarge, undergo central necrosis, and may become the site of rupture, since few if any tendon fibrils are left in continuity. Nodules are generally thought to be more common in the extensor tendons, but this is probably because these tendons are more easily examined. Bäckdahl and Strandberg found nodose tendinitis in 48% of 391 patients with rheumatoid disease. The incidence in the flexor tendons was three times higher than that in the extensor tendons of the fingers. In most patients the more active hand was attacked, and the incidence at the metacarpophalangeal joint level in the index, long, and ring fingers was similar, whereas the small finger was less commonly involved and the thumb was involved only one fifth as frequently as the large fingers. During the 6-year observation period they did not see one case of rupture of the flexor tendons in any of their patients.

Nodules that occur in the flexor tendons in the palm can cause a restriction of active (compared with passive) flexion, a state that Wissinger has described as digital flexor lag. Brewerton has pointed out that this cause for lack of tight grip is frequently overlooked or dismissed as the result of "arthritis." When the nodule is large enough, the finger tends to lock in flexion in the sense that the patient cannot fully extend the

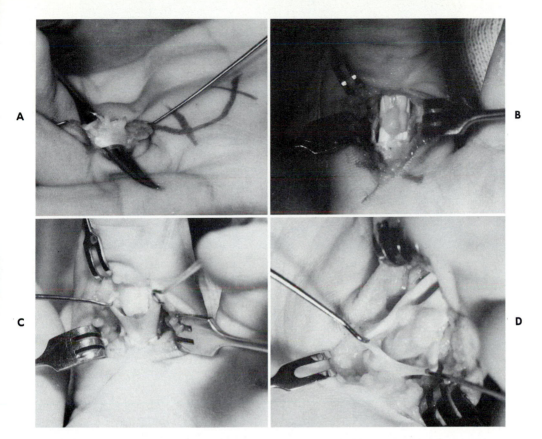

Fig. 5-13. Flexor tendon nodular disease. Nodules of the flexor tendons within the finger are confined to the profundus tendon. **A,** Ragged irregular nodule, which produced a creaking sensation on finger flexion. **B,** Edematous juicy nodule, which caused occasional triggering. **C,** Large, hard discrete nodule, which locked in the decussation of the superficialis tendon. **D,** Massive irregular nodule, which completely prevented flexion of the finger.

finger but can usually fully flex it (Fig. 5-13). Occasionally the nodules are sufficiently proximal in the flexor tendons to cause a trigger wrist. Davalbhakta and Bailey have described two patients in whom nodules were present on the profundus tendons within the carpal tunnel when the fingers were extended. Flexion of the fingers produced pain and a clicking sensation in the wrist at the level of the proximal edge of the flexor retinaculum. Synovectomy and nodule excision gives excellent relief.

The nodules that occur in the flexor tendons in the palm and cause the trigger, or snapping, finger are not always rheumatoid nodules. The catching is commonly caused by a synovitis and a swelling of the actual tendon sheath. A secondary reactionary nodule may develop in the tendon in response to these primary external changes. These changes may respond favorably to an injection of hydrocortisone into the tendon sheath. Such an injection can almost be regarded as a diagnostic test, since, if the condition does not improve after injection, it is probable that a true rheumatoid nodule is present in the tendon.

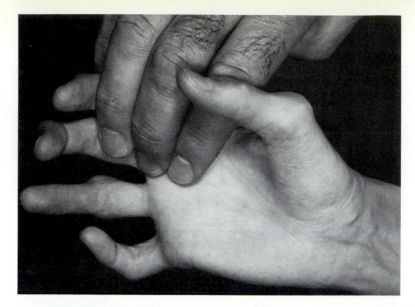

Fig. 5-14. Flexor tendon nodular disease. When a finger is "triggering," three fingers must be used to palpate a sufficient length of tendon to identify whether the nodule lies in the palm or the area of the shaft of the proximal phalanx where the superficialis tendon decussates.

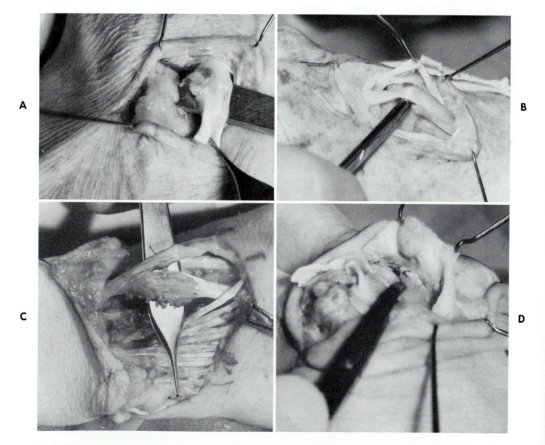

Fig. 5-15. Extensor tendon nodular disease. Nodular disease in the extensor tendons is probably more often multiple than solitary. **A,** Large solitary nodule on a single tendon. **B,** Discrete nodules within the length of several extensor tendons. **C,** Area of ragged diffuse involvement in the extensor pollicis longus and the extensor carpi radialis brevis. **D,** Nodule on the deep surface of an extensor tendon at the point where it crosses the metacarpophalangeal joint. The nodule lies at the top of the picture between two skin hooks.

This test can be deceptive, since a rheumatoid nodule can be associated with a concurrent acute synovitis, which might respond favorably to an injection of hydrocortisone. I do not hesitate to operate and relieve the constricting tendon sheath if the snapping finger does not respond to a hydrocortisone injection. Nodular disease within the finger is virtually confined to the profundus tendon, but unfortunately the nodule frequently occurs near the site of division of the superficialis tendon. These fingers tend to lock in extension in the sense that profundus action is present when the finger is held extended, but as flexion to the midposition or beyond occurs, the distal joint becomes flail because of trapping of the nodule in the tendon decussation. The nodules can be discrete or ragged, as well as single or multiple (Fig. 5-13). Because nodules can occur on the flexor tendons from the level of the distal palmar crease to the middle of the proximal phalanx, it is necessary to palpate the area with three fingers (Fig. 5-14). To use the customary single finger over the entrance to the digital sheath would miss a nodule triggering in the decussation of the superficialis.

In the extensor tendons the nodules can occur on the dorsum of the hand or in relation to the metacarpophalangeal joint. All sizes and shapes can be found, and there can be single or multiple tendon involvement (Fig. 5-15). A very early nodule is illustrated in Fig. 5-9 and an old nodule in which necrosis has led to rupture of the extensor pollicis longus is shown in Fig. 6-10, p. 126. Obvious nodules should be excised from a tendon, but judgment must be used because removal of very large nodules may so weaken the tendon that it could subsequently rupture. On the flexor aspect of the hand, nodules that protrude on the working surfaces of grip and pinch should be removed.

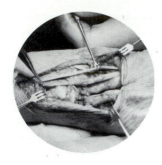

CHAPTER 6

Soft tissue disease— operative treatment

Radical synovectomy of both the flexor and extensor tendons has proved to be a useful procedure. These tendons pass through their synovial sheaths on either side of the wrist and are susceptible to nodular disease in these areas. Meticulous removal of all the synovial tissue and careful dissection of any nodules will give consistently good results. Backhouse and Kay have pointed out that thorough radical surgical clearance may leave tendons that appear in imminent danger of postoperative rupture. Their follow-up studies show that such tendons almost always recover and, given support, take up any slack that may be left. By removing diseased synovium before secondary changes have occurred in surrounding structures, the surgeon can prevent many deformities and disturbances of function.

EXTRINSIC TENDONS
Extensor tendon synovectomy

The synovial sheaths surround the tendons as they run in separate compartments beneath the extensor retinaculum. The only effective treatment of disease in this area

110

is synovectomy. Treatment by an injection with some corticosteroid preparation is illogical because, even if multiple injections could reach all the diseased areas, the steroid preparations are not curative.

The extensor carpi ulnaris tendon runs in its own individual synovial sheath, which does not always show involvement at the same time as the sheaths surrounding the extensor tendons of the fingers. The total procedure should include synovectomy of the extensor carpi ulnaris tendon because it commonly becomes involved at some stage in the disease. Isolated involvement of this synovial sheath also occurs. Synovectomy should not be postponed until the finger extensors are also involved. It is not inevitable that this involvement should occur, and postponement of the synovectomy may allow sufficient stretching of the tendon sheath of the extensor carpi ulnaris for the pull of the tendon to become aberrant and produce a gross disturbance of wrist action.

To be effective the operation must be thorough, and nothing short of a complete synovectomy should be attempted. The approach is through a skin incision of the lazy-S type centered on Lister's tubercle (Fig. 6-1). Some believe a straight vertical incision gives adequate exposure; a slightly curved compromise is acceptable. Two skin flaps are mobilized to expose the extensor retinaculum. Great care should be taken to protect the sensory branches of the radial nerve as they cross the area. Tender neuromas are in particular likely to form on the radial nerve if it is damaged. The dorsal veins draining the hand are also exposed by this incision, and equal care should be taken to protect them. It is probable that a few veins will have to be tied and cut. The dorsal veins are relatively scarce, and as few as possible should be destroyed so that the venous return of the fingers is not impaired.

In advanced stages of disease the extensor retinaculum may be perforated and partially destroyed by expansion of the diseased synovium (Fig. 6-2). An attempt should always be made to unroof the extensor tendons by raising the retinaculum as one piece hinged on either the ulnar or radial side. When the whole length of synovial covering of the tendons has been exposed, a meticulous excision of all diseased tissue must be performed. This is a slow, tedious, and seemingly unrewarding process. It is impossible to be sure that all diseased tissue has been removed, particularly on the deep surface of the tendons, because of the frequent involvement of the synovium of the carpal joints. After the best clearance possible has been carried out around the tendons and on the dorsum of the wrist, the distal end of the ulna and the inferior radioulnar joint must be inspected. If there is gross dislocation of the joint or severe dorsal subluxation of the ulna, the distal end of the ulna is excised.

The extensor retinaculum should then be passed under the tendons so that it lies directly on the carpal bones. By placing the retinaculum deep to the tendons, a barrier is provided against probable future invasion of the tendons by disease from the carpal area. The retinaculum is held in place by a few catgut sutures anchored in the carpal tissues. No attempt need be made to provide an alternative retinaculum for the extensor tendons. No functional disturbance results from this procedure. The tendons do not bowstring across the dorsum of the wrist because in most rheumatoid patients the wrists are held in neutral position or in flexion. The extreme extension

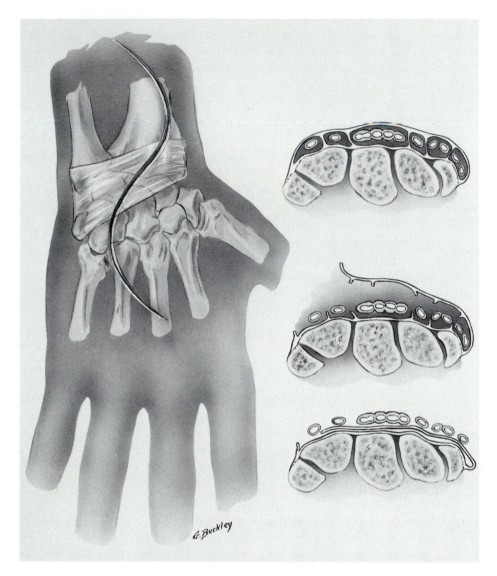

Fig. 6-1. Extensor tendon synovectomy. The tendons are approached through a lazy S-shaped incision. It has become fashionable to use a straight, vertical incision at this site. This is permissible only if the incision is of sufficient length to tolerate the lateral traction that will be needed to obtain adequate exposure. The cross-sectional drawings of the carpus show how the extensor retinaculum is raised up on a hinge on one side and, after removal of the diseased synovium, placed beneath the extensor tendons to serve as a barrier between the carpus and the extensor tendons.

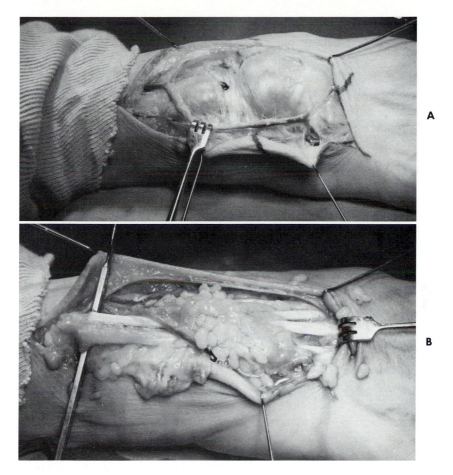

Fig. 6-2. Extensor tendon synovitis. **A,** The expanding synovitis has gradually destroyed much of the extensor retinaculum. The tension beneath the remnants of the retinaculum can be judged from the swelling at its proximal and distal edges. **B,** After the retinaculum has been reflected, many rounded fibrin rice bodies are revealed, and diffuse disease can be seen in the tendons passing over the retractor handle. (From Flatt, A.E.: Consultant **6**:36-39, July-Aug., 1966.)

necessary to produce a degree of bowstringing sufficient to cause a functional disturbance is hardly, if ever, seen.

Subcutaneous sutures are unnecessary, and the skin is closed by interrupted sutures of a nonabsorbable material such as nylon or wire. Fluffed-up dressings and a compression bandage are applied.

Postoperative care is concentrated on maintaining the general mobility of the patient. Bed rest should be discouraged, but the hand should be elevated for the first 24 hours after the operation. The compression bandage can be greatly reduced in size after 48 hours, and therapeutic exercises can be started.

RESULTS

I continue to be pleased with the long-term results of synovectomy of the extensor tendons and rarely see a recurrence of synovial swelling in the area. Straub has shown slides demonstrating impeccable results many years after extensor tendon synovectomy. This is contrary to the experience of Bäckdahl, who has commented that synovectomy of the finger extensor tendons had shown a surprisingly high number of recurrences when one considers the easy approach to the operative field.

Backhouse and colleagues have reported a careful study of 30 patients in whom extensor tendon synovectomies were done in the dominant hand only. Only 6 of these patients had a pure synovectomy performed; the remaining 24 had an excision of the distal end of the ulna combined with synovectomy. Eight patients also had tendon repairs, and 3 patients had synovectomies of one or two metacarpophalangeal joints. The nondominant hand was kept as a control, and the results showed that 21 of the patients preferred the surgically treated hand. In general there was a decrease in pain, some decrease in joint range in wrist and digits, and an increase in grip strength. As the follow-up continued over a period of 3 years, the full extent of the initial increase in strength did not appear to be maintained.

It has been suggested that actual clearance of diseased synovium is not necessary—decompression by removal of the extensor retinaculum will be sufficient. Abernathy and Dennyson have reported complete resolution of synovitis in 81.5% of a group of 54 wrists that were treated with mechanical decompression of the tendons by relocation of the retinaculum. Regardless of the degree of synovitis or involvement of the tendons, the synovium was not excised. They suggest that simple decompression of the tendons produces an unknown change in the local environment that evokes a satisfactory resolution of synovitis in the majority of cases. I have never tried this surgical approach and am impressed by their results. I agree that decompression is essential, but to conserve, or fail to remove, the diseased synovium around the tendons does not seem, to my mind, to be a logical procedure.

Carpal tunnel decompression

Symptoms of median nerve compression are frequently one of the first clinical warnings of tenosynovitis in the flexor compartment. It is a moot point whether or not one is ever justified in performing median nerve decompression by itself. It is probably more sensible to combine the decompression with a total synovectomy, thereby removing a source of potential trouble. The operation should therefore be planned so that the incision can be adequately lengthened, both proximally and distally, to allow a total synovectomy of the flexor compartment.

The operation can be done using direct local anesthesia, but I much prefer to do it using axillary intravenous block anesthesia, since I can then extend the incision as far as necessary.

The skin incision crosses the wrist crease at right angles. It runs parallel with and to the ulnar side of the thenar eminence crease in the palm and extends proximally into the forearm in an ulnar direction for 1 or 2 inches. Formerly this operation was done through a transverse wrist incision. This is a faulty approach, since it is impossible to visualize the distal edge of the transverse carpal ligament where it lies deep in the palm. All patients with the diagnosis of recurrent median nerve compression whom I have seen had been previously operated on through the transverse incision.

All were found to have an intact distal edge of the transverse carpal ligament when the wrist was reexplored through a longitudinal incision.

The incision proximal to the wrist is explored first. The median nerve will be found between the tendons of the palmaris longus and flexor carpi radialis muscles just deep to the palmar carpal ligament and the deep fascia of the forearm. When the median nerve has been properly identified, the distal portion of the incision can be deepened. The branches of the superficial cutaneous branch of the median nerve may cross the area of the incision, and branches of significant size should be saved. When the superficial surface of the transverse carpal ligament has been exposed, it is incised in a proximal to distal direction. It is my practice to pass a pair of fine, curved, blunt-ended scissors beneath the retinaculum to make certain that the median nerve is not adherent to its deep surface. The scissors are left in place, and a sharp knife is used to cut down through the ligament to the scissors underneath. The incision should be made to the ulnar side of the nerve so that any risk of cutting the thenar motor branch of the median nerve is avoided.

The incision must be carried sufficiently distal to cut the thick distal edge of the ligament. After the nerve has been exposed throughout its length, any tightly adherent synovium is carefully dissected with blunt scissors. The area of compression usually shows as a narrow waist of flattened nerve, which may be injected with many tiny vessels (Fig. 6-3). Occasionally the median artery can be clearly seen proximally and distally, but it will be obliterated in the compressed area. After the nerve has been satisfactorily decompressed, a piece of synovial tissue should be taken for biopsy and the decision made whether or not a total synovectomy is to be done.

The transverse carpal ligament need never be resutured, and a small piece (3 mm wide) should be excised along the ulnar line of the incision. No attempt need be made to close the subcutaneous tissues, and the skin is closed with interrupted mattress sutures. Horizontal mattress sutures are advised because it is vital to obtain good eversion of the skin edges so that primary healing will be assured in the thick palmar skin. These sutures have an undeservedly bad reputation. When inserted properly and tied with normal tension, they will give excellent eversion of the thickened keratin and correct approximation of the deeper epithelial tissues.

Postoperative care is simple. The hand is elevated for 24 hours and the compression dressing kept in place for about 48 hours. Its bulk can then be greatly reduced and the patient encouraged to start using the hand within the limits of comfort. The sutures are removed after 14 days and the patient allowed to use the hand normally, except strong traction with a flexed wrist should be avoided for at least 6 weeks.

Flexor tendon synovectomy in the wrist and palm

Because of the strong volar carpal and transverse carpal ligaments, swelling of the synovium surrounding the flexor tendons frequently produces symptoms of median nerve compression before any obvious physical signs of synovitis appear.

Despite this lack of physical signs, the disease is often extensive and a total clearance of the flexor compartment is necessary. The incision used for median nerve decompression is employed, but it is extended in both directions (Fig. 6-5, *B*). Often

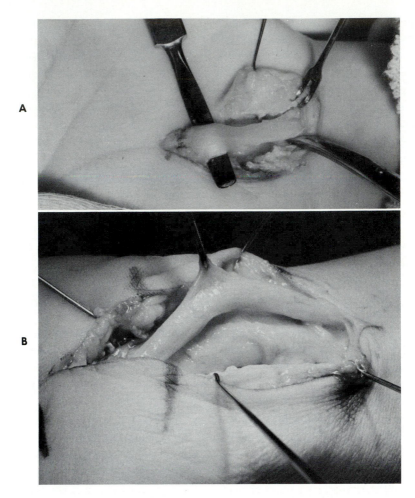

Fig. 6-3. Median nerve decompression. Two types of involvement of the median nerve can occur. **A,** Typical hourglass constriction of the nerve produced by pressure from the swollen synovium within the carpal tunnel. **B,** More uncommon adhesive type of synovitis, which tends to strangle the nerve. (**A** from Flatt, A.E.: Geriatrics **15:**733, 1960.)

the incision needs to be started 10 cm proximal to the wrist crease just to the ulnar side of the palmaris longus tendon. It should curve across the wrist, parallel the thenar crease, and then curve in an ulnar direction as far as the proximal palmar crease. This extensive incision is necessary to adequately expose the synovial sheaths of the flexor tendons.

The most important structure in this area is the median nerve. It can be found at the wrist, deep to the palmar ligament between the tendons of the palmaris longus and the flexor carpi radialis muscles. The superficial palmar cutaneous branch of the nerve arises about 4 cm proximal to the wrist and runs distally to supply the palmar skin. The nerve can often be seen in the middle third of the incision just deep to the skin and should be preserved.

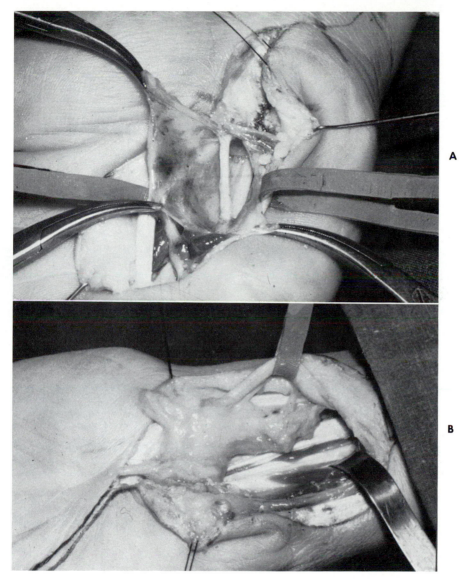

Fig. 6-4. Flexor tendon synovectomy. **A,** Typical early disease of the synovium with areas of injection and even frank hemorrhage. **B,** More chronic type of disease in which the synovium is swollen and creamy white in appearance.

The thickened synovium will be clearly seen after incision of the deep fascia of the forearm, the palmar carpal ligament, and the transverse carpal ligament. The stage of the disease determines the state of the synovium; it is always thickened and somewhat adherent to the tendons. If the disease is active, the synovium will be very edematous and frequently will show areas of injection or frank hemorrhage (Fig. 6-4, *A*). In more chronic disease the synovium usually becomes creamy white in color, but it occasionally can be somewhat grayish in hue (Fig. 6-4, *B*).

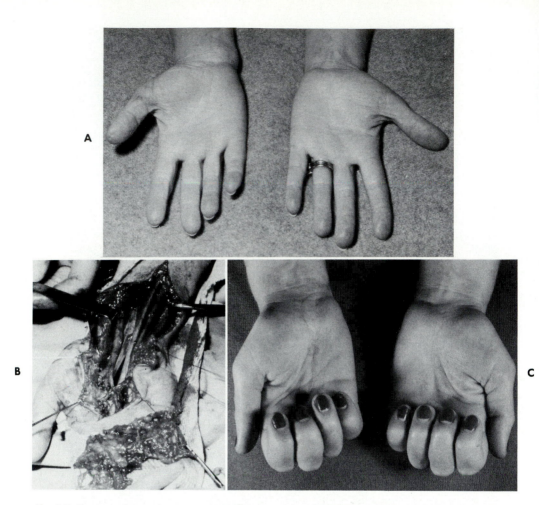

Fig. 6-5. Flexor tendon synovectomy. **A,** Small amount of swelling that is present just proximal to the wrist crease in the right hand of this patient. **B,** Extensive incision necessary for complete synovectomy of the flexor compartment. The diseased tissue that has been removed from the flexor tendons lies on the palm of the hand. **C,** Good flexion possible 7 years after synovectomy. (**B** from Flatt, A.E.: Ann R. Coll. Surg. Engl. **13:**283, 1962.)

The synovium is removed in a proximal-to-distal direction by blunt dissection, having been separated from the tendons by spreading of the scissor points. It will be necessary to cut the synovium away piecemeal from the separate tendons as it is stripped distally toward the wrist crease. Great care must be taken to identify and protect the median nerve. It also will be surrounded by thickened synovium, which must be meticulously removed. The median artery can usually be seen on the anterior, or flexor, surface of the nerve. It is a useful guide for determining the depth to which the nerve is cleaned, since the artery must be left intact on the surface of the nerve.

As the clearance proceeds distal to the wrist, it is wise to define the limits of the median nerve and its branches completely (Figs. 6-5 and 6-6). If it has been con-

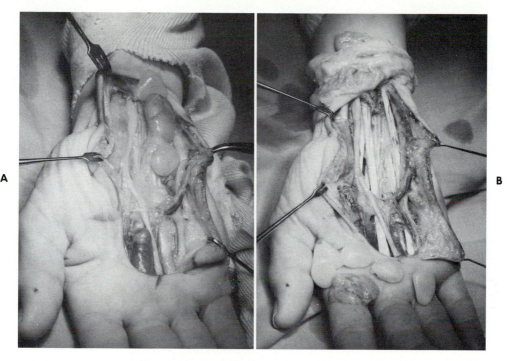

Fig. 6-6. Flexor tendon synovectomy. The presence of fibrin rice bodies greatly increases the pressure on the median nerve within the carpal tunnel. **A,** Extensive disease exposed by the palmar incision. **B,** Flexor tendons and the lumbricals have been cleared of synovium, and the superficial palmar arch can be seen lying across the tendons. Some synovium and fibrin bodies lie on the distal palm.

stricted beneath the carpal ligament, the synovium will be particularly adherent in this area and must be carefully removed so that the blood supply of the nerve can return to normal. The vital thenar motor branch of the median nerve usually arises from its anteroradial surface and must always be clearly identified before the synovium is cleared from this area.

In the palm the final clearance becomes difficult because of the presence of the superficial palmar arch and because the synovium around the flexor digitorum profundus tendons merges with the surface of the lumbrical muscles. The intrinsic muscles often appear edematous and occasionally discolored. The normal reddish brown color of the muscles loses its brightness, becoming drab and even slightly grayish in color.

During this operation it is not uncommon to find dense adhesions between the flexor digitorum superficialis and profundus tendons. These adhesions must be removed at the time of synovectomy, since they alter the amplitude of tendon movement and thereby restrict the action of the profundus tendon. Occasionally it is necessary to excise the involved section of the superficialis tendon to restore full range to the profundus tendon. If the profundus tendon is not diseased, this procedure gives excellent results.

Total removal of every portion of synovial tissue cannot be accomplished, but every effort must be made to remove all visible tissue even though it may appear to be normal. Complete removal of this tissue will prevent future invasion of normal tendons and will not interfere with future function (Fig. 6-5, *C*). Unless this operation is thorough, spread of synovial disease is inevitable.

The postoperative complications of this operation are few, and patients usually volunteer that they feel an increase in strength after surgery, presumably because of the relief of pain. Savill commented that his results with radical synovectomy of the flexor tendons were so satisfactory that he performed this operation regularly. Jackson and Paton also comment that the results of extensive flexor tendon synovectomy are usually excellent or good. Ranawat and Straub have reviewed 60 flexor compartment synovectomies after an average follow-up of 3½ years. They classed as satisfactory an operation that yielded complete relief of pain, almost complete active flexion of the fingers, no recurrence of synovitis, and an improvement of sensation over the median nerve distribution. Eighty-three percent of their results were satisfactory to good. Of the failures, two patients with a severe adhesive tenosynovitis were unable to flex their fingers to within 3 cm of the thenar eminence either before or after surgery. All the other complications were associated with persistent paresthesias of the median nerve or neuroma formation on its palmar cutaneous branch.

Flexor tendon synovectomy in the digits

Tenosynovitis within the fingers causes pain, swelling, stiffness, and occasional triggering with resultant loss of function and manual dexterity. Surgical treatment yields good results but injection of steroids into the tendon sheath may be helpful. Gray and colleagues have reported the use of steroid injections in tenosynovitis in the fingers of 46 patients with proven rheumatoid disease and 38 nonrheumatoid patients. The steroid was given with an equal volume of lidocaine and was repeated at 1- to 4-week intervals as indicated. Ninety-three percent of the rheumatoid patients and 89% of the nonrheumatoid patients showed early improvement. A mean of 1.3 injections was required for flexor tenosynovitis resolution. It seems, therefore, that such injection treatment of digital tenosynovitis could be tried before resorting to surgical clearance. Surgical clearance of the synovium from the flexor aspect of a finger is not difficult and should be done using the Bruner or palmar zigzag incision (Fig. 6-7). The skin incision may not need to be extended distal to the proximal interphalageal joint because the profundus tendon can be pulled proximally into the wound.

Preservation and even reconstruction of the pulleys retaining the flexor tendon against the phalanges is vital. They should be trimmed of disease but retained at all sites; it is particularly important to retain the A1 and A2 pulleys as a restraint against ulnar drift (Fig. 6-8). Nodular disease of the profundus tendons may be discovered during the synovectomy and the nodules should be excised both from the surface and from within the tendons. Ferlic and Clayton point out that further decompression of the flexor tendons can be obtained by detaching the ulnar slip of the superficialis from its insertion and removing it as far as the palm. Passive tendon range must be checked to ensure smooth movement and that the proximal cut end of the superficialis does not catch on the A1 pulley. The other half of the superficialis insertion is preserved to

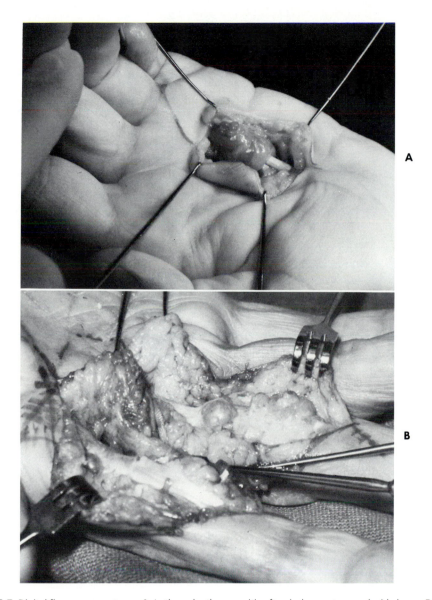

Fig. 6-7. Digital flexor synovectomy. **A,** In the palm the synovitis often bulges out as a palpable lump. **B,** The finger should be approached through a zigzag Bruner incision, which allows wide exposure. The index finger at the bottom of this illustration has been cleared of synovitis. The long finger in the middle of the illustration shows the bulging synovitis prior to removal.

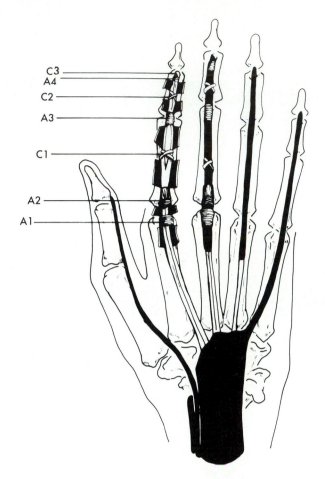

Fig. 6-8. Preservation of flexor pulleys. It is vital to preserve or to even reconstruct the "A" pulleys in the flexor tendon sheath during synovectomy. If this is not done, the tendons will increase their ulnar torque and induce ulnar drift. (From Ferlic, D.C., and Clayton, M.L.: Flexor tenosynovectomy in rheumatoid finger, J. Hand Surg. **3:**364-67, 1978.)

prevent development of swan-neck deformity. Early postoperative motion is advisable.

The results of this operation are uniformly reported as satisfactory, the only adverse reports being from the association of the proximal interphalangeal joint with synovitis and arthritis.

Trigger finger release

The tendon nodule in most trigger fingers occurs at the level of the proximal opening of the flexor tendon sheath. The surface marking of this level is the line of the distal palmar crease. In the thumb the common level is the flexor crease over the metacarpophalangeal joint. If the snapping of the digit has not responded to a hydrocortisone injection, permanent relief can be obtained by sectioning the proximal portion of the flexor sheath.

The operation can be done under local anesthesia, using 1% lidocaine (Xylocaine) without epinephrine. The solution is injected into the skin directly over the nodule and then infiltrated into the deeper tissues. A short transverse skin incision at right angles to the line of the tendon over the nodule is usually sufficient exposure. The deeper fibrofatty tissues are spread apart by the end of a pair of scissors or hemostats, and the tendon sheath is exposed. The distal end of the tendon sheath is incised longitudinally just to one side of the midline, and the nodule exposed. The length of tendon sheath that has to be opened can be gauged by asking the patient to flex and extend the digit completely. When the tendon can travel freely, the middle third of the circumference of the sheath is excised to ensure that subsequent healing does not allow the condition to recur. A small pressure dressing is applied for not more than 24 hours, and digital movement is encouraged immediately. The skin sutures are removed in 7 to 10 days.

Multiple trigger finger releases in the same hand can cause severe biomechanical problems. This problem is discussed in Chapter 10 (p. 262).

Nodules that occur in the profundus tendon within the finger are usually at the level of the decussation of the superficialis tendon (Fig. 5-13, p. 107). Hydrocortisone injections do not usually relieve the symptoms, and operative removal of the nodule is the best treatment.

The operation is done under local anesthesia through a transverse skin incision centered over the nodule when the finger is held extended. The nodule can usually be removed by dissection with the point of a knife or by cutting it off with curved or flat scissors. Caution must be used, since total clearance of all diseased tissue would usually leave a transected tendon. Occasionally when large multiple nodules are present, I have trimmed the tendon to roughly its normal shape and then removed one or the other of the slips of insertion of the flexor digitorum superficialis. By this means the tight, V-shaped yoke is removed, and the irregularly shaped profundus tendon can glide freely within the finger.

Postoperative care is the same as that for the more common palmar trigger finger.

Repair of diseased tendons

Diseased tendons may be discovered during a synovectomy, they may be diagnosed because of nodule formation within their length, or they may be noticed because of the gross disturbance of function that follows rupture. Despite variations in the basic pathological process, restoration of function can be achieved in several ways. Nalebuff has published an excellent review of the various options available.

END-TO-END SUTURE

If a very short length of tendon is involved, it may be possible to excise the diseased area and suture the tendon ends. This direct end-to-end suture should be reserved for limited lesions such as nodule formation.

Even in such circumstances it may be impossible to do an end-to-end repair after excision of the necrotic tissue. An intramuscular tendon slide can be done, and Backhouse and Kay recommend this procedure, particularly for the flexor digitorum profundus and flexor pollicis longus tendons.

The first stage in end-to-end repair is to cut across the tendon through normal tissue just distal to the nodule. A No. 4-0 braided wire suture with two straight needles swaged onto the ends is passed through the distal tendon after the manner of Bunnell. The proximal end of the tendon can be pulled distally by a hemostat clamped to the nodular tissue and the distal end of the tendon pulled proximally by the wire suture. When a normal part of the tendon reaches the level of the cut distal end, an empty Keith needle is passed through a more proximal portion of the tendon and surrounding tissues. Transfixing the tendon in this way overcomes the proximal pull of normal muscle tone and makes the completion of the end-to-end suture relatively simple.

The sutured tendon should be protected by appropriate splinting for 3 weeks before active motion is allowed. This splinting must be judiciously applied, since it is never wise to immobilize the whole hand of a rheumatoid patient.

When disease is present over a considerable length of a tendon, or when the tendon ends are ragged and diseased, attempts to restore continuity by direct end-to-end suture are fruitless. Power must be restored by bridging the gap with a tendon graft or by transferring motor power by utilizing a muscle-tendon unit that can be spared.

FREE GRAFT

I always prefer transferring muscle power to using a free graft. I believe it is illogical to place a free graft onto a bed of diseased tissue from which the graft is destined to receive its blood supply. Surgical synovectomy of the graft bed can never be absolute and thus cannot permanently prevent involvement of the graft by the rheumatoid tissues. I have occasionally used free grafts to replace lengths of diseased tendons with satisfactory short-term results. I cannot believe that a free graft will give such satisfactory long-term results as tendon transfers, and I use a free graft only as a last resort. However, it should be reported that Backhouse and Kay believe that "grafts, contrary to some reports, do well in rheumatoid arthritis."

The graft of choice is from the palmaris longus from the same limb. If the palmaris longus is absent, I prefer to use the plantaris. My third choice is a toe extensor tendon. The graft is a cable graft replacing only the length that is diseased or missing (Fig. 6-9). If the tendon is ruptured, care must be taken to pull the proximal end distally, thereby restoring normal muscle tone before completing the graft insertion.

Postoperative care is essentially the same as that for end-to-end tendon suture. The graft should be protected by appropriate splinting for 3 weeks. After removal of the splint, active movements are encouraged. Passive movements may put too great a strain on the graft and should be avoided.

TENDON TRANSFER

The most satisfactory treatment in all cases of tendon rupture is to transfer motor power by utilizing a motor-tendon unit that can be spared. On the dorsum of the hand

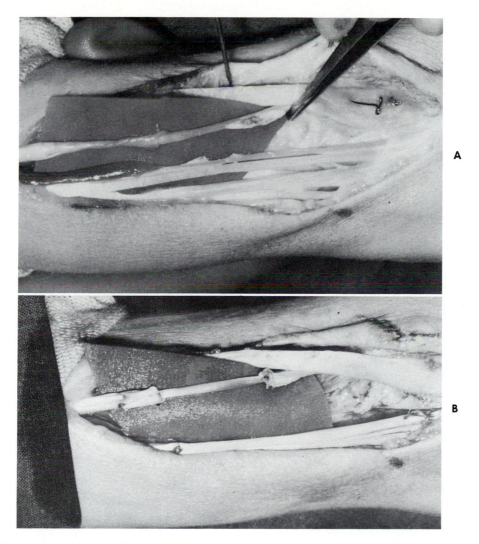

Fig. 6-9. Free graft. **A,** Localized area of attempted repair in a diseased tendon lying on the piece of rubber dam with the forceps pointing to the normal distal end. **B,** Short cable graft replacing the excised ruptured ends of the tendon.

the unit of choice is the extensor indicis proprius. Additional units that can be used are the extensor carpi radialis longus, the extensor carpi ulnaris, or the brachioradialis. On the flexor surface there is no unit that can always be spared. The choice will usually be between a flexor digitorum superficialis tendon and one of the wrist flexors or, occasionally, the brachioradialis. The brachioradialis has acquired an undeserved reputation as being responsible for bad results when used in tendon transfer because of its poor amplitude of excursion. If the tendon of insertion is deliberately stripped up from the radius for several centimeters in a proximal direction, it will be found that the muscle will have a perfectly adequate excursion.

If more than one tendon is ruptured, the best results are obtained by performing multiple tendon transfers. It is possible to sew two distal tendons into a single prox-

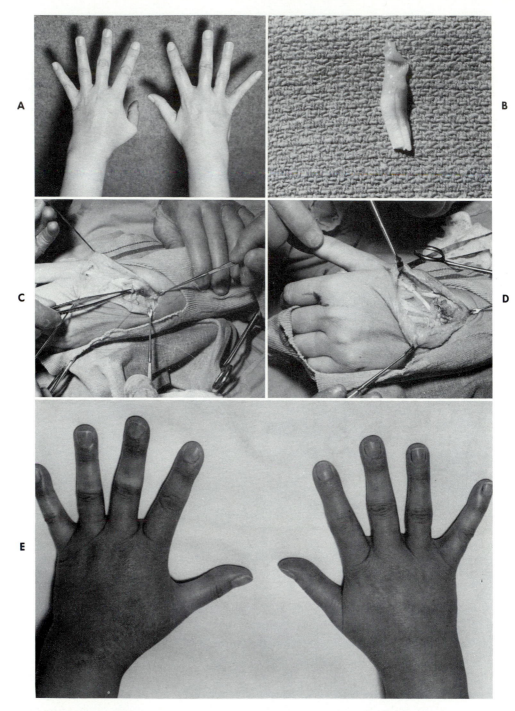

Fig. 6-10. Tendon transfer. **A,** Typical flexion deformity of the metacarpophalangeal joint of the thumb after rupture of the extensor pollicis longus tendon. **B,** Portion of the tendon with the nodule that caused the rupture. **C,** Site of rupture in relation to Lister's tubercle on the dorsum of the wrist. **D,** Transferred extensor indicis proprius tendon sutured into the distal end of the extensor pollicis longus tendon. **E,** Voluntary extension possible 1 month after the operation.

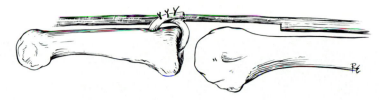

Fig. 6-11. The extensor loop operation. This procedure to centralize the extensor tendon and provide a counterforce to progressive subluxation has been advocated by Harrison and colleagues in their paper "Repair of Extensor Pollicis Longus Using the Extensor Pollicis Brevis in Rheumatoid Arthritis." (Modified from Harrison, S., Swannell, A.J., and Ansell, B.M.: Ann. Rheum. Dis. **31:**490-492, 1972.)

imal motor tendon, making a Y junction. This procedure usually leaves a slight lag in distal tendon function, particularly if the extensor tendons of the fingers are those involved. This extensor lag is more obvious immediately after surgery and tends to improve during the next 6 months.

Several different methods of tendon junction can be used. Since most of the tendons that rupture are comparable in size to those that are used as transfers, I prefer to do an end-to-end suture using buried No. 4-0 braided wire. The motor unit tendon is pulled distally about two thirds of its total travel distance so that it is joined to the distal tendon under considerable tension. It should not be so tight that it resembles a tenodesis, but I have found that the most satisfactory results are obtained with those patients in whom the transfer is relatively taut.

Extensor tendons. On the radial side of the hand the extensor pollicis longus tendon is the most commonly ruptured. It is usual for the extensor indicis proprius tendon to be transferred to restore thumb extension (Fig. 6-10).

Harrison and co-workers advocate the use of the extensor pollicis brevis. They select this tendon because it supplies a needed element of abduction for the rheumatoid thumb and because the extensor indicis proprius is thus spared for use elsewhere. The potential loss of metacarpophalangeal extension is counteracted by passing a loop of half of the distal end of the extensor pollicis longus through the base of the proximal phalanx. This provision of an insertion into the base of the proximal phalanx also centralizes the extensor tendon and provides a counterforce to progressive subluxation (Fig. 6-11).

The restoration of extension in the more ulnar fingers after rupture is usually accomplished by the use of the extensor carpi ulnaris tendon as the proximal motor. This operation was introduced by Vainio in 1954, and the procedure has certainly stood the test of time. I do not have any detailed range-of-motion follow-ups of this particular operation, but the results have been uniformly satisfactory in the sense that the hand can be opened at the level of the metacarpophalangeal joints. It may take many months of postoperative exercises to gain the maximum range of extension. I usually warn my patients not to expect the full result for 6 months and not to expect to regain the full range of motion present before the tendons ruptured. Both Nalebuff and Bäckdahl have commented that the excursion of the extensor carpi ulnaris is short compared with that of the finger extensors, and they therefore recommend use of the

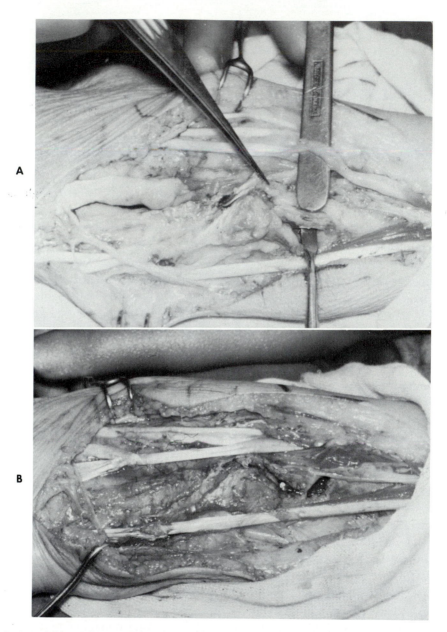

Fig. 6-12. Multiple tendon rupture. **A,** State of disease over the dorsum of the wrist. The proximal end of the extensor tendon to the ring finger lies on the scalpel blade, and the forceps holds the diseased synovium over the distal end of the ulna. **B,** In the repair the extensor carpi ulnaris was used as an independent extensor for the small finger, and the intact long finger tendon has been used to form a Y junction with the distal end of the ring finger tendon. **C** and **D,** Two months after surgery there is a slight extensor lag but a good fist can be made.

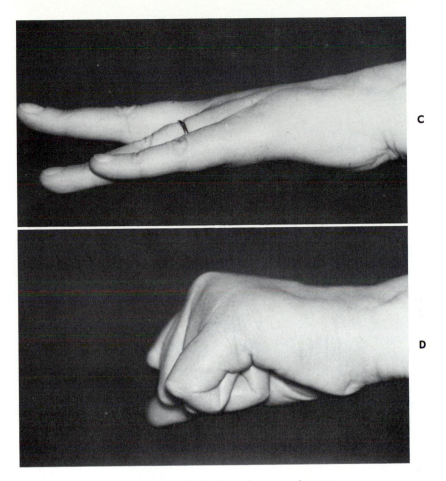

Fig. 6-12, cont'd. For legend see opposite page.

extensor indicis proprius, particularly for the solitary loss of small finger extension. Savill was particularly disappointed in the results of his repair of ruptured extensor tendons by transference. He commented that although the ability to extend the fingers may have been restored, he often found some degree of tenodesis, which limited metacarpophalangeal joint flexion. Because of the tenodesis effect, Savill suggested that conservative management by the use of functional dynamic bracing may avoid the problem of tenodesis. He stated that the distal part of the ruptured tendon will, in time, become adherent to a neighbor.

I have no experience with this conservative method of treatment. Although I, too, have seen occasional limitation of full anatomical range of flexion of the metacarpophalangeal joints, I have yet to see a patient whose hand function did not show overall improvement after operative restoration of extensor action (Fig. 6-12).

When three or even four extensor tendons are ruptured, an excellent motor tendon is the flexor digitorum superficialis, which can be transferred through the interosseous membrane. The small finger superficialis can be used alone or in combination with the extensor indicis proprius or the superficialis of the long finger. Use of these combinations will give greater independence of extension, but such dexterity is not often needed by the rheumatoid patient. Nalebuff has given a detailed description of the procedure and stresses that the correct tension is obtained by attaching the transfer with maximum tension when the fingers are in flexion and the wrist is in slight dorsiflexion.

Flexor tendons. Rupture of the thumb flexor or a profundus tendon is usually recognized by the patient, but the weakness of grip caused by the rupture of a superficialis tendon is more commonly dismissed as "due to arthritis."

Isolated rupture of the thumb flexor can be treated by fusion of the interphalangeal joint, by transfer of a superficialis tendon, or by a tendon graft. The choice is primarily influenced by the dynamic balance in the carpometacarpal and metacarpophalangeal joints. The simplest and usually most satisfactory treatment is fusion of the interphalangeal joint, but if instability of the more proximal joints is best treated by fusion, then movement of the interphalangeal joint is essential and is best provided by tendon transfer. I rarely, if ever, use a graft for the thumb flexor in a rheumatoid patient.

Isolated rupture of a profundus tendon is best treated by fusion of the distal interphalangeal joint. When both flexors of a finger are ruptured I prefer to try to restore direct action of the superficialis by local repair with either the superficialis or profundus motor unit and fusion of the distal interphalangeal joint. If this approach is not possible, then my usual choice is to transfer an adjacent superficialis tendon into the distal profundus stump; the anastomosis should be made in the distal palm whenever possible.

INTRINSIC MECHANISM

Swan-neck deformity is most frequently caused by tight intrinsic musculature. However, mobile swan-neck deformities may or may not be associated with intrinsic muscle tightness. When the intrinsic muscles are normal the imbalance is usually caused by a synovitis of the proximal interphalangeal joint that stretches out the palmar plate. The treatment for this type of swan-neck deformity consists of synovectomy of the joint and tenodesis in mild flexion using one slip of the insertion of the flexor superficialis.

When the deformity is solely caused by tight intrinsic muscles, their release will restore normal posture to the finger. Fixed swan-neck deformity can be caused by contracture and adhesions of the proximal interphalangeal joint, which is frequently associated with tightness of the intrinsic muscles. The intrinsic muscles must, therefore, be released, but gentle manipulation of the joint into 90 degrees of flexion is also necessary. Nalebuff has shown that the most satisfactory way to maintain this correction and to avoid dorsal skin necrosis is by passing a Kirschner wire across the joint, and by releasing the skin over the joint. An oblique skin incision just distal to the joint relaxes the skin tension and secondary healing, without skin grafting, rapidly occurs. The Kirschner wire should be removed within a month and hand therapy started.

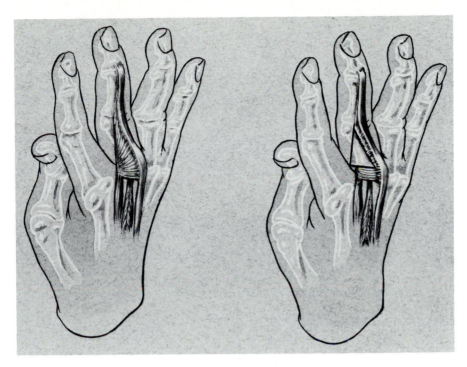

Fig. 6-13. Intrinsic release. The operation of intrinsic release is designed to remove a triangle of tissue from the side of the finger. This triangle includes the oblique fibers of the intrinsic insertion together with the free edge of the hood. The hands in this drawing are traced from the casts of the hand shown in Fig. 6-15.

Intrinsic contracture release

Bunnell originally described an operation to neutralize the overaction of the intrinsic muscles by relieving the muscle tension. He suggested stripping the interosseous muscles from their metacarpal origins and displacing them distally. This operation is a major procedure, produces a great deal of hemorrhage, and does not influence the contracture that may be present in the lumbrical muscles. An operation that has become generally adopted is described by Littler, in which the same result is achieved by a simple excision of the distal insertions of the intrinsic muscles.

As the tendons of the intrinsic muscles pass to their insertion into the extensor mechanism, the fibers fan out from a proximal vertical portion through a series of oblique fibers into the free edge of the intrinsic hood. The free edge is thicker than the vertical or oblique fibers and passes dorsal to the axis of the proximal interphalangeal joint to join the extensor mechanism on the dorsum of the middle phalanx.

Before the operation is begun, lateral x-ray films of the proximal interphalangeal joints are always taken because a simple soft-tissue release is doomed to failure if gross changes have occurred in the articular surfaces. The operation is planned to remove the extensor pull of the oblique fibers and the free edge of the hood on the middle and distal phalanges. The proximal vertical fibers of the insertion are left intact to provide flexion of the metacarpophalangeal joint (Fig. 6-13).

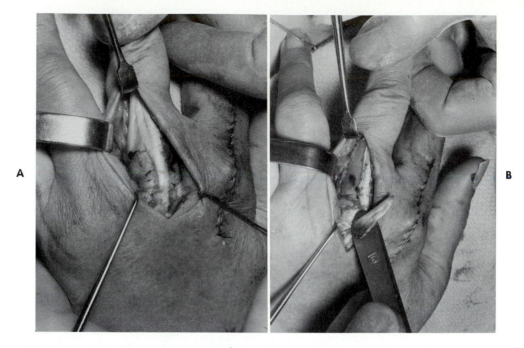

A

B

Fig. 6-14. Intrinsic release, single finger. **A,** Intrinsic fibers passing up the side of the finger and onto the dorsum of the proximal interphalangeal joint. The triangle and the free edge of the hood can be seen between the blades of the two retractors. **B,** Triangle of tissue removed and lying on the handle of the scalpel.

Intrinsic contracture in a single finger is rare, but when present, it can be released through a short midline dorsal incision over the proximal two thirds of the proximal phalanx (Fig. 6-14). Usually all fingers are involved, although to a varying degree. The approach for the release of all four fingers is through a transverse dorsal incision centered over the metacarpal heads (Fig. 8-3, p. 184).

The two portions of the intrinsic hood that are to be removed lie over the sides of the proximal half of the proximal phalanx. In excision from a single finger, the skin and subcutaneous tissues separate easily from the underlying hood and extensor tendon. When using the transverse skin incision, the hood is approached by lifting the skin and subcutaneous tissues with a long-bladed narrow retractor.

The free margin of the hood is defined by slipping a blunt hook under the edge and passing it proximally and distally. After the hood has been freed from any deep-lying adhesions, the area where the vertical fibers begin to fan out obliquely should be identified. A hemostat is placed on the free edge of the hood at this site, and with a small scalpel an incision parallel to the vertical fibers is made proximal to the hemo-stat and carried to the outer edge of the extrinsic tendon. At this point the incision is turned at right angles and continued parallel to the extrinsic extensor tendon. The incision is continued distally until the free edge of the hood and the outer edge of the extrinsic extensor tendon converge. By pulling on the hemostat, the surgeon can demonstrate the hyperextension force of the intrinsic tendons. The removal of the

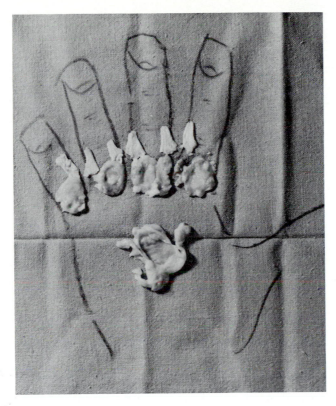

Fig. 6-15. Intrinsic release, all fingers. This photograph shows the position from which the triangles are removed during intrinsic release of all fingers. Because of the difference in anatomical arrangement, triangles of tissues are not removed from the outer borders of the index and small fingers. Synovectomies of the metacarpophalangeal joints were also carried out through the transverse skin incision, and an additional synovectomy was done on the extensor tendons over the dorsum of the hand.

triangular piece of tissue is completed by turning the knife edge laterally and pulling the free edge of the hood against it via the hemostat.

Because of the difference in the anatomy of the intrinsic insertions into the ulnar side of the small finger and the radial side of the index finger, a true hood release cannot be done on these borders of the hand (Fig. 6-15). After all the triangular pieces of tissue have been removed, the test for intrinsic contracture should be repeated. Usually a great improvement over the preoperative state will be found. In some long-standing cases of intrinsic contracture the presence of periarticular and intraarticular adhesions will prevent a gain in range. In these instances gentle manipulation is usually sufficient to overcome the adhesions, and a good range of movement is obtained. Even a gain of only a small range of flexion can be of great importance to the function of the hand. If the proximal interphalangeal joints can now be flexed at the beginning of grasp, the proper sequence of motion has been restored and prehension will be greatly improved.

Firm resistance to passive pressure should be accepted and no violent force applied. This resistance indicates that the operation has been done too late for full correction and that gross periarticular and intraarticular changes have occurred in the proximal interphalangeal joint.

The incision is closed by interrupted nylon sutures, and a compression bandage is applied while the fingers are slightly flexed at all joints.

It is pointless to do this operation if the postoperative course of treatment cannot be properly controlled. Early postoperative movement is important. It is started before the sutures are removed and must be performed under trained supervision for at least the first week. The fingers should always remain in flexion; full extension and particularly hyperextension must be avoided. The patients have usually developed habits of hand usage that are adapted to the hyperextension deformity, and, unless they are broken of these habits, the operation will be fruitless and the deformity will recur. Experience in prescribing physical and occupational therapy is required, since different forces must be developed over the joint surfaces. The extrinsic extensor tendon must be trained to take over the extensor action of the interphalangeal joints, and the extrinsic flexor tendons have to "take up" sufficiently to hold the proximal interphalangeal joint in neutral position or a few degrees of flexion. The most satisfactory position is therefore one in which the metacarpophalangeal joint is straight or very slightly flexed and the proximal interphalangeal joint is free to flex but unable to hyperextend.

Exercises and controlled use of the hand are often necessary for several months before the full benefit of the operation is obtained (Fig. 6-16).

Potter has pointed out that the free edge of the lateral bands should move palmarward during flexion of the proximal interphalangeal joint. This shift usually does not occur in swan-neck deformity because of adhesions to the deep surface of the intrinsic mechanism. Operating with the area under local anesthetic, he mobilizes the lateral bands by careful dissection, paying particular attention to the preservation of Landsmeer's ligament. He reports gratifying results in over 75 patients.

Modified intrinsic contracture release

Release, or destruction, of the extensor mechanism insertion of the intrinsic muscles gives excellent results when done early in the disease. As originally described, the operation was designed to relieve the excessive pull of intrinsic muscles contracted by localized disease. The operation has been adopted for use in rheumatoid patients without sufficient recognition of the additional problems created by this generalized disease.

The operation cannot provide complete extension of the metacarpophalangeal joints if the intrinsic contracture has allowed a secondary flexion contracture to develop at these joints. When this secondary contracture is present, I have often extended the excision of the more proximal part of the intrinsic insertions by including some the vertical fibers that are responsible for flexion in the normal metacarpophalangeal joint.

This removal of extra intrinsic tissue must be done judiciously. Wholesale removal of all the vertical fibers would destroy the yokelike mechanism holding the extrinsic extensor tendon in its normal central position.

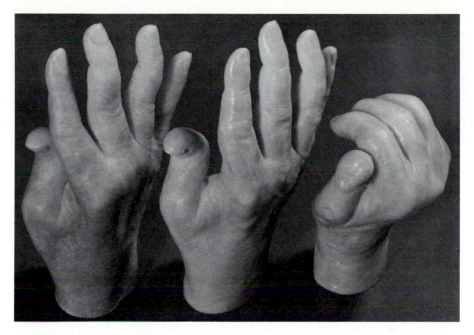

Fig. 6-16. Intrinsic release. The three casts in this picture show the typical swan-neck deformity, which is seen in patients with rheumatoid disease. The hand on the left is a cast taken before surgery; the cast in the center was taken 2 weeks after surgery and shows that the hyperextension deformity has been reversed. The cast on the right shows the function obtained 2 months after operation following intensive exercises. (From Flatt, A.E.: Rheumatism **16**:90, 1960.)

In patients with long-standing intrinsic contracture, the flexion deformity of the metacarpophalangeal joint will improve after this removal of the more distal vertical fibers of the intrinsic hood. Frequently, however, the deformity does not completely disappear. There are two reasons for this lack of full correction: (1) the tissues of the palmar plate have contracted secondarily, and (2) the bony insertions of the intrinsic muscles are still a deforming factor.

Excision of the vertical fibers of the hood provides a good view of this bony insertion into either side of the base of the phalanx. If these bony insertions prevent full extension of the metacarpophalangeal joint, the insertions will be seen to tense when the joint is passively extended. In such circumstances I do not hesitate to detach the bony insertions completely, which usually gives an excellent correction of the deformity. Occasionally, however, the contracture of the membranous portion of the palmar plate has to be relieved by spreading a pair of fine blunt scissors between the dorsal surface of the flexor tendons and the flexor surface of both the metacarpophalangeal joint and the neck of the metacarpal.

I believe that these additions to the original operation are extremely useful. The general and progressive nature of the disease demands a more ruthless approach than the standard operation. Since I adopted these additional measures, I have obtained much more satisfactory results.

Zancolli has suggested that a similar release of both wing and bony insertions of the interossei can be more easily accomplished by transecting the muscles at the site where they lie dorsal to the intermetacarpal ligament. This is a neat and attractive operation—and it works. Caution is necessary in its use because the frequent adhesions between the deep surface of the wing tendons and the proximal phalanx will not be relieved. Since these adhesions are distal to the site of interosseous transection, they may still prevent the restoration of a functional arch in the finger. If passive testing of the finger does not show good flexion at the proximal interphalangeal joint, the adhesions must be sought and destroyed.

Crossed intrinsic transfer

A modification of the intrinsic release operation has been suggested by Straub for some years in an attempt to supply a radially deviating force to counteract the tendency to ulnar deviation. The principle of this operation is to perform an intrinsic wing or lateral band release on the ulnar side of the index, long, and ring fingers. Instead of excising the triangle of tissue, it is left attached proximally to its muscle belly, passed ulnarward onto the radial side of the next adjacent ulnar finger, and attached to this finger's radial intrinsic wing or lateral band.

By this means the ulnar-sided intrinsic of the index finger becomes a radial deviator and extensor of the long finger. The equivalent muscle of the long finger acts on the ring finger, and that of the ring finger tends to pull the small finger in a radial direction. It is usually necessary to release the abductor digiti minimi muscle to allow full radial correction of the small finger.

The operation is principally used in patients with early ulnar drift of the fingers and differential tightness of the ulnar intrinsics. Demonstration of the differential tightness of the ulnar intrinsics, as opposed to the radial intrinsics, can be done by fixing the metacarpophalangeal joint in extension and passively flexing the proximal interphalangeal joint, with the digit first in radial deviation and then in ulnar deviation (Fig. 6-17). Tightness present in radial deviation implicates the ulnar intrinsics and vice versa.

Some have criticized the procedure on the grounds that the insertion of the tight ulnar intrinsic muscle into the radial side of the adjacent finger is liable to produce a swan-neck deformity in the recipient finger. In 1966 Straub reported 47 instances of this crossed intrinsic transfer that had been followed for at least 3 years without development of swan-neck deformity in any finger. My experience has not been so satisfactory. Swan-neck deformity frequently occurred in patients in whom the released ulnar intrinsic tendon was transferred to the radial wing tendon. I have examined this problem in the laboratory and feel confident in recommending that the transfer be attached to the distal end of the radial collateral ligament of the metacarpophalangeal joint.

The operative approach is through a dorsal transverse incision, and for each finger the extensor hood and capsule are incised longitudinally on the radial side of the extensor tendon, a synovectomy is done in the usual manner, and the insertion of the radial collateral ligament into the proximal phalanx is identified. Then on the ulnar aspect of the adjacent radial digit the insertion of the ulnar interosseous tendon into

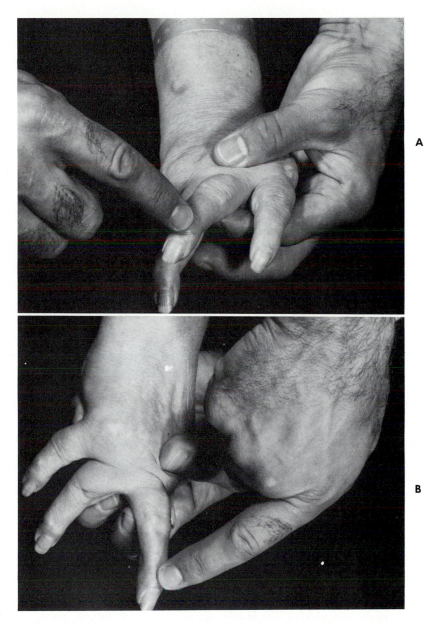

Fig. 6-17. Selective ulnar intrinsic tightness. If there is differential tightness between the ulnar and radial intrinsic muscles in a finger, the amount of passive interphalangeal joint flexion will be less when the ulnar intrinsics are the tighter. **A,** Finger tested in ulnar deviation, thus tightening the radial intrinsics. **B,** The ulnar intrinsics are stressed by putting the finger in radial deviation. Since there is more passive flexion in **A** than in **B,** there is greater relative tightness in the ulnar intrinsics.

the extensor expansion of this digit is identified. Beginning distally this insertion is detached from the extensor hood by sharp dissection, and the tendon is dissected proximally to its musculotendinous junction. Free excursion of the interosseous muscle-tendon unit must be demonstrated at the completion of this dissection (Fig. 6-18, A).

The distal end of the detached ulnar interosseous tendon is then sutured to the previously exposed radial collateral ligament of the other finger near the distal insertion of the ligament on the phalanx (Fig. 6-18, B). Several interrupted sutures of No. 4-0 unabsorbable sutures swaged on a small vascular needle are used to secure the transfer. The tension of the transferred tendon should be such that the ulnar drift is corrected while the hand is held in the "rest" position. The dorsal expansion is also repaired with interrupted No. 4-0 sutures in such a manner that the extensor tendon is repositioned in the dorsal midline of the metacarpophalangeal joint.

I find it convenient to begin the dissection and definition of tendons at the index finger and proceed in sequence to the small finger. I then begin the transfers and repair at the small finger and work backward toward the index finger. At the small finger, the abductor digiti minimi is selectively released by separating it from the flexor digiti minimi and dividing its tendon so that the ulnar-deviating effect of the hypothenar muscles is eliminated but the flexor component necessary for power grip is preserved. At the index finger, the first dorsal interosseous tendon is replaced into its normal position if it has sagged palmward.

The skin is then closed with interrupted No. 5-0 nylon mattress sutures, and the hand is dressed and immobilized with the metacarpophalangeal joints in a few degrees of flexion. Postoperative elevation is important and should be continued for 2 or 3 days.

Three days postoperatively, the original dressing is removed and the wound is inspected. A light dressing is applied, and the wrist and metacarpophalangeal joints are supported in a neutral position for 3 weeks on a palmar plaster splint with an ulnar flange. Thereafter the splint is removed during the day and active exercises are begun. I recommend the continued use of the splint at night for an additional 3 weeks.

Ellison and associates have published the results of our early studies on this operation; we have not seen the subsequent development of a swan-neck deformity, which appears to be a frequent complication of the original operation.

Correction of swan-neck deformity

Intrinsic release operations will remove deforming factors that tend to pull the proximal interphalangeal joint into hyperextension. If the hyperextension deformity has been present for some time, laxity or disruption of the palmar plate will still allow the deformity to occur. Associated with this deformity must be a stretching or disruption of the oblique retinacular ligaments, redescribed by Landsmeer. These ligaments help to prevent the hyperextension deformity and restore the capacity for coordinated finger flexion and extension. Littler has published an ingenious operation designed to restore this ligament by using the free edge of a lateral band in the

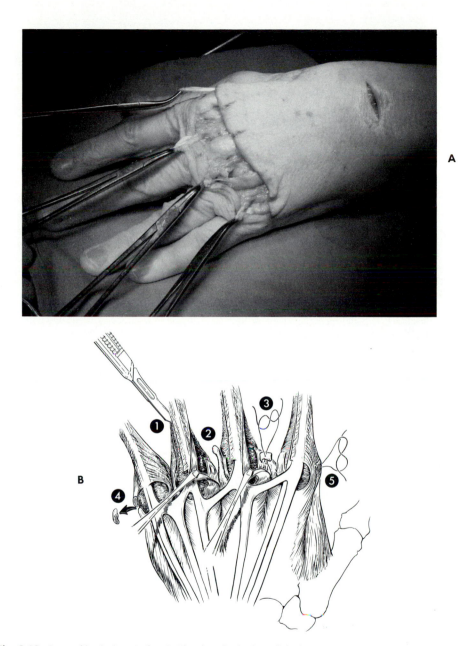

Fig. 6-18. Crossed intrinsic transfer. **A,** The detached wing of the interosseous tendon must be dissected back proximally enough to allow free excursion. Three hemostats are on the freed-up ulnar intrinsic tendons; at the top of the figure the extensor indicis proprius tendon is shown in a hemostat for those who wish to continue to use this transfer. **B,** Crossed intrinsic transfer. *1,* Release of the ulnar intrinsic tendon. *2,* Its mobilization to the musculotendinous junction and the slit in the radial collateral ligament of the adjacent finger through which the transfer should be passed. *3,* The sewing in of the transfer. *4,* Abductor digiti minimi release. *5,* Repositioning of the first dorsal interosseous.

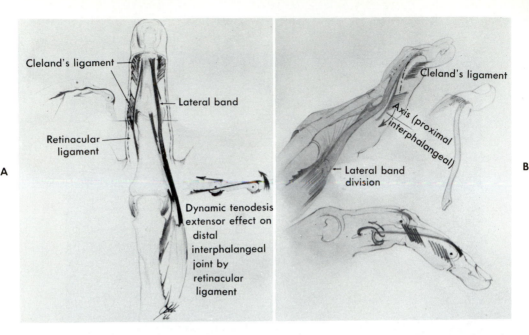

Fig. 6-19. Restoration of Landsmeer's ligament. **A,** Retinacular ligament is relaxed in flexion and tightened in extension of the proximal interphalangeal joint. As it tightens, it assists extension of the distal interphalangeal joint. Cleland's ligaments attach to the oblique retinacular ligament on either side of the finger. **B,** Incision and separation of the edge of the lateral band. It is passed palmar to Cleland's ligaments and attached to the proximal phalangeal flexor tendon pulley. (From Littler, J.W.: Restoration of the oblique retinaculum ligament for correcting hyperextension deformity of the proximal interphalangeal joint. In La main rhumatismale, Paris, 1966, L'Expansion Scientifique Francaise.)

affected finger. He recommends that the ulnar-sided intrinsic be used. It should be sectioned proximally at the musculotendinous junction, split longitudinally as a cord away from the wing apparatus, but left attached at its distal insertion (Fig. 6-19). The band is then passed proximally but on the flexor side of Cleland's ligaments and anchored to the proximal phalangeal flexor tendon pulley. Before the band is sewn in place its tension must be adjusted to control hyperextension of the proximal interphalangeal joint.

I use this operation frequently but usually employ the radial intrinsic band, since I thereby retain the option of using the ulnar band for a crossed intrinsic transfer.

The side of the finger is approached through a curvilinear incision that finishes distally just short of the dorsum of the distal interphalangeal joint. During the dissection of the lateral band it is essential not to destroy the horizontal Cleland's ligament beneath which the freed lateral band must be passed (Figs. 6-20, *C,* and 6-21). The adjustment of tension in the transfer is difficult, and it is better to err on the side of tightness rather than risk a recurrence of hyperextension. The postoperative care follows the same general principles as those for a crossed intrinsic transfer.

When the problem is confined to the proximal interphalangeal joint and additional correction of the distal interphalangeal joint is not needed, a simpler operative procedure is sufficient.

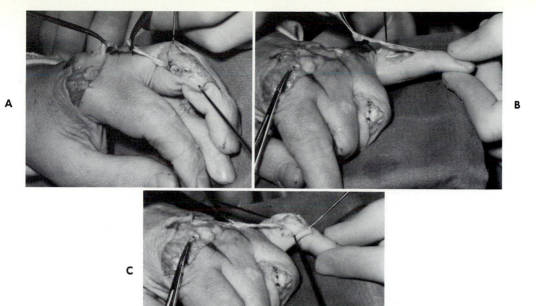

Fig. 6-20. Swan-neck correction. **A,** The transferred lateral band has been sutured in place and the proximal interphalangeal joint is held in about 40 degrees of flexion. **B,** Mobilization of the radial band of the small finger. **C,** The radial band has been transferred beneath Cleland's ligament, and the joint is held in the correct degree of flexion.

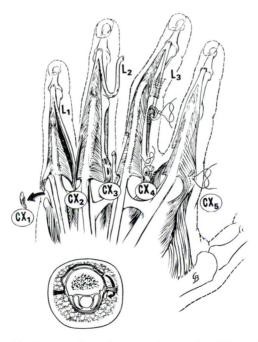

Fig. 6-21. Combined crossed intrinsic transfer and swan-neck correction. This combined procedure can be done at one operation, but it is not one for the inexperienced. The *CX* series illustrate the same procedures as are described in Fig. 6-18, *B,* and the *L* series, those in Fig. 6-20. The cross sectional inset drawing emphasizes L_3, in which the lateral band must be passed beneath Cleland's ligament.

Tenodesis of the joint in 20 degrees of flexion using one slip of the superficialis tendon is an excellent procedure. Either slip of the tendon can be used and is brought out of the sheath through a hole in the area of the cruciform pulley at the level of the joint. The distal insertion of the selected slip is left intact and is cut off proximally at the decussation. It is then passed through a hole in the A_2 pulley (Fig. 6-8) and sutured back on itself.

Exercises can be started in 3 or 4 days both into flexion and extension.

Combined crossed transfer and swan-neck correction

I have found that in a Landsmeer ligament reconstruction, in which the radial wing tendon is used instead of the ulnar as originally described by Littler, it is possible to do crossed intrinsic transfers at the same operation. Correction of deformity at two joint levels is therefore possible, but this extensive operation is not for the inexperienced (Fig. 6-21).

An intact central extensor tendon is essential for each finger, since the operation reroutes both wing tendons of each finger. The index finger is the exception, since the lumbrical extension on the radial side of the finger is not disturbed. In this finger the ulnar wing tendon is used both for crossed transfer and for retinacular ligament reconstruction. There is sufficient length to accomplish both procedures but each portion of the tendon has little to spare!

Hypothenar muscles release

Because of their size and anatomical arrangement, the hypothenar muscles have long been considered a powerful etiological factor in ulnar deviation and even dislocation of the small finger at the metacarpophalangeal joint. It might seem logical to detach the insertion of these muscles to remove such a deforming force. Such a procedure has to be done in cases of late deformity to bring the small finger back into line with its metacarpal. In our patients with less deformity, application of this idea led to symptomatic and functional postoperative complications.

If synovectomy of the metacarpophalangeal joint of the small finger is performed without release of the hypothenar muscles, a satisfactory range of flexion is often maintained in the finger but it may still lie in ulnar deviation. If the hypothenar muscles are detached, many patients seem to experience an undue amount of pain. Because of this discomfort, they have difficulty in moving the joint, regardless of which postoperative day the therapy is started. It usually takes 2 or 3 weeks for the pain to subside completely, and during this time considerable range of motion is lost. Full restoration of range demands many weeks of intensive exercises and frequently does not occur even then.

When total hypothenar release is performed, lateral rotation and the ability to oppose the small finger are lost. Cupping of the ulnar side of the hand is compromised, and the power of flexion of the metacarpophalangeal joint is greatly reduced. This loss of mobility and grip was demonstrated in my follow-up study of synovectomy of the metacarpophalangeal joints. Table 4 shows that in eight patients the average loss of flexion in the small finger metacarpophalangeal joint was 27 degrees. Depri-

Table 4. Hypothenar release, showing range of motion in the metacarpophalangeal joint

	Extension			Flexion		
	Minimum	**Average**	**Maximum**	**Minimum**	**Average**	**Maximum**
Preoperative						
Small finger (8 patients)	0	13	45	60	78	97
Small finger (8 patients)	25H	5	17	0	51	85

Note: The minimum and maximum show the spread of the ranges from which the average was computed.
H Hyperextension.

vation of this range of motion proved to be a great problem in adjustment for those patients who had such function before their operation. I believe now that it is important to separate the abductor and flexor digiti minimi muscles; the former is released and the latter left intact, thereby retaining good flexion for power grip. Tightness in these muscles is best assessed after anesthesia is satisfactory. When the abductor digiti minimi is cut, care must be taken to avoid the ulnar neurovascular bundle, which runs very close to the muscles at the level of the metacarpophalangeal joint.

Backhouse has told me that he often utilizes the released abductor digiti minimi as an additional crossed transfer. He states that by passing the released tendon and distal muscle substance across the dorsum and to the radial side of the small finger, he can repair even 90-degree ulnar deviations of the small finger. I have no personal experience in using this additional transfer.

Repair of boutonniere deformity

The correction of boutonniere deformity caused by trauma is difficult. The correction of boutonniere deformity caused by rheumatoid disease is virtually impossible. The fully developed boutonniere deformity has three essential components: (1) hyperextension of the metacarpophalangeal joint, (2) flexion of the proximal interphalangeal joint, and (3) hyperextension of the distal interphalangeal joint. This position is the result of imbalance of the tendon mechanism within the finger. The ideal treatment is the restoration of the normal alignment of the finger joints and the normal arrangement of the tendon mechanism over the dorsum of the proximal interphalangeal joint. If the deformity has been caused by recent trauma, it may be possible to restore the mechanism by simple suture of the cut parts. In rheumatoid disease, however, the onset of the deformity is insidious, and all the structures over the dorsum of the joint are involved. The disease destroys some parts of the tendon mechanism and allows others to stretch. This complete derangement cannot respond to simple suturing, and more complicated surgical procedures are necessary. The fact that many procedures are described to treat this deformity indicates that none is entirely satisfactory; the most satisfactory results are obtained in those fingers that can be fully extended passively.

Nalebuff and Millender suggest that the treatment of this deformity be considered

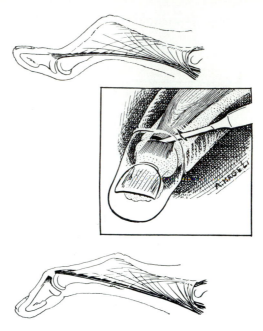

Fig. 6-22. Boutonniere to mallet. Tenotomy of the extensor tendon over the distal interphalangeal joint will relieve the extreme flexion of the proximal interphalangeal joint and the hyperextension of the distal interphalangeal joint. This operation, which is suitable for patients with late stages of the deformity, tends to restore a more normal arch to the finger.

in three stages: mild, moderate, and severe. This classification is based on the degree of deformity, the presence of passive correctibility, and the status of the joint surfaces.

MILD DEFORMITY

The functional loss for these patients is minimal, since they have only a slight lag of extension at the middle finger joint and may or may not have hyperextension of the distal joint. Tightness of the extensors over the distal joint is best tested for with passive flexion of the joint while holding the proximal interphalangeal joint in full extension. If no tightness is present, no surgical treatment is indicated. If, however, there is marked resistance to passive flexion, then a tenotomy of the extensor tendon should be considered.

The operation can be done under local anesthesia in the outpatient operating room. The purpose is to detach the extensor tendon completely from its attachment to the dorsum of the distal phalanx (Fig. 6-22). The skin over the dorsum of the joint is infiltrated with 1% lidocaine or a similar local anesthetic. A small scalpel or tenotomy knife is introduced through a very small stab wound and passed across the dorsum of the joint. Firm pressure toward the bone will cut through the extensor tendon. Conversion of the hyperextension deformity into a mallet type of deformity shows that the whole extensor tendon has been cut across.

Some prefer to do the tenotomy over the dorsum of the middle phalanx and to, in effect, allow a lengthening of the tendon to occur by dividing the tendon obliquely. Nalebuff points out that by doing the operation over the middle phalanx, the retinacular ligaments (Fig. 6-19) are left intact to supply extension of the distal interphalangeal joint. The only post-operative dressing needed is a small adhesive bandage, and immediate use of the finger should be insisted on. I have been greatly encouraged by the results obtained by this procedure and do not hesitate to advise it for patients with mild boutonniere deformities. It is advisable to also use dynamic splinting for extension of the proximal interphalangeal joint, thereby restoring digital balance.

MODERATE DEFORMITY

These patients usually have a 30- to 40-degree flexion deformity of the proximal interphalangeal joint. To maintain function they compensate for the deformity by adopting a hyperextension of the metacarpophalangeal joint. As long as the deformity of these two joints is passively correctible, surgical reconstruction of the extensor mechanism over the proximal interphalangeal joint is justified. For the dorsal tendons to act properly the articular surfaces and supporting structures of the proximal interphalangeal joint must be normal. The restored tendon mechanism cannot be expected to overcome secondary contractures, subluxations, or even dislocations of the joint.

Repair of extensor communis digitorum. If full, normal passive movement is present, a modification of the method described by Kaplan for use in acute trauma can be used. The terminal central portion of the extensor communis digitorum tendon is usually elongated, and sufficient length must be excised just proximal to the insertion for the proximal end to be under moderate tension before it is reattached to the base of the middle phalanx. It is usually necessary to incise the oblique fibers near the joint so that a better balance is restored in the lateral bands in relation to the tension in the central slip. The bands must be resutured to the oblique fibers to ensure their retention above the axis of the joint.

Several operations have been described for repair of long-standing deformity in which the lateral bands are used in various ways to reconstitute the central extensor tendon. The three main methods are the side-to-side suture of the bands, a crossing over of the bands, or an overlapping of the bands. All these methods would appear to be reasonable, but in fact the normal muscle tension will tend to pull the lateral bands away from this unnatural position. An additional problem is that these methods increase the tension in the intrinsic muscles, because the lateral bands are forced through a course that is longer than that of their normal lateral position. I believe that these factors are serious drawbacks to these procedures, and for this reason I prefer to use a free graft to replace the central extensor tendon.

Free graft. Full passive range of the digital joints must be present if the use of a free graft for replacement of the extensor mechanism is planned. Secondary involvement of the proximal interphalangeal joint with intraarticular adhesions of joint surface destruction is an absolute contraindication for free grafting.

The graft can be taken from the palmaris longus or from the plantaris. I have a strong personal preference for the former and would regard any other alternative, such as toe extensor tendons, to be a very poor third choice. My reason for preferring the palmaris longus is that a suitable length can easily be obtained with its accompanying paratenon. In addition, adjacent deep fascial tissues can be taken in one piece with the graft. This additional deep fascial tissue is, I believe, essential to the success of the procedure, since it is used to replace the oblique fibers that normally retain the lateral bands in their correct relationship to the joint.

The area is approached by a right-angled, S-shaped incision centered over the dorsum of the proximal interphalangeal joint. After the two flaps have been developed and reflected, the extrinsic extensor tendon must be identified. It is dissected back proximally to the middle of the proximal phalanx. If the tendon shows no signs of disease, one end of the graft is attached at this level. Distally the tendon usually disappears into a mass of ill-defined diseased tissue over the dorsum of the joint. It is uncommon to find normal tissue at the tendon insertion into the base of the middle phalanx. Therefore the site of junction of the two lateral slips over the dorsum of the middle phalanx is lifted free from the bone so that the distal end of the graft can be joined to this area (Fig. 6-23).

The two lateral slips will usually be found lying far down on the flexor aspect of the sides of the joint. They are freed by blunt dissection and mobilized sufficiently to lie above the axis of the joint.

By the time the three tendon components have been mobilized the joint cavity will have been entered. Inspection will show whether or not the joint surfaces are sufficiently normal to justify the grafting operation. If all is well, the adjacent diseased tissue is removed and the necessary length for the graft measured when the finger is held straight at all three joints.

The palmaris longus graft is taken under direct vision through an S-shaped skin incision. This relatively large exposure is necessary because sufficient deep fascial tissue will have to be removed on each side of the tendon to replace the oblique retaining fibers. The exact size and shape of the graft is outlined by a sharp knife and the tissue removed en bloc. By this means the smooth gliding tissues surrounding the actual tendon will not be disturbed. The first part of the graft to be inserted is the distal end. It is joined to the site of junction of the lateral bands over the middle phalanx. The end of the tendon is sutured to the inside of the tendinous V junction, and its surrounding paratenon is spread over the deep and superficial surfaces of the junction site. I use either No. 4-0 black silk or No. 4-0 braided wire sutures for both ends of the graft. The sutures are buried, and no pullout wires are used.

The proximal end of the graft is then joined to the distal end of the extrinsic extensor tendon. The finger is held extended to all three joints. Adequate tension must be put on the motor tendon before the tendon graft is sewed into place.* After the tendon portion of the graft has been secured the lateral wings of deep fascia are passed deep to the freed lateral bands and then pulled up around the lateral bands until they lie in their correct position. The bands are held in place by a series of

---

*I use the term "adequate tension" deliberately. I regard it as being in the same category as the chef's "season to taste"—impossible to define but essential to success.

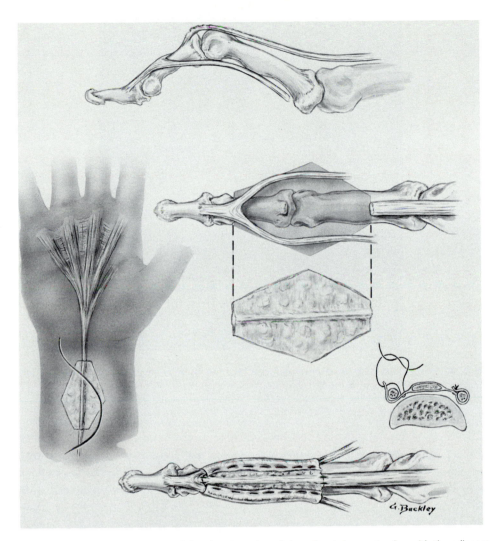

Fig. 6-23. Free graft in boutonniere deformity. A portion of the palmaris longus tendon with the adjacent tissues is used as a free graft to replace the diseased central slip overlying the proximal interphalangeal joint. The lateral bands must be mobilized and brought back into their proper relationship to the axis of this joint. The free edges of the palmaris graft should be looped beneath the lateral bands to hold them in place.

interrupted synthetic, absorbable sutures (Fig. 6-23). Excess deep fascia can be excised or sutured back onto itself to aid in retaining the lateral bands in position.

The skin wounds are closed with interrupted fine nylon sutures, and the grafted finger is splinted straight at all three joints for at least 14 days. The rest of the hand is padded with fluffed-up dressings and wrapped in the functional position. From the fourteenth day gentle movement may be permitted, but full movement should not be allowed for 3 weeks.

Whether the extension mechanism has been directly repaired or a graft used, it is often useful to add the decompression or tenotomy of the distal interphalangeal joint described with the mild deformity.

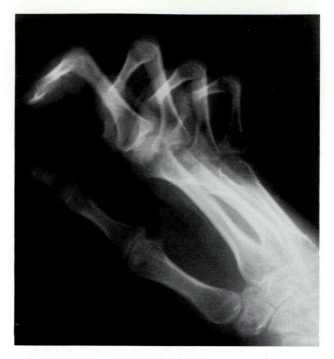

Fig. 6-24. Dislocation of the proximal interphalangeal joint. This x-ray film shows chronic dislocation of the proximal interphalangeal joints in the hand of a juvenile rheumatoid arthritic patient. A new articular surface has formed on the flexor aspect of the neck of the proximal phalanx. The only satisfactory treatment for such gross deformity is fusion of the joints in a more functional position.

Both methods of repair should be protected for about a month by passing a Kirschner wire across the fully extended proximal interphalangeal joint. An extension night splint should then be used supplemented by a reverse knuckle bender splint during the day.

SEVERE DEFORMITY

The only operation of predictable use in patients with very late neglected deformity, in whom only a jog of even passive movement is possible, is fusion of the joint in a more functional position. This indication is reinforced if a palmar dislocation of the base of the middle phalanx has occurred on the head of the proximal phalanx (Fig. 6-24). This deformity is seen quite frequently in the hands of juvenile rheumatoid arthritic patients after they reach adult life.

Implant arthroplasty of the proximal interphalangeal joint is performed by some very experienced surgeons for these severe deformities. Considerable experience and excellent judgment are needed to obtain satisfactory results because bone resection, palmar plate release, reattachment of the central slip, and relocation of the lateral bands must all be precisely integrated to yield an acceptable result. Occasionally, I have obtained a satisfactory result.

Fusion can be done for all four fingers, but the angles should vary from about 25 degrees of flexion for the index finger to 40 degrees for the small finger. The posture of the metacarpophalangeal joint must also be considered; any hyperextension must be reduced into a flexion position. If manipulation followed by soft-tissue release is inadequate, excisional arthroplasty must be done to allow full benefit to be obtained from the restoration of the proximal interphalangeal joints into their functional position.

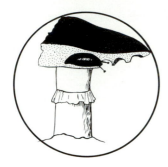

CHAPTER 7

Digital joint disease— general considerations

Rheumatoid disease changes the thin, shining synovium into an aggressive, expanding, tumorlike mass of tissue that is capable of penetrating tendons, ligaments, or bone and of destroying articular cartilage. When the synovial lining of a joint is diseased, the synovium will expand, and it is inevitable that the surrounding joint structures will be affected. The rising intraarticular pressure, increased vascularity, and any direct effects of the disease will cause thinning and eventual destruction of the capsular structures, the collateral ligaments, and the extensor mechanism of the metacarpophalangeal and interphalangeal joints. The flexor tendons, because of the interposed strong palmar plate, are protected from direct involvement by the diseased joint synovium.

Moberg and colleagues have published an excellent review of the pathological changes caused by rheumatoid disease and have stressed that in the early stages the expanding joint synovium tends to burrow beneath and affect the ligamentous attachments. The circular illustration heading this chapter is taken from their paper,* in which they state: "The granulation 'snail' is eating the bony structures from behind. This gives a good impression of what the early lesions in rheumatoid arthritis are like."

This cavitation beneath the collateral ligaments occurs early and rapidly destroys the mechanical stability of the joint. The deeper ligamentous fibers are attacked first; the degree of destruction, even in early disease, is dramatically shown by the scanning electron microscope (Fig. 7-1).

---

*Moberg, E., Wassen, E., Kjellberg, S.R., et al: The early pathologic changes in rhemautoid arthritis, Acta Chir. Scand., suppl. 357, pp. 142-147, 1966.

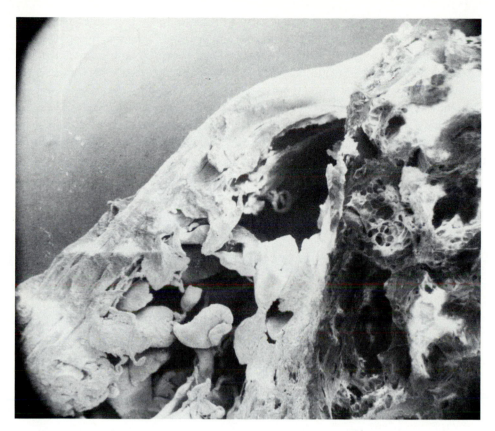

Fig. 7-1. Collateral ligament disease. This scanning electron microscope picture dramatically illustrates the cavitation between the deep surface of the ligament on the left of the picture and the site of its bony attachment on the right.

Patients with acute synovial disease of joints are usually treated with systemic medicinal preparations or by local injection of adrenocortical steroids. Such treatment may give symptomatic relief but cannot be considered curative. In fact, repeated intraarticular injections of adrenocortical steroids may be dangerous, since there is good evidence that these injections may contribute to intraarticular destruction.

Removal or destruction of the diseased synovium is a more rational method of treatment. It is of particular value when done as a preventive measure before secondary changes have occurred in the joint structures. Surgical synovectomy is a useful operation, making possible the removal of a remarkable amount of diseased tissue from the metacarpophalangeal and proximal interphalangeal finger joints. These joints do not always react favorably to surgical intervention; therefore, some restriction of range may occasionally follow synovectomy. However, in view of the inevitable joint deterioration that will occur if the diseased synovium is left undisturbed, I consider this minor restriction of range a small price to pay. Synovectomy should always be considered as an additional measure whenever other surgical procedures are performed on a digital joint.

I have been particularly interested in the effects produced by very early involvement of the synovial pouch lying between the attachment of the metacarpophalangeal ligament and the metacarpal head. My biomechanical experiments have shown that loosening or detachment of this key ligament leads to profound disturbance of the mechanical balance of the joint. Biopsies have been taken from the deep surface of these ligaments during synovectomy in very early disease. To the naked eye the only change that could be seen was a slight pearly opacity in the ligament's surface appearance, and no real mechanical laxity could be demonstrated in these joint restraints. The ultrastructural changes, however, are significant and have been reported by

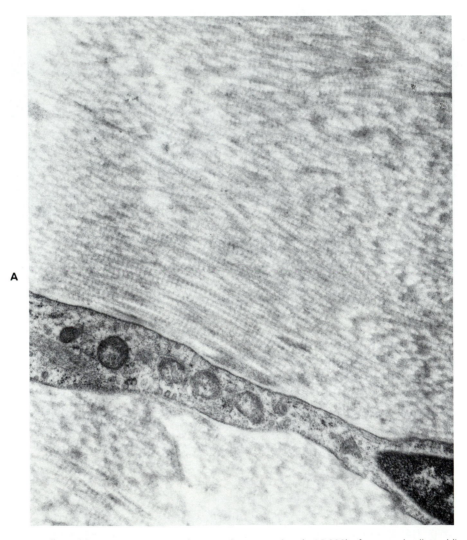

Fig. 7-2. Collateral ligament disease. **A,** Electron microscope view (×16,000) of a normal collateral ligament. **B,** An early diseased ligament (×24,000) showing fragmented disarrayed and jumbled collagen fibrils. (From Mickelson, M., and Cooper, R.R.: Iowa Chapter, Arthritis Foundation Med. Info. Bull. **12**[3-4]: 13-16 and **12**[5-6]:9-11, 1971.)

Mickelson and Cooper. They demonstrated that many of the ultrastructural vascular and cellular changes seen in rheumatoid synovium are also seen in the collateral ligaments. These ligaments are characterized by areas of collagen fibril fragmentation and degeneration and by cellular changes, including evidence of a vascular and mast-cell response. They found that compared to the normal, all diseased ligaments contained varying degrees of abnormal collagen (Fig. 7-2). Although the fibrils remained normal in diameter and periodicity, they became fragmented and disarrayed, and no longer remained in an orderly parallel arrangement. They concluded that the disruption and degeneration of collagen may account for the ligamentous laxity subsequently found in progressive disease.

If, as I believe, these changes in the collateral ligaments occur very early and are progressive, when should synovectomy be advised?

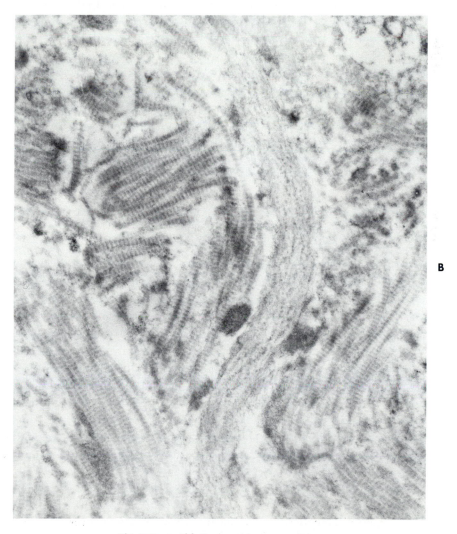

B

Fig. 7-2, cont'd. For legend see opposite page.

NATURAL HISTORY

All the digital joints are affected by rheumatoid synovitis, and tradition has it that the distal interphalangeal joints are not as commonly involved as the more proximal joints. Gatter and McCarty have shown that the distal joints are commonly involved but that their symptoms and signs are usually less distinct and of shorter duration than the larger digital joints.

Rheumatoid disease of the distal interphalangeal joints should not be confused with erosive osteoarthritis. Peter and his colleagues have described this condition as an inflammatory erosive degenerative osteophytic arthritis of the interphalangeal joints that is typically found in middle-aged postmenopausal women (Fig. 7-3). The histology of the synovium has been reported as ranging in compatibility from degenerative arthritis to that of rheumatoid disease. In the patients I have seen with this condition the diagnosis of degenerative disease has not been difficult, since all signs, symptoms, and tests for rheumatoid disease have been negative. In the acute inflammatory phase of the disease the synovial reaction may resemble that considered consistent with rheumatoid disease.

The indications for surgical synovectomy of the metacarpophalangeal and proximal interphalangeal joints are absolute if one believes that diseased synovium is the common denominator of every deforming process of the rheumatoid hand. Such narrow reasoning, however, cannot be applied in wholesale fashion to the problem of synovitis of the digital joints, since conservative and medicinal measures must be given an opportunity to relieve the painful swollen joints. It is equally important to relate the disease to its natural history. The general types of disease process have been described by Smyth and are illustrated in Fig. 1-4 (p. 8). He has also stressed that the course of disease in the two more proximal joints of the digit is different and that if the physician ignores this fact, "many synovial membranes may be needlessly sacrificed upon the operating table."

April Kay followed 33 rheumatoid patients for 2½ years and showed that synovitis of the metacarpophalangeal joints is common and persistent but that there was a 63% remission rate of synovitis of the proximal interphalangeal joints. Synovial involvement tended to occur earlier in the dominant hand but ultimately there was no significant difference between the two hands. It is of interest that the multiaxial metacarpophalangeal joints of the thumb and of the index and long fingers showed a frequent and persistent involvement, whereas the uniaxial proximal interphalangeal joints, primarily used in power grip activity, showed a high remission rate.

This selective involvement of the more mechanically unstable metacarpophalangeal joints is a common clinical finding and can reasonably be related to the many forces acting over the joint.

It was Steindler who first proposed that the joint deformities in rheumatoid disease were produced by imbalance of muscular stresses acting across inflamed and weakened joints. The inflamed joints are eventually pulled into the end position created by the predominant antagonists that cross them; the capsule is stretched on the side of the weaker antagonists, and permanent contracture results.

These mechanical influences will determine the ultimate direction of deformity

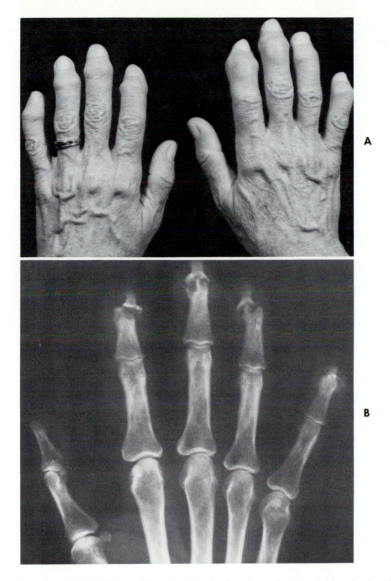

Fig. 7-3. Erosive osteoarthritis. This condition is said to be largely confined to the hands of middle-aged, postmenopausal women. **A,** Swelling of the distal interphalangeal joints is often painful. **B,** Destruction of the articular surfaces can lead to gross instability.

but they are not the primary factors. In the early stages of disease these forces act on the disease-weakened ligaments and produce deformities that are still correctable.

McMaster has reviewed the destruction seen at the metacarpophalangeal joints of 31 patients and showed that the sites and extent of the initial joint erosions correspond with the sites and size of the synovial pouches (Fig. 7-4). The areas of joint cartilage degeneration were related to the degree of flexion, ulnar deviation, and subluxation of the proximal phalanx on the metacarpal head (Fig. 2-17, p. 35).

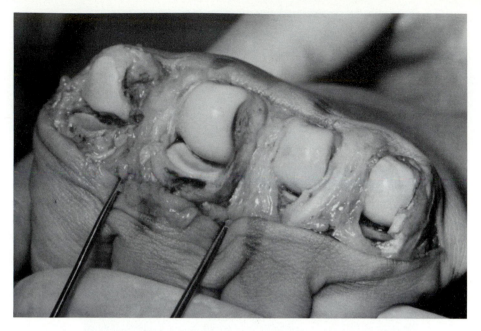

Fig. 7-4. Early synovial joint disease. This patient's hand at surgery showed erosions on both sides of the index metacarpal head and the base of its proximal phalanx. The base of the long finger proximal phalanx between the two blades of the forceps clearly shows the dorsal erosion at the site of synovial reflection.

Ehrlich has stressed that "early" synovectomy is not necessarily a function of time. The term refers to operating before irreversible damage has been done to the joint by the invasive synovium. In some patients there may be multiple transient attacks on a joint, and "early" might be years after the initial attack. In other patients the onset is more savage, and irreversible damage threatens within a short time after the onset of disease.

When the patient is being seen in concert by surgeon and rheumatologist, a mutually agreed-on period of time can be allotted to conservative treatment directed at the relief of pain and restoration of function. The period of time cannot, and should not, be exactly defined; it will depend on many factors and particularly on the length of history and the previous treatment of the patient. The important factors to monitor are progression of disease, deformity, and muscular imbalance. At the metacarpophalangeal joint the vital test is for integrity of the collateral ligaments. In the normal hand these ligaments tense and supply stability during flexion in grasping. Their integrity can therefore be tested only with the joint held in 90 degrees of flexion (Fig. 7-5). In the normal hand passive ulnar deviation is not possible in this position. Even in early disease, if laxity is present, the fingers can be moved ulnarward with little passive force.

Imminent mechanical disaster such as boutonniere deformity must be regarded as a strong indication for synovectomy even though the period of observation may have been short. Demonstrable increasing laxity of supporting ligaments is also a strong

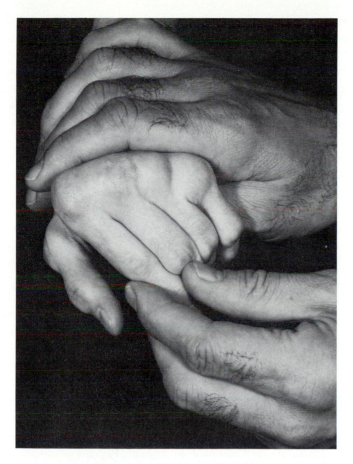

Fig. 7-5. Metacarpophalangeal joint laxity. Integrity of these collateral ligaments can only be tested with the joint passively held at 90 degrees. This patient's hand demonstrates destruction of the radial collateral ligaments because the fingers can be readily moved to 45 degrees in an ulnar direction.

indication for surgery. My colleagues and I have found that it is reasonable to try properly controlled conservative treatment for 3 or more months. This does not mean that our patients are seen only at 3-month intervals; patients whose hands show borderline signs of impending disaster are examined at much shorter intervals of time. Even a monthly visit lasting only a few minutes is worthwhile if it can substantiate worsening of the physical signs and thereby indicate surgery before irreparable harm has been done.

SYNOVECTOMY
Chemical synovectomy

Since the synovium is the target tissue for rheumatoid disease in the hand, it must also be the target for the treating physician. Surgery should always be avoided where possible, and it would be ideal if it were possible to perform a "chemical" synovectomy by intraarticular injection. No ideal substance has yet been identified, but the literature consistently reports trials of a variety of substances. The pathological synovium can be destroyed either by a caustic substance or by a radioactive product. Menkes and his colleagues at the Hôpital Cochin in Paris have reported the use of beta-emitter isotopes. They make an important distinction between the use of these substances in large joints, such as the knee, and the digital joints. They stress that yttrium 90 or even gold 198 should never be injected into finger joints because of the risk of skin necrosis. Erbium 169 is said to have limited penetration, and they consider it suitable for digital joint injection. They believe the wrist joint can be treated with either gold 198 or, better still, rhenium 186. Rhenium has the special advantage of not provoking reactions in patients previously sensitized to nonradioactive gold salts. In contrast to gold 198, which emits significant quantities of gamma rays, rhenium is an almost pure beta emitter.

Menkes and his colleagues conclude that their experience indicates the use of radioactive isotope injections as a replacement for early surgical synovectomy. The results are better in digital joints than in the wrist because of the difficulty in attaining uniform radiation of the many folds of the wrist synovium.

Among the caustic substances that have been used are sodium morrhuate, osmic acid, and the two alkylating agents nitrogen mustard and thiotepa. Osmic acid is usually reserved for use in large joints; experimental studies have shown that it can slow the growth rate of cartilage and epiphyseal bone.

I have had personal experience only with the alkylating agents. These agents combine with nuclear protein components necessary for the formation of DNA. By preventing nuclear growth, the drugs inhibit cell division and can therefore be considered for use against the heavy population of white cells in the synovial membrane. Nitrogen mustard has been used for some time as both a systemic and a local agent in the treatment of patients with rheumatoid disease. Reports concerning its use have varied in their conclusions, but there seems to be little doubt that the alkylating agents do have a specific destructive effect on the plasma cells and lead to a recession of the joint systems over a varying period of time. Riordan has revived, and continues, the intraarticular use of nitrogen mustard for chemical synovectomy.

I have used thiotepa (triethylenethiophosphoramide) for intraarticular injections into the digital joints for over 20 years. I selected it for trial, since it is related chemically and pharmacologically to nitrogen mustard but is considerably easier to handle in the small doses needed for intraarticular injections of the digital joints.

Fearnley has compared the injection of thiotepa into 58 joints within the hand against 53 joints injected with methylprednisolone. At the end of a month there was a significant increase in grip strength in both groups; at the end of a year there was no significant difference in grip strengths. There was no clinical evidence of permanent remission in any of the injected joints, and there was a gradual tendency for both symptoms and signs to relapse. No significant side effects were observed and in no case did the white blood cell count fall below 3000/mm^3 after injections of the same strength that I use.

In a double-blind comparison of intraarticular thiotepa, methylprednisolone acetate (Depo-medrol), and procaine in the joints of the hand, Gristina and colleagues could not demonstrate a satisfactory "medical synovectomy." Joints injected with procaine alone showed about the same general improvement as those injected with thiotepa alone. They did, however, conclude that there is some therapeutic effect from the use of thiotepa.

The literature seems to bring in the verdict, acceptable in Scottish courts, of "not proven"; roughly translated, this means, "We know you did it but we can't pin it on you." My use of thiotepa leads me to the same conclusion. When used in small doses, it appears to do no harm to the patient, and in an unpredictable number it will have a beneficial effect for 6 to 9 months. Thiotepa is not painful when injected into joints and may be used as outpatient therapy, with no more than the usual precautions necessary for any injection procedure.

TECHNIQUE FOR INJECTION OF THIOTEPA

Thiotepa is supplied in powder form in 15 mg vials. Three milliliters of sterile water are injected into the vial, making a solution in which 0.5 ml contains 2.5 mg of thiotepa. The manufacturers state that such a solution may be kept for 5 days in a refrigerator without substantial loss of potency.

The only technical problem in the injection is ensuring that the needle point is intraarticular. It is wise to use a syringe containing some innocuous fluid to flush the joint and to determine the position of the needle point. I use 1% lidocaine as the fluid, since it will prevent any immediate pain reaction. It is probably unnecessary to use a local anesthetic to flush out the joint. Lidocaine is essential only when nitrogen mustard is being used, since this injection can cause considerable pain. I have occasionally used physiological saline solution instead of lidocaine and have not encountered any complaints of pain. An infrequent accidental injection of thiotepa into the periarticular tissue has caused no adverse reaction.

After adequate skin preparation a No. 25 needle on a 5-ml syringe containing 1% lidocaine is passed into the joint (Fig. 7-6). Both the metacarpophalangeal and proximal interphalangeal joints are best approached from the dorsolateral side, with the needle penetrating the softer tissues between the extrinsic extensor tendon and thick collateral ligament. The needle should slant obliquely through the tissues to prevent the thiotepa from leaking out after the needle is withdrawn. To test if the needle point is within the joint cavity, two fingertips are placed on either side of the joint. If the needle point is truly intraarticular, the tension within the joint can be felt to rise and fall as the plunger of the syringe is pushed home and withdrawn. If several joints are to be injected, the needle is left in situ and the syringe containing the lidocaine is used to place the other needles.

A second syringe is filled with the thiotepa solution, and each joint is then injected with as much solution as it will comfortably hold. The average digital joint will accept about 0.5 ml of solution and therefore receives about 2.5 mg of thiotepa. The needle is withdrawn immediately after the injection and the joint is massaged. Early movement must be encouraged.

RESULTS OF THIOTEPA INJECTIONS

Dr. Arthur Brooks of Vanderbilt University has an extensive experience in the use of intra-articular injections of thiotepa combined with steroids. He tells me that he

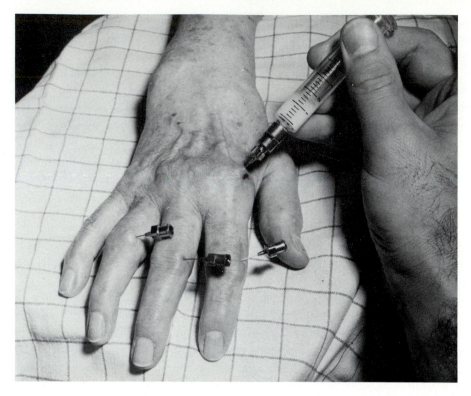

Fig. 7-6. Alkylating agent injection. A No. 25 needle should be passed obliquely into each joint; then the syringe containing the alkylating agent is connected in turn to each needle.

has found that the response to injections is directly related to the severity of the disease. The patient with severe unremitting disease shows a high recurrence rate of synovitis after injection. Joints that show early involvement but no mechanical derangement will always do well, regardless of the type of disease, if given a sufficient number of injections.

My original trial of thiotepa was reported in 1962, and in 1971 we published a further long-term report. Thirty patients with established rheumatoid disease were studied for an average follow-up period of 4.8 years. In these patients a total of 123 digital joints had been injected only once (Table 5). I did not include those patients who had more than one injection in the same joint.

Only one complication occurred as a result of thiotepa injection in the patients we studied. In one patient who had three proximal interphalangeal joints treated, a painful cutaneous vesicle developed at the injection site in each joint. The lesions appeared 5 days later and were accompanied by a generalized cutaneous eruption of "hives." The local and generalized reaction responded to oral diphenhydramine hydrochloride (Benadryl) regressing systemically in a period of 72 hours but persisting locally for 3 weeks. Later skin tests with dilute thiotepa confirmed the clinical impression of a true drug allergy.

Table 5. Digital joints injected with thiotepa

Joint	Number
Finger	
Metacarpophalangeal	41
Proximal interphalangeal	66
Distal interphalangeal	10
Thumb	
Interphalangeal	1
Metacarpophalangeal	5
TOTAL	123

The results were assessed in four areas: symptomatic pain relief, clinical response to injection, postinjection radiographic state of the joints, and postinjection progression of clinical deformity. Only 7 of my 30 patients showed good results in all four objective assessments, but 53% reported subjective improvement. In Currey's trial of thiotepa he reported that a symptomatic improvement occurred in a control series injected with procaine. He rightly suggests that this improvement may be the result of the patients' awareness of, and curiosity in, the trial, stimulating increased exercising of the injected joint.

Half of my patients showed continuing clinical and radiographic progression of disease. In all these patients active systemic illness persisted after injection. This suggests that no benefit was derived from the injection, since progression in these treated joints was largely commensurate with that in adjacent, untreated joints. The seven patients in whom a beneficial response to the injection was obtained failed to demonstrate any consistent clinical parameter that might be used to effectively predict this response. Because of the favorable response to injection locally, none of these joints was subsequently explored surgically and examined histologically.

Biopsies from other patients in the series were compared with noninjected controls, and this examination failed to substantiate my earlier hope that some consistent histological difference exists after the injection of thiotepa. In each instance the tissues were similar in regard to cellular populations and other histological characteristics.

The value of intraarticular thiotepa without additional steroids is thus, at best, unpredictable in terms of potential benefit. At this time I tend to use it in preference to surgical synovectomy for patients who are considered poor candidates for anesthesia and for the patient with a single joint involvement. I also use it more frequently than surgical synovectomy in the juvenile rheumatoid.

In the operating room it is largely used for the patient with multiple joint involvement. Surgical synovectomy may be done at one joint level and thiotepa used in other joints, thereby avoiding excessive operating procedures on the hand and keeping the tourniquet time within reasonable limits.

I do not believe that there is, even now, sufficient evidence to justify the routine use of intraarticular alkylating agents, but I will continue to use them on selected patients.

Surgical synovectomy

The major problem in deciding on the timing of joint synovectomy is the impossibility of accurately defining the degree of joint involvement from external inspection. It is a consistent finding during surgery that the changes in the joint surfaces are always worse than the clinical signs might lead one to believe. Even relatively mild degrees of synovial swelling can conceal far-advanced degrees of joint destruction.

Synovitis can occur in all three digital joints and, if left untreated, will eventually cause irreversible changes. Detection of early involvement cannot be done by one- or two-finger palpation of a joint; three-finger palpation is necessary. Each digital joint resembles a miniature knee joint in the sense that there is a "suprapatellar pouch" on the dorsum of the head and neck of the proximal bone in each digital joint (Fig. 8-4, p. 184). Small amounts of swelling or fluid can be detected by placing a finger on either side of the dorsal edge of the pouch. As these fingers press gently inward, the third finger presses down on the dorsum of the joint; if fluid is present, it will rebound against the two lateral fingers (Fig. 7-7). Using two fingers merely sloshes the fluid around in the cavity, and no judgment can be made on its volume.

X-ray films of the hand are of little value in determining the extent of early changes in the joint surfaces. Destruction of articular surfaces must be far advanced before such a relatively coarse test as x-ray examination will reveal any change. McMaster has shown that opinion based on radiographic findings alone will not be truly representative of all the pathological changes within the joint. A thorough clinical examination will reveal more than x-ray examination can show in the early stages of the disease. Young has described the first changes that are seen on x-ray films, but in relation to the disease, the changes must be considered late and irreversible. An important point concerning interpretation is made by Young when he states that density changes alone do not provide reliable criteria of early pathological change. The additional changes of bone destruction and/or new bone formation are necessary to establish a radiological diagnosis of rheumatoid disease.

An important feature to look for in x-ray films of the hands is evidence of early cortical loss and erosion. This is usually seen on the lateral portion of the metacarpal head. It is caused by the mass of rheumatoid pannus, which develops in the crypt between the collateral ligament and the metacarpal head. If the pannus is not cleaned out of this crypt during surgical synovectomy, destruction of the metacarpal head and collateral ligament attachment will continue.

Brewerton has introduced a very useful tangential x-ray projection that discloses early destruction in the peripheral crypts near the attachments of the capsule and ligaments to the bone (Fig. 7-8). In this method the dorsum of the fingers is placed flat on the cassette, with the metacarpophalangeal joints flexed through 65 degrees, the thumb fully extended, and the beam angled 15 degrees from the ulnar side (Fig 7-9). I have adopted this view for routine use in radiography of the rheumatoid hand, eliminating the customary oblique view but retaining the posteroanterior and lateral views.

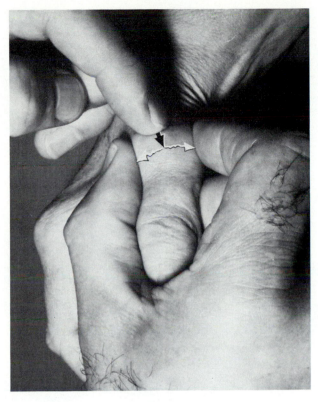

Fig. 7-7. Detection of digital joint synovitis. Pressure from three digits is necessary to detect small degrees of swelling in a digital joint. The metacarpophalangeal joint of this patient's thumb is being examined. The examiner's thumb and index finger tips are pressing the sides of the joint; the second index finger presses vertically downward, and the transmitted force is felt between the other index finger and the thumb.

At the distal interphalangeal joint the swelling of the synovium will affect the insertion of the extensor tendon. The tendon will stretch, become thinned, and may even rupture, allowing the joint to lapse into the flexion deformity characteristic of mallet finger. It is technically possible to perform synovectomy of the distal interphalangeal joint, but the operation is seldom attempted. Synovectomies of the proximal interphalangeal joint and the metacarpophalangeal joint can be easily accomplished and yield highly satisfactory results. Synovectomy at these two joints is usually combined with other procedures. Most patients come to surgery too late for synovectomy alone to be sufficient.

It is a fundamental fact that the natural history of digital joint synovitis has a direct bearing on the indications for surgery and the quality of results. Earlier generalized enthusiasm for "prophylactic" synovectomy has been distilled into several careful analyses of factors influencing the results. There is general agreement with the views of Backhouse and colleagues that in patients with early rheumatoid disease synovial involvement occurs more frequently in the metacarpophalangeal joints than in the proximal interphalangeal joints. However, spontaneous remission of the synovitis occurs five times more frequently in the proximal interphalangeal joints than in the

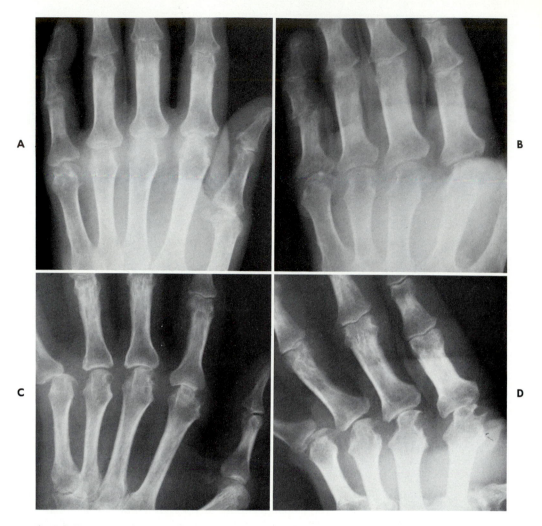

Fig. 7-8. Brewerton x-ray projection. A comparison between the usual anteroposterior view and the Brewerton view. **A,** Moderate disease in the anteroposterior view. **B,** Same hand in the Brewerton position. **C,** Severe disease in the anteroposterior view. **D,** Extent of the destruction shown in the Brewerton view.

metacarpophalangeal joints. This variability in behavior of the synovium at different joint levels is well known to rheumatologists and may account for the reluctance of some to accept the concept that surgical synovectomy has a place in the care of the rheumatoid hand. This variation in the natural history of the disease is largely responsible for the continuing debate on the timing of surgical intervention in any particular patient. Early synovectomy has been advocated by most surgical investigators in the field, but the term *early* means different things to different observers. Most would agree, however, that for maximum benefit, synovectomy should be done before the x-ray appearance of bone erosion and narrowing of the joint space, and before mechanical changes make their appearance. Mason suggests that the best results are obtained in cases without x-ray changes and in which the duration of the disease in the

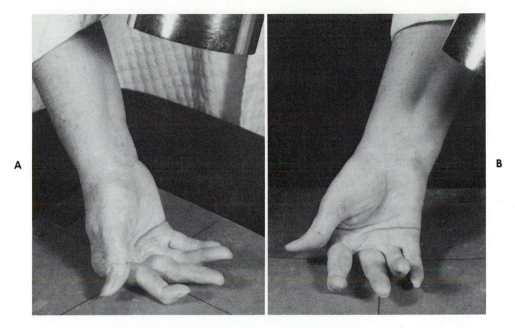

Fig. 7-9. Brewerton x-ray projection. **A,** Thumb is fully extended to avoid obscuring the fingers. The metacarpophalangeal joints of the fingers are flexed through 65 degrees. **B,** Tube is angled from a point 15 degrees to the ulnar side of the hand.

joint to be operated on is less than 5 years. All should agree that surgical intervention is indicated only when it has been demonstrated that conservative measures are ineffective in controlling the disease process in an individual joint.

How long should one wait to determine if conservative treatment is to be effective? Lipscomb suggested at least 6 months. He further suggested that surgery should be done when the synovium is in a "chronically thickened and boggy state." Preston suggested 4 months; others suggest different timing. Gschwend has pointed out that ultimately only the operative findings allow us to define whether the operation is an early or late synovectomy.

I believe it is essential to consider the general disease state of the patient in determining the time for surgical intervention. In severe active stages of the systemic disease, a hand may completely deteriorate in 6 months, and the optimum opportunity for prophylactic surgery will then have passed (Fig. 7-10). A patient in a quiescent state of disease can be observed for a longer period because mechanical deterioration will not be so rapid.

There is no point in delaying surgical intervention in a patient with a history of persistent swelling, exacerbations of disseminated involvement, and constant pain. The persistence of pain between exacerbations of the disease is a sure indication that the process is progressive and that mechanical disruption is likely to occur.

The degrees of involvement of joints proximal and distal to the joint under consideration for synovectomy must be carefully considered. I have previously pointed out that the reciprocal interaction between joints must be considered when operative

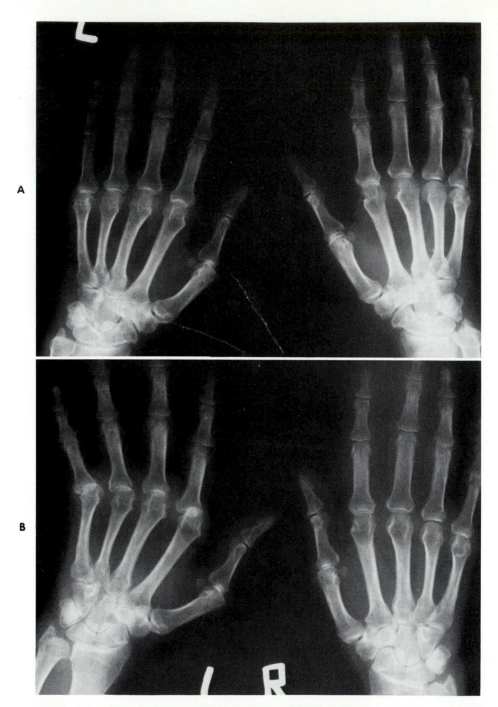

Fig. 7-10. Synovectomy in severe disease. X-ray films of the hands of a 53-year-old woman with severe progressive disease. **A,** Minimal x-ray changes in both hands immediately prior to synovectomy of right metacarpophalangeal joints. **B,** Four months later the left metacarpophalangeal joints have severely deteriorated; synovectomy of both metacarpophalangeal and proximal interphalangeal joints was done at this time. **C,** Three years later x-ray films show continued deterioration in all the joints operated on. This postoperative progression is typical in patients with continued active disease. (From Ellison, M.R., Kelly, K.J., and Flatt, A.E.: J. Bone Joint Surg. **53-A:**1041-1060, 1971.)

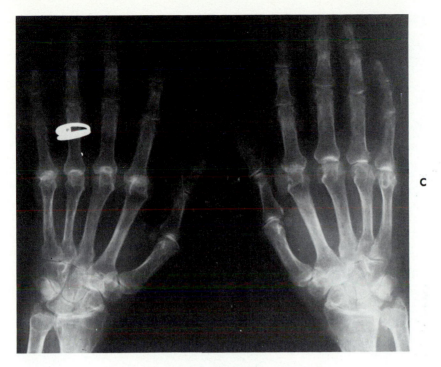

C

Fig. 7-10, cont'd. For legend see opposite page.

procedures for the hand are designed. I extend this reasoning to include involvement at the wrist. Many well-intended surgical procedures at the metacarpophalangeal and proximal interphalangeal joints have been defeated by severe and continuing wrist disease.

When the disease has been present for some time and architectural changes have occurred in the joints, more drastic procedures are needed to restore function. The greatest problem in the restoration of function to the rheumatoid hand is still instability at the metacarpophalangeal joint (Fig. 7-11). The instability is usually associated with ulnar drift and palmar dislocation. Ultimately, collapse of both the longitudinal and the distal transverse arches of the hand occurs. Disease at the proximal interphalangeal joint usually causes varying degrees of stiffness and deformity rather than instability. The combination of instability at the metacarpophalangeal joint and stiffened deformity at the proximal interphalangeal joint is particularly unfortunate because it destroys virtually all normal power of grasp.

The three operations of fusion, arthroplasty, and prosthetic replacement are available to correct these deformities. None of these operations is suitable in all conditions, and varying combinations are used according to the circumstance.

FUSION

Fusion operations have been used for many years in rheumatoid disease but are not routinely acceptable within the hand for several reasons. Most important is the fact that rheumatoid disease is a progressive condition in which the state of the dis-

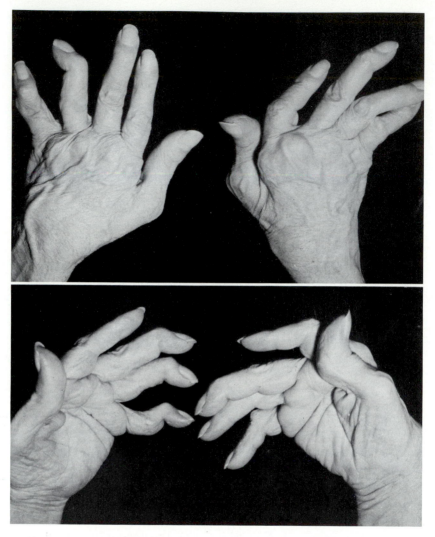

Fig. 7-11. Instability of metacarpophalangeal joints. Destruction of the integrity of the metacarpophalangeal joints, causing instability and dislocation such as that seen in these hands, is the greatest problem in the restoration of function to the rheumatoid hand.

ease changes from year to year. Long-term follow-up has shown that this progression of the disease may so alter the condition of the hand that fusions that previously yielded increased function may become a liability and thereby actively hinder function of the hand at a later date. Firm bony union is often hard to achieve, and the prolonged immobilization needed to encourage fusion is bad for the rheumatoid hand. Fusion of a single digital joint can be used, but its widespread use across the hand is unwise. It is equally unwise to fuse the metacarpophalangeal and the proximal interphalangeal joints of the same finger, since the finger is then quite unable to curve around an object being grasped.

In totally burned-out disease and in digits with grotesque combinations of flexion and hyperextension deformities, fusion may be the only operation that can provide any increase in function. Under such conditions one has to accept a simplification of the normal mechanism of the hand and restore the basic arch formation of the digits so that minimum prehension is possible. If both hands are involved, the operative plan should attempt to provide a different type of activity for each hand with, if possible, the more precise actions being built into the dominant hand.

ARTHROPLASTY

Because of the problems associated with fusion and because retention of movement in a joint is always desirable, many varieties of excisional arthroplasties have been described. The majority of these operations are designed for use at the metacarpophalangeal joint. Late results of many of the earlier arthroplasty operations at the metacarpophalangeal joint were disappointing because the palmar dislocation of the base of the proximal phalanx recurred. More recently, operations have been designed to prevent this recurrent dislocation, and the results are more satisfactory.

At the proximal interphalangeal joint, excisional arthroplasty can be of great benefit in the long and ring fingers. Good support is provided for the fingers if the collateral ligaments are intact. Additional and essential lateral support is supplied by the two border fingers, the index and small fingers. Arthroplasty is inherently unstable in these two fingers, even if the collateral ligaments are intact, since the support of neighboring fingers is missing on one side of each finger.

The fundamental problem of arthroplasty operations is the degree of instability created in the joint. The joint is deliberately excised to provide flexion and extension. This movement tends to occur as a combination of gliding and angulation after excision of the bone. Unfortunately this excision of the joint also allows undesirable movements in lateral and rotational planes. It is interesting that the most satisfactory function is obtained from arthroplasties that provide a relatively small range of movement. In effect, these operations are supplying sufficient stability at the expense of movement to counteract the dislocating forces.

PROSTHETIC REPLACEMENT

Because of the grave functional liabilities associated with multiple fusions of the digital joints and the poor long-term follow-up results associated with excisional arthroplasty operations at some joints, many surgeons perform prosthetic replacement of digital joints.

There are basically only three reasons justifying prosthetic replacement of a digital joint: (1) no joint present, (2) joint surfaces destroyed, and (3) joint restraints destroyed.

These fundamental requirements are frequently present in the rheumatoid hand, but prosthetic replacement of a diseased finger joint cannot be considered as an isolated undertaking. It must be related to the function of the other two joints of the finger and of the hand as a whole. In the normal hand there is a functional relationship between the movements of the metacarpophalangeal and proximal interphalangeal joints. In the diseased finger this interrelationship is of vital importance.

Adequate muscle control is a prerequisite to any form of joint reconstruction, including prosthetic replacement. In rheumatoid disease of the hand there is frequently an imbalance between the flexor and extensor muscles of the fingers. The extensor mechanism is usually weaker because it is commonly involved by disease, whereas the flexor mechanism is protected by the tough palmar plate.

There is no functional contraindication to prosthetic replacement of several finger joints within the same hand. Both metacarpophalangeal and proximal interphalangeal joints have been replaced in the same hand, and in recent years techniques have been developed allowing replacement of these two joints in the same finger. Replacement of the distal interphalangeal joint of the fingers has been tried to a limited degree in recent years. In the thumb the carpometacarpal and the metacarpophalangeal joints have been replaced by a prosthesis, but I do not attempt to replace the interphalangeal joint because of the short length of the distal phalanx.

Compound deformities have usually been allowed to develop at the level of the metacarpophalangeal joint of the fingers before the patient is referred for surgery. The most common deformities are ulnar drift, palmar displacement, rotation of the digit, distortion of the hood mechanism, and dislocation of the extensor tendons. It is impractical to place a prosthesis in one or more of these joints without, at the same time, correcting the accompanying deformities and those of the adjacent joints. At the proximal interphalangeal joint the condition of the intrinsic muscles is of fundamental importance. It would be futile to replace a destroyed joint with a prosthesis if no correction was applied to a concurrent intrinsic contracture.

Under ideal conditions a prosthesis will supply the stability of a fusion combined with the movement of an arthroplasty. I believe that the provision of such stable movement is essential in a hand subject to progressive rheumatoid disease. Nearly 20 years ago I wrote: "No prosthesis exists which can approach the stability and versatility of movement of a normal joint. All mechanical devices so far produced are inadequate substitutes and most have severe drawbacks." Time and experience allow me to soften the severity of the language, but I honestly believe that the era of perfect spare-parts surgery for digital joints has still not arrived.

Sir Herbert Seddon has written, "A great deal of surgical activity has misfired—the patients being the losers—because it never occurred to the clinicians to consult an engineer before embarking on some ingenious venture."* At least in the design of finger prostheses surgeons and engineers are now active partners, and design problems are being studied in a rational manner. Linscheid and Chao have demonstrated the importance of this cooperation in their biomechanical assessment of finger function in prosthetic joint design.

If the prosthesis is to be a satisfactory joint substitute, it should conform to the following requirements:

1. Restores functional range of motion
2. Provides appropriate stability
3. Provides a mechanical advantage equivalent to the normal

---

*From Seddon, H.: Br. Med. J. 2:36, 1966 (Book review.)

4. Seats firmly and resists rotational stresses
5. Provides easy implantation
6. Accommodates anatomical size variations

The proximal interphalangeal joint is a simple fixed-axis hinge joint, and its replacement with a hinged prosthesis is not a major technical problem. It is the multiaxial carpometacarpal joint of the thumb and the metacarpophalangeal joint of the finger that defy the best efforts of all the current research work.

Design problems

Still unresolved is the fundamental question of whether in this work we should strive for a mechanical reproduction of the human joint—a true prosthesis—or whether we should supply a spacer that separates the bone ends and provides a form around which scar can grow. My preference is for a prosthesis, but no matter which device is used, there are two basic problems that have not yet been solved. The first is whether or not the stems need a firm fixation in the body tissues, and the second is the establishment of the best form of axis through which movement is to take place.

The double-stemmed metallic hinge made of SS 316, which I used during the late 1950's and early 1960's, provided excellent stability and resisted the powerful subluxating force of the flexor tendons. It allowed a high proportion of the tendon force to be translated into grip strength. However, a study of the results showed major problems with lateral migration of the stems in the medullary canal and fatigue fracture at the junction of the stems with the hinge (Fig. 7-12).

In the early 1960's Swanson introduced the use of silicone rubber. A cruciform bar of Silastic supplied support across the joint and held the raw bone ends apart. Thousands of these implants have been used, and despite the development of a far tougher rubber, fractures still occur in the stems; however, the patients' function does not seem to be adversely affected.

Neibauer devised a true prosthesis made of a Dacron-reinforced silicone rubber. The stems were covered with a mesh into which fibrous tissue could grow, thus effectively locking the stem in place. Although several modifications have been made in the original design, the thin hinge still shows fractures after prolonged use.

In the 1970's the apparent success of various total hip replacement mechanisms stimulated the production of a variety of ingenious "total" finger joints. These third-generation devices employ basically the same materials as the total hip replacements, high-density polyethylene and stainless steel alloys, scaled down and modified in design to resemble the metacarpophalangeal joint of the human finger.

Unfortunately, there are fundamental errors in this simplistic approach. The hip joint is a large ball-and-socket articulation deeply seated in the pelvis, surrounded by large ligaments and supported by a massive musculature. By contrast, the human metacarpophalangeal joint is a shallow skin-deep articulation supported by relatively small ligaments. A variety of tendons passes over the four sides of the joint, supplying dynamic support when it is in action.

Although the actual magnitude of forces passing through the hip joint must be greater than in the metacarpophalangeal joint, the proportion of force per unit size of

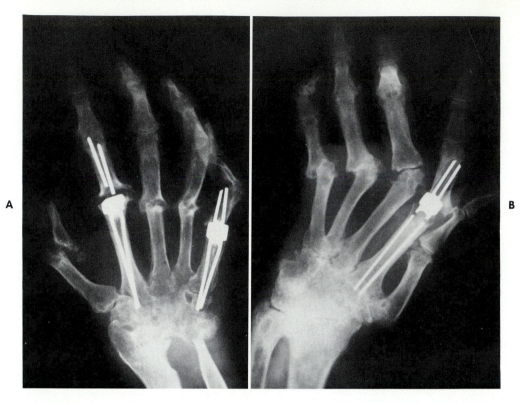

Fig. 7-12. Fractured metal prostheses. **A,** Eight years before this x-ray film, prostheses were placed in the index and small fingers. The index finger prosthesis has fractured, whereas in the small finger the prosthesis has settled in both the phalanx and metacarpal. **B,** This prosthesis was inserted in the left index finger of this 50-year-old man 5 years before this x-ray film. The metacarpal prongs are fractured, the phalangeal prongs have shifted in the phalanx, and the finger is pronated. (From Flatt, A.E.: J. Bone Joint Surg. **54-A:**1317-1322, 1972.)

the materials used is probably much greater in the hand. Direct force measurement in human joints is not yet possible, but material failure has been reported in the total hip and certainly occurs in all the various total finger joints currently available. An important additional problem is that all these devices have to be fixed to the host tissues if they are to work effectively. Methyl methacrylate is currently used as the fixative or "glue." In fact, this material is really only a packing or filler. While it may bond to the synthetic material, it does not effectively join to human tissue. Eventual loosening of these devices is being reported with increasing frequency in both the hip and the hand. A serious short-term problem has been the delayed appearance of infection in the glue. Despite careful precautions, *Staphylococcus epidermidis* and other organisms may appear as pathogens 1 or 2 years after insertion of the prosthesis.

For effective use of any joint, there must be accurate control of the tendon forces passing over it. In the normal joint anatomical restraints maintain the moment arms of these tendons so that the joint is effectively controlled. An artificial substitute for a human joint provides a freely movable articulation but usually does not accurately reproduce the mechanical features of the original. It cannot supply the subtle anatomical restraints needed to maintain the line of action of the tendons.

In any joint, weakness in a ligamentous support, deviation in a tendon's line of action, or permanent alteration in its strength will inevitably disturb the equilibrium of forces passing over the joint. Imbalance will occur, and frequently intolerable forces will build up in the joint or in a synthetic substitute.

If these problems are not recognized, it is probable that a prosthesis will be an ineffective joint substitute and, because of lack of equilibrium in the tendon forces, may well move into an end position.

The metacarpophalangeal joint of the fingers is the joint most commonly replaced in the human hand. Unfortunately, it also is a joint with a great demand for accurately controlled movement in all three planes—most often in a combination of several planes at the same time. Because this joint demands such freedom of motion, the third-generation total joints appear to be attractive alternatives for diseased or destroyed joints. In clinical practice these devices have shown material or biomechanical shortcomings, and several have been returned to the drawing board.

We have examined the biomechanical behavior of a variety of metacarpophalangeal joint substitutes implanted in fresh cadaver fingers. The center of rotation, range of motion, tendon excursion, and fingertip force were determined on the fingers before and after implanting Swanson, Niebauer, Steffee II, St. George-Buchholz, Schultz, and modified Strickland prostheses (Fig. 7-13). Their biomechanical behavior varied considerably, and none duplicated the normal metacarpophalangeal joint. Each has design characteristics that may be clinically advantageous as well as disadvantageous. Irrespective of the design, it was found that the silicone rubber implants buckled with tendon loading. This deformity created a significant mechanical flexor advantage and a mechanical disadvantage in extension. We also found that the third-generation articulated prostheses required a precise implantation technique. Errors in technique resulted in significant alterations in their biomechanical behavior.

This study was done in the laboratory; it suffers from the limitations of any such in vitro work, and any correlation with clinical behavior should be made with reservation. This may be particularly true of the Swanson and Niebauer implants, which rely on the patient's postoperative healing mechanisms. In contrast to the precise placement necessary for the stems of third-generation prostheses the Swanson implant is very forgiving. Implanting it correctly or even upside down made little difference in the fingertip force studies.

Materials used

I always warn my patients that the replacement of their finger joints cannot carry a lifetime guarantee. Fatigue is a problem in any material subjected to repeated stress, and they should be prepared for possible failure after years of use.

The metal prostheses that I used were made of SS 316, extra-low carbon vacuum melt. Fatigue of the stems becomes a definite problem the longer these prostheses remain in my patient's hands (Fig. 7-12). Because of this, the silicone rubber devices have a definite technical advantage over the original metal prostheses. They are easy to handle, and implantation is less difficult than when rigid metal or third-generation devices are used. The major reservation I continue to have is in relation to the dura-

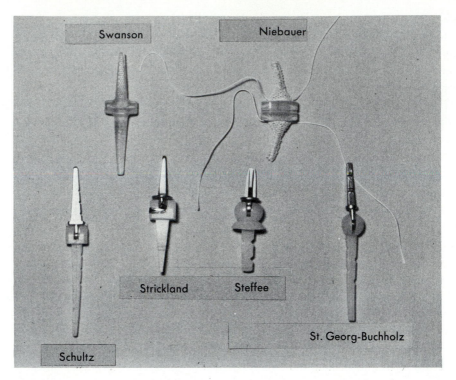

Fig. 7-13. Metacarpophalangeal joint substitutes. The two devices in the top row are made of silicone rubber. The four prostheses in the bottom row are made of dissimilar materials and must be "glued" into the finger bones.

bility of all the various materials used. The two types of silicone rubber prostheses have both been subjected by their developers to extensive mechanical fatigue testing outside the human body with satisfactory results, but there are reported failures of both during clinical trials. Swanson feels that among the probable causes of fracture of his implant are inadequate release of subluxating forces and inadequate resection of bone. It may be that these forces tend to produce a shear line at the junction of the stem and central bar because of damage from either instruments or tiny spikes of bone present at the amputated surface of the metacarpal or phalanx.

On the basis of 20 years of clinical and experimental work, I believe that prosthetic replacement of digital joints in the rheumatoid hand is a reasonable, and better, alternative to fusion of these joints.

It must be understood that no matter what type of prosthesis is used, it cannot reproduce the precise action provided by the intricate anatomical arrangement of a normal metacarpophalangeal joint. Precision can never be supplied. If, however, the prosthesis supplies stability, has sufficient integrity to resist the forces put through the hand, and, in addition, has an arc of motion that will supply function, then a satisfactory result can be anticipated.

The overall improvement provided by the joint substitutes in the weakened rheumatoid hand is so marked that I intend to continue using them whenever indicated.

Indications

As knowledge has increased, the indications for prosthetic replacement have become more clearly defined.

The majority of my patients receiving prostheses have been female; less than 30 men needed prosthetic insertion. The great majority of the women were housewives, a few worked in offices, one was a nurse, and one was a professional harpist who returned to full-time employment in an orchestra after metal metacarpophalangeal prostheses had been placed in eight fingers. The occupations of the men varied from a professor of education and politicians to barbers and executives. In no instance was heavy manual labor the prime occupation of the patient, although one man with Swanson implants in the metacarpophalangeal joints of both hands drives a dump truck.

If the tendon mechanism of a digit is intact, even though it may be displaced, prosthetic replacement of the metacarpophalangeal joint should be considered if the following are present:
1. Gross joint destruction
2. Palmar and proximal dislocation of the base of the phalanx
3. Marked ulnar drift combined with joint destruction or palmar dislocation

Simple ulnar drift without dislocation or joint destruction is not considered an indication for prosthetic replacement, since soft-tissue operations yield acceptable results.

If the tendon mechanism is intact at the proximal interphalangeal joint, the indications for prosthetic replacement are as follows:
1. Gross joint destruction
2. Persistent swan-neck deformity
3. Ankylosis in a nonfunctional position

Indications for replacement of the distal interphalangeal joint in the fingers are not yet well established. A few surgeons are using joint replacements, and reports on the use of Swanson implants have been published. The operation is technically demanding and tends to be used in early erosive or degenerative joint disease.

In the thumb, prosthetic replacement can be performed only at the carpometacarpal and metacarpophalangeal joints. I do not believe that the indications are as clearly defined as for the fingers. The principal use of a prosthesis is to stabilize a metacarpophalangeal joint in which the proliferating synovitis has so destroyed the integrity of the joint that the thumb has become in effect "double-jointed" at its most important joint. Gross flexion of the joint associated with hyperextension of the interphalangeal joint has also been found to be a reasonable indication for the use of a prosthesis.

Contraindications

The mere presence of a feature cited as an indication does not necessarily justify an operation. The overall function of the hand and its use by the patient are the important factors to consider. Postoperative cooperation by the patient is vital, and it is useless to advise surgery for a passive patient who has expressed no interest in obtaining an improvement in function.

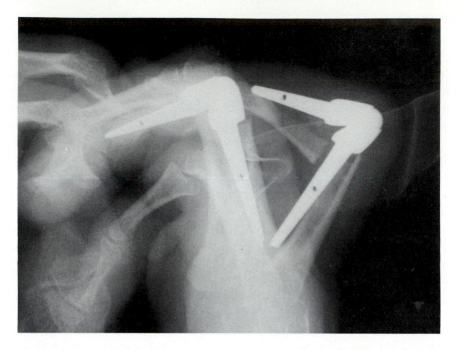

Fig. 7-14. Interphalangeal joint prosthesis complication. The bones in the hands of patients with juvenile rheumatoid disease are so small that it is extremely difficult to insert even a single-stemmed prosthesis. In this patient both phalanges of the ring finger were fractured when a prosthesis was inserted. (From Flatt, A.E.: J. Bone Joint Surg. **43-A:**753, 1961.)

Juvenile rheumatoid disease frequently produces severe deformities of the hand. Unfortunately the disease inhibits growth of the hands so that in adult life the phalanges and metacarpals are much smaller than the average adult size. Attempts at prosthetic replacement in these small fingers have been uniformly unsuccessful, and I rarely, if ever, attempt prosthetic replacement in these patients (Fig. 7-14).

Caution must be used in advising prosthetic replacement of the metacarpophalangeal joints in patients who have extensive carpal arthritis. Many of these patients have such severe involvement of the carpal and carpometacarpal joints that all movement is lost at these levels. In addition, a narrowing of the width of the hand frequently occurs at the metacarpophalangeal joint level. As a result of these changes, great difficulty may be experienced in placing the prostheses within the metacarpal shafts. Another problem produced by narrowing of the hand is that the fingers will lie very close together and may sometimes impinge on each other, since all abduction/adduction movement is absent in the prostheses.

There are two major contraindications to prosthetic replacement of the proximal interphalangeal joint. Both are related to the state of the extensor tendon mechanism. Long-standing boutonniere deformity must be regarded as a contraindication because of the difficulties in reconstructing the distorted extensor mechanism. Attempts at reconstruction of the extensor mechanism at the time the prosthesis was inserted have not yielded good results. In the majority of patients the deformity has recurred.

The only benefit to the patient has been the loss of the constant aching pain that was present in the joint before excision.

Persistent flexion deformity of the proximal interphalangeal joint presents the same reconstructive problem as long-standing boutonniere deformity. Imbalance between the flexor and extensor muscles is present, and the constant pressure of the flexed joint against the deep surface of the extensor mechanism weakens and stretches the extensor tendon. Experience has shown that reconstruction of this extensor mechanism is just as difficult as that in boutonniere deformity. In both conditions, fusion in the optimum position will yield better functional results than prosthetic replacement.

Digital joint replacement in the rheumatoid hand is now an accepted procedure. Similar replacement for individual joints destroyed by degenerative or posttraumatic arthritis is becoming more common, but I do not believe the indications are yet concisely defined.

The greatest problem is that the concept of joint replacement is seductively simple, and the lay mind has difficulty in accepting the many problems inherent in the procedure. The second generation of silicone substitutes has provided several improvements over the original metal design. The third generation, now under development, in which the sound engineering principle of using dissimilar materials for articulating surfaces has been applied, may eventually prove to be a further improvement.

But I must still close this chapter by repeating that I do not believe the millennium is near; the perfect finger joint substitute has not yet been devised.

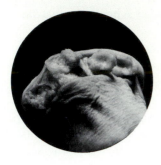

CHAPTER 8

Joint disease— operative treatment

Surgery on the joints of an arthritic hand cannot restore normal anatomical function. All operative plans are based on compromise; movement may be sacrificed to relieve symptoms and stability sacrificed to restore motion. Dislocations can be corrected, but only at the expense of full function. The basic problem in surgery of the joints is the balancing of the functional disturbance created by the joint disease against the degree of function that can be restored by the operation. Surgery should be advised if a significant increase in function can be achieved or further destruction prevented.

Anyone undertaking this work should pay heed to Dr. Paul Lipscomb's wise and provocative paper, "Is Early Synovectomy of the Small Joints of the Hand Worthwhile?"* He ends his discussion by stating: "In the past we have perhaps tried to play God. We must realize that we are only human and are not capable of remaking and reproducing the intricacies of joints and their accompanying neuromuscular tendinous components."

DIGITAL JOINT SYNOVECTOMIES

The expanding synovium within a digital joint is contained by the capsular and ligamentous structures joining the two bones. As the pressure increases, the weakest areas will yield a synovial "blowout," or hernia, will occur (Fig. 8-1). At the proximal interphalangeal joint level these hernias are sometimes misdiagnosed as rheumatoid nodules. At the metacarpophalangeal joint the eccentric swelling is said to contribute to the lateral displacement of the extensor tendon on the dorsum of the joint.

Excision of the synovium from any large joint usually causes temporary mild stiffness, which is overcome by exercises and active use. Digital joints are even more sensitive to this postoperative stiffness, and it may be at least 6 months before the maximum range of movement is achieved. Patients must be warned of this stiffness, since most of them tend to expect immediate and miraculous benefits from the operation. It must be made clear that the object of the operation is not the cosmetic improvement of the swollen joint but the prevention of future, more drastic troubles by removing the primary site of the disease.

No synovectomy can be complete; however, the more synovium removed the better the long-term results. There is an indefinable but well-recognized amount that has to be removed before any benefit is obtained. No less than 75% of the total synovial tissue should be excised for a satisfactory result. If only about 60% of the synovium is removed, the remaining 40% will be sufficient to cause rapidly recurring symptoms. When 80% or more is removed, the results may be excellent. The patient judges the result of the operation by the final range of movement; the physician assesses the result by the degree of ablation of the disease as well as by the stability and range of movement.

---

*Lipscomb, P.R.: Is early synovectomy of the small joints of the hand worthwhile? In Cramer, L.M., and Chase, R.A., editors: Symposium on the hand, vol. 3, St. Louis, 1971, The C.V. Mosby Co.

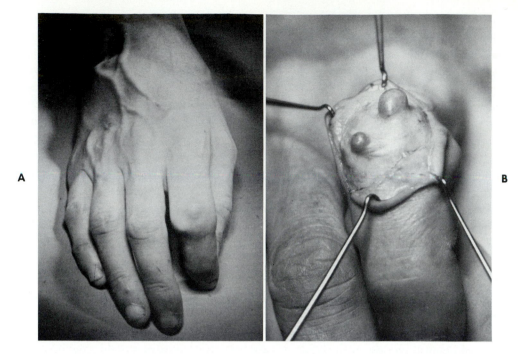

Fig. 8-1. Proximal interphalangeal joint synovitis. **A,** Protrusions of synovium from the joint are sometimes misdiagnosed as rheumatoid nodules. **B,** At surgery these hernias are found to extrude on either side of the central extensor tendon. (From Flatt, A.E.: Consultant **6**:36-39, July-Aug., 1966.)

Distal interphalangeal joint

It is uncommon for the distal interphalangeal joint to be operated on, but technically it is perfectly possible. A dorsal transverse incision is made from the line of one neutral border of the finger to the other. The skin edges are retracted, and two small incisions are made on either side of the terminal extensor tendon. The diseased synovium can be removed piecemeal through these incisions, and it is unnecessary to suture them after the synovectomy. The skin wound is closed with interrupted nylon sutures and movement encouraged as soon as the postoperative soreness has worn off.

A much more common operation at this joint is excision of a mucous cyst. These cysts are ganglia, containing synovial fluid, that occur beneath the dorsal skin between the distal interphalangeal joint and the eponychial fold. As the cyst increases in size, it presses on the nail root area, producing distortion of the nail as it appears beneath the eponychial fold. These cysts usually occur in the middle-aged with hypertrophic arthritis of their joint; they are therefore more common in women.

There is general agreement that these cysts arise from the joint synovium and that the inciting cause is a dorsal spur or osteophyte at the joint margin. To prevent recurrence of the cyst, its pedicle and any osteophytes should all be excised. It is sometimes difficult to demonstrate the full extent of the cyst but Newmeyer, Kilore, and Graham have shown that the palmar injection of methylene blue into the joint cavity will demonstrate the cyst and any occult satellite cysts (Fig. 8-2). These authors recommend using a 27- or 30-gauge needle passed through the joint crease in the midline into the joint. They recommend a mixture of methylene blue, diluted with saline solution or lidocaine, and hydrogen peroxide. The hydrogen peroxide facilitates movement of the dye into the cyst through its stalk. The joint may need to be distracted to permit entry of the needle and will accept only 0.1 to 0.2 ml of the fluid.

Proximal interphalangeal joint

An approach that is becoming increasingly popular is to make a curved dorsal incision on one or the other side of the joint. The ends of the incision reach the dorsal midline of the finger, allowing the flap to be raised and providing access to the joint. An alternative approach that I have used for years is a curvilinear dorsal incision centered over the joint line. The two skin flaps are developed sufficiently to allow exposure of the dorsum of the joint. Longitudinally running veins will be encountered; they should be preserved if their presence does not interfere greatly with the subsequent procedures. The joint cavity is opened on one side through the interlacing fibers by a longitudinal incision placed halfway between the extrinsic tendon and the lateral band. Frequently, small herniations of diseased synovium will be seen protruding through the interlacing fibers joining the lateral bands to the central slip of the extrinsic extensor tendon (Fig. 8-1). It is often possible to modify the line of the incision to include any small herniation holes. It does not matter which side of the joint is opened. If the swelling of the synovium has produced uneven expansion of the capsular tissues, I prefer to make the incision in the more swollen side, since the tissues can be overlapped during the subsequent repair. It may not be necessary to open both sides of the joint, since the capsule is usually so expanded that clearance may be accomplished through a single incision.

Removal of the synovium from the dorsal part of the joint is easy, but excision from the lateral and flexor aspects of the joint is difficult. Attempts must be made to clear any pockets of tissue that lie between the collateral ligaments and the sides of the phalanges where the ligaments are attached to the bone. Additional synovium lies between the flexor edge of the collateral ligament and the palmar plate; this synovium should be removed and can usually be reached after lateral retraction of the collateral ligament. The joint must then be passively flexed and the articular surfaces inspected. Any pannus or loose pieces of articular cartilage are removed. A pocket of synovium is often present between the palmar plate and the flexor aspect of the head and neck of the proximal phalanx; this synovium should also be removed.

The incision in the interlacing fibers is closed by interrupted, fine, absorbable sutures. It is usually possible to overlap the two sides of the incision because the dorsal tissues are relatively slack after excision of the synovium. The position of the lateral bands in relation to the axis of the joint must always be inspected; they may lie on the flexor aspect of the joint after the synovium has been removed. If allowed to remain in this position, they would tend to produce a boutonniere deformity. Therefore, when the incision in the interlacing fibers is being closed, sufficient overlap

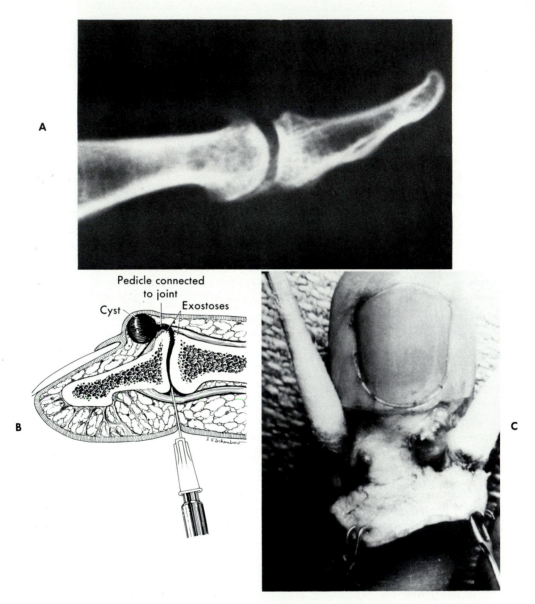

Fig. 8-2 Mucous cyst. **A,** The dorsal osteoarthritic spur frequently associated with a mucous cyst. **B,** Injection of methylene blue into the joint to fill the dorsal cyst or cysts that are present. **C,** Dissection at surgery showing a large cyst and also the presence of a small, hidden, and undiagnosed smaller cyst. (**A** and **C** Courtesy of Eugene Kilgore, II, M.D. **B** From Newmeyer, W.L., Kilgore, E.S., and Graham, W.P.: Mucous cysts: the dorsal distal interphalangeal joint ganglion, Plast. Reconstr. Surg. **53:**314, 1974.)

must be used to maintain the lateral band in its normal position dorsal to the axis. The opposite lateral band must also be inspected, and it is often necessary to reef the interlacing fibers on this side to make sure that this lateral band is also positioned to act as an extensor of the joint. If a large amount of tissue needs to be reefed, it is usually more satisfactory to incise the interlacing fibers and formally overlap the tissues rather than make a bulky roll of tissue that would lie immediately beneath the skin.

The skin incision is closed by interrupted nylon sutures and the finger bandaged in slight flexion. After the first few days, when the soreness has worn off, movement should be encouraged. It must be stressed to the patient that only active movements are to be used and that it may take many weeks to regain the maximum range of joint movement.

There are other approaches that can be used to clear the synovium from the joint. In the past Vainio has advocated a midline splitting of the central extensor tendon as far distally as its insertion. I have not used this approach, and, on theoretical grounds, it might be thought potentially dangerous because of the risk of interfering with the intratendinous blood supply in a vital area. Vainio comments that this dorsal approach makes it difficult to clear the synovium between the neck of the phalanx and the palmar plate.

Vainio has also advocated a curved skin incision on the lateral side of the joint, with the convexity toward the palmar surface. The synovium is approached by lifting up the free edge of the lateral extensor slip. This exposure gives a good view of most of the joint and is one that I use in patients who do not have severe synovial hernias.

Metacarpophalangeal joint

The synovium of the metacarpophalangeal joints is almost invariably involved early in rheumatoid disease and is frequently the first sign of disease within the hand. If, as rarely occurs, a single joint is involved, a longitudinal curvilinear incision centered over the dorsum of the joint is the correct approach. Usually all the finger joints are involved to some degree. Several types of incisions have been advocated to approach all four joints. I believe the best is a straight transverse incision just proximal to the line of the joints when the fingers are extended (Fig. 8-3). My experience with a serpentine dorsal incision has been bad (Fig. 8-3); I have not tried the dual curved incisions used by Crawford. These two incisions, which are each about 3 cm long, slant obliquely across the dorsum. The radial incision begins distally on the dorsoradial side of the base of the index proximal phalanx and proceeds proximally and transversely around the metacarpal head. It then continues across in the concavity proximal to the distal-ulnar border of the diaphysis of the long finger metacarpal. The ulnar incision begins distally at the dorsoradial margin of the proximal phalanx of the ring finger and passes proximally parallel to the radial incision in an ulnar direction.

Whichever approach is chosen, the skin flaps should be mobilized by blunt dissection, accomplished by gently spreading the scissors' points. The longitudinally running veins must not be damaged, or persistent edema of the fingers may develop.

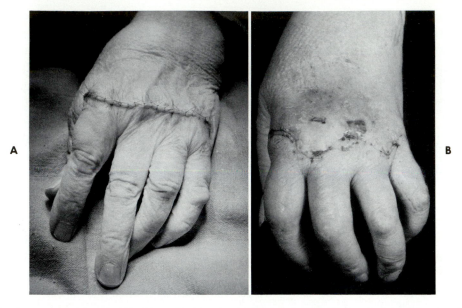

Fig. 8-3. A, Dorsal transverse incisions. The best approach for the variety of procedures performed at the metacarpophalangeal joint is the transverse incision. Great care must be taken to preserve the longitudinal veins, which run immediately beneath the skin. **B,** Serpentine incision. Some advocate this approach but my experience with it has been bad. Delayed healing is frequent, as in this patient's hand shown 17 days after operation. (**A** from Flatt, A.E.: J. Bone Joint Surg. **43-A:**753, 1961.)

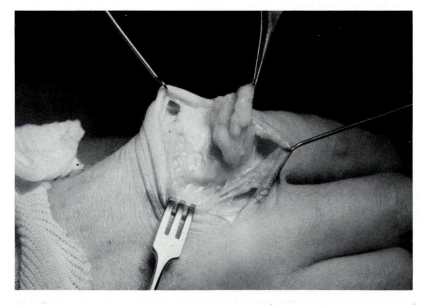

Fig. 8-4. Metacarpophalangeal joint synovectomy. There is a large dorsal and proximal pouch of synovium that must be stripped up from the neck and head of the metacarpal before the true joint cavity is entered.

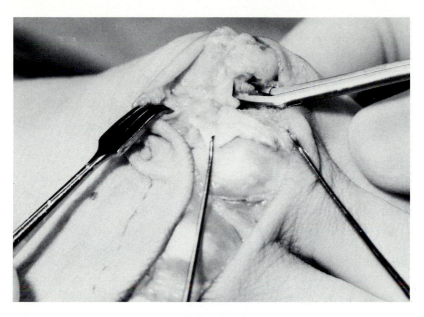

Fig. 8-5. Metacarpophalangeal joint synovectomy. A pituitary rongeur is a very useful instrument for removing the tongue of synovium that lies between the collateral ligament and the side of the metacarpal head.

Each joint is approached on the radial side of the hood through an incision parallel with the extrinsic extensor tendon and 3 to 5 mm away from it. The hood fibers can be separated easily from the underlying diseased synovium, and both sides of the hood are completely elevated. The extrinsic extensor tendon is then dislocated to the ulnar side of the joint and the synovium exposed. The synovium extends as a pouch for an appreciable distance on the dorsal surface of the head and neck of the metacarpal. It is comparable in its attachments to the suprapatellar synovial pouch of the knee. The superficial surface of the synovium rolls underneath and attaches loosely to the neck of the metacarpal; it is attached firmly to the bone only at the edge of the articular cartilage. The synovectomy is started by peeling back this pouch of tissue until the margin of the articular cartilage is reached. The attachment to the articular cartilage is incised and the joint entered (Fig. 8-4).

The synovium also attaches to, and reflects over, the dorsum of the proximal phalanx. Erosion occurs in this area between the margin of the articular cartilage and the attachment of the capsule. A careful clearance must be done here; otherwise the remaining synovium will continue to invade the bone and may separate the subchondral cortex from the main shaft of the phalanx.

Next, the two collateral ligaments are defined, and the synovium is stripped, where possible, from their deep surfaces. Particular care must be taken to remove the tongue of synovium, which lies between the collateral ligament and the neck of the metacarpal. A narrow-jawed pituitary rongeur is often useful in reaching into this small space (Fig. 8-5). The synovium must be removed from this area, since its behavior at this point is almost "malignant" because of its strong invasive ability. It erodes the bony attachment of the collateral ligament and undermines the articular cartilage with its subchondral cortical bone from the side. Flexion and distraction of the joint will allow the articular surfaces to be inspected and any loose flakes of articular cartilage removed. The pouch of synovium lying beneath the neck of the metacarpal can also be excised from this approach.

The hood is closed by interrupted sutures, with sufficient overlapping of the two radial layers of the hood to hold the extrinsic extensor tendon in the midline on the dorsum of the joint. As in the interphalangeal joint, it may be necessary to reef any excess tissue of the hood on the opposite, or ulnar, side of the joint in order to retain the extensor tendon in the midline. If a considerable amount of reefing seems necessary, it is usually wiser to make an incision similar to that used on the radial side and to double-breast the hood tissues on both sides of the joint.

The skin wound is closed with interrupted nylon sutures and a drain is frequently used. A large compression dressing is placed on the dorsum of the hand and a palmar plaster slab extending beyond the metacarpophalangeal joints is incorporated in the bandages. The hand is elevated for 24 hours and movement of the extensors encouraged as soon as the postoperative discomfort subsides.

Usually on the third postoperative day the palmar slab can be removed and a dynamic extensor splint placed on the dorsum of the forearm and hand. The metacarpophalangeal joints should be held in full extension and slight radial deviation. The patient must be trained to flex actively against the finger slings for short periods many times a day. The splint should be worn full time for 3 weeks, and then the patient should be gradually weaned from it during the next 2 or 3 weeks. Many more weeks of regular exercising may be necessary before the extensor muscles "take up" sufficiently to support the fingers in full extension.

Results of digital synovectomy

Total removal of all the synovium of a digital joint is technically impossible unless the joint is completely disarticulated. Because of this, synovectomy has acquired an undeservedly poor reputation particularly among those who believe that surgical results should be permanent. I believe it is wrong to assess the results of such a localized surgical procedure without relating it to the state of the disease in the patient as a whole. I therefore related a review of 67 patients for whom I had performed digital joint synovectomy in 390 joints over a 10-year period to a dynamic classification of the general disease state of the patient. We used the American Rheumatism Association terms *early, moderate,* and *severe* to indicate the degree of systemic activity of the disease and the terms *incipient, intermediate,* and *late* to depict the stage of involvement of one specific joint or of all the involved joints of the hand at the time of synovectomy. At the time of synovectomy, 25 patients (37%) fell into the early group, 30 (45%) were in the moderate category, and the remaining 12 were classified as severe. Reassessment of the patients at the time of follow-up revealed that the joints of only 13 patients had remained in the early stage. In 40 patients the joints had progressed either into the next stage or had progressed within the confines of the category in which they had been classified when synovectomy was performed.

Recurrent postoperative synovial swelling was much more common in my patients operated on in the late stages of their disease and also was more common in those whose systemic disease activity persisted postoperatively. This seems logical, because the stimulus responsible for the original synovial involvement should not be altered by localized excision of a single target area, and continued progression should, and did, occur in other nonoperated joints. Ansell and colleagues, in their report on synovectomy of the proximal interphalangeal joint, showed that recurrence occurred in their patients with severe active seropositive disease.

Branemark and co-workers have operated on 12 patients for recurrent synovial swelling. In all 12 patients they found tissue that was clinically and histologically identical to that which had been excised at the first operation. Brown had a similar experience with 5 patients at reoperation. In 3 of my patients with recurrent disease the excised synovial tissue was similar grossly and microscopically to that originally removed. I believe all this is convincing evidence that local excision of synovial tissue does not completely protect a joint from reinvolvement if the patient's systemic disease continues in an active state.

It is of interest that the onset of pain in those joints showing synovial recurrence usually does not occur until at least 6 months after surgery. The ultrastructural studies of Goldie and Wellisch have shown that at 1 year the nerve endings are fully regenerated in the new synovium.

Proximal interphalangeal joint. Synovectomy of the proximal interphalangeal joint is properly indicated in joints in which the swelling is so gross that mechanical disturbance of function is present. The operation is also indicated if the swelling is unlikely to resolve before mechanical derangement occurs. The high rate of resolution of synovitis in this joint prohibits prophylactic synovectomy in the early months of the disease.

The greatest technical problem in operating on this joint is that imbalance between flexor and extensor forces usually results from the surgical decompression of the enlarged joint capsule. Attempts to repair the attenuated dorsal extensor mechanism are not routinely successful, and boutonniere deformity is the most commonly reported postoperative complication.

In my series of 79 joints operated on, 4 joints subsequently developed boutonniere deformity. Three of them had additional operations designed to correct the deformity. All failed. Wilde reports a series of 98 joints in which no boutonniere deformity developed as a result of his operative technique. Only one boutonniere deformity developed postoperatively, for a 2.9% incidence in his adult patients—a far better figure than the incidence of 39.2% that follows the medical treatment of adult rheumatoid disease.

Recurrent synovitis appeared in 24% of the joints I operated on; Ansell and associates record a 19% recurrence. Wilde, however, reports a 30% incidence of recurrent synovitis that doubled with a follow-up into the 3- to 5-year period.

We have also been unsuccessful in our attempts to retain motion in this joint after surgery. Our patients showed an average loss of range of 22 degrees in all digits (Table 6). Wilde's patients showed an average postoperative loss of motion of 4 degrees, whereas Ansell and colleagues recorded that the range of motion had not changed at

Table 6. Total postoperative motion in proximal interphalangeal synovectomy.*

Digit	Average preoperative motion (degrees)	Average early post-operative motion (degrees)	Average late post-operative motion (degrees)	Average preoperative and postoperative difference (degrees)	Number of joints
Index					
Metacarpophalangeal	67	64	65	− 2	
Proximal interpha-					26
langeal	84	67	67	−17	
Long					
Metacarpophalangeal	72	61	62.6	− 9.4	
Proximal interpha-					14
langeal	83	74	60	−23	
Ring					
Metacarpophalangeal	78	79	67	−11	
Proximal interpha-					24
langeal	84	59	58	−26	
Small					
Metacarpophalangeal	85	78	69	−16	
Proximal interpha-					15
langeal	83	80	61	−22	
Average loss in all proximal interphalangeal joints operated on				−22	79
Associated average loss in all metacarpophalangeal joints not operated on				− 9.6	

*From Ellison, M.R., Kelly, K.J., and Flatt, A.E.: The results of surgical synovectomy of the digital joints in rheumatoid disease, J. Bone Joint Surg. **53-A:**1041-1060, 1971.

the 1-year follow-up in 83 of 114 joints operated on. Seventeen patients showed an improved range; only 14 were worse. Because of the importance of reciprocal inter-action in digital joints to hand function, we also studied the range of motion of the metacarpophalangeal joints of fingers in which the proximal interphalangeal joint had been operated on. Table 6 shows that there is also an associated loss of motion in the more proximal digital joint of nearly 10 degrees.

A large carefully controlled study of the prophylactic value of synovectomy of this joint was published by Raunio in 1977. In his patients the operation produced com-plete relief of pain in 60% of the joints. He judged that a little over 50% of the joints eventually showed a recurrent synovitis. In general there was an improvement in range of motion after the operation. The evidence showed that the normal deterio-ration of flexion is retarded by synovectomy.

The results of synovectomy of the proximal interphalangeal joint are therefore at best mixed. However, I agree with Nalebuff that persistent proximal interphalangeal joint synovitis should be removed by surgery. I believe the discomfort and possible reduction in motion to be a small price to pay in comparison with the severe, and often irreparable, mechanical disruptions that can occur in this very important middle digital joint.

Metacarpophalangeal joint. The significant factor common to all papers that report reasonably long-term follow-up studies of synovectomy of this joint is the adverse influence of demonstrable preoperative radiological changes in the joints.

Nicolle and associates have reviewed a group of 102 synovectomies performed in the early 1960's. The 168 unoperated joints of their patients provided a control group for the follow-up study. At this time the indications for surgery were conservative, and surgery was performed only on those joints with obvious signs or symptoms. They demonstrate the degree of this conservatism in operative indications in the early 1960's by analyzing the duration of symptoms before synovectomy. The average duration of symptoms before 1966 was 14.7 years, whereas for those treated in 1966 it was only 3.8 years.

Functional and symptomatic improvements were clearly demonstrated, and recurrent synovitis occurred in only 6 of the 102 joints. The authors were also able to show that those joints without radiological changes before surgery continued to show no change 4 to 8 years after synovectomy. However, 25% of the joints with minimal changes before synovectomy progressed to moderate or severe changes in the same length of time.

Aptekar and Duff have reviewed the results of synovectomy performed on 88 metacarpophalangeal joints in which disease had been present for even longer periods of time. The average duration was 20 years in a range of 9 to 35 years. They stress that in none of these joints was early or prophylactic synovectomy done and that in many joints, additional procedures such as tendinoplasty or arthroplasty were performed.

Although most of their patients experienced temporary benefits, the recurrence rate of synovitis proved to be 36% in the long-term follow-up. Minimal radiological changes were present in one patient who obtained an excellent result in both hands, but they believed that the surgical procedures were less effective in the hands in which the disease had already eroded the joint.

Thompson and colleagues have published the results of their controlled trial of metacarpophalangeal synovectomy at a 2-year follow-up time. Fifty-two patients were allocated to the operation group and 48 to the control group according to a previously compiled random series contained in numbered and sealed envelopes. All the operations were done by one surgeon to ensure uniformity of technique. The differences between the two groups were reduced to the surgical procedure alone by the use of the same postoperative regimen for the same lengths of time.

There was a significant difference in favor of the surgically treated hand by all the clinical methods of evaluation when the two groups were compared. The operation conferred significant and sustained clinical improvement in terms of pinch grip, baggage grip, joint tenderness, and the patient's opinion. During the 2 years of the study the x-ray films showed slight deterioration that was approximately equal in all groups, and these authors comment that further long-term radiographic studies are needed to determine whether the operation can favorably influence the natural course of the disease.

Theoretically, a thorough synovectomy in a joint showing early x-ray changes might arrest destruction and even allow healing of the lesion. Strang and Hueston have recorded and illustrated such healing in the metacarpophalangeal joints of the left hand of a nurse 2 years after synovectomy. In my own series of 390 synovectomies of the digital joints in 67 patients, only 20 patients showed no progression of x-ray lesions after surgery. Fourteen of these patients were operated on in an early stage of disease in these joints, and 3 each during intermediate or late stages. In all 20 patients, the systemic illness was mild or under medical control, or complete remission occurred postoperatively. X-ray examination showed that there were no lesions with sufficient healing changes to warrant an excellent rating.

In a large percentage of my patients who were operated on in the intermediate or late stages of disease, x-ray examination showed progression of the destruction, and in all these patients, active systemic disease of varying severity was present postoperatively. Savill's experience was similar to mine, and he reported postoperative progression in 56% of his patients.

The incidence of recurrent synovial swelling after synovectomy is high in my series, compared with the incidence in other reports. This disparity is probably related to the lack of uniformity in the criteria for what constitutes recurrence. I chose to include as a recurrence every instance of postoperatively visible and palpable swelling of the synovium, regardless of its immediate clinical significance.

Twenty patients had recurrence of synovitis in one or more of the joints operated on at the time of follow-up examination. One of my patients had a recurrence, was operated on again, and showed a recurrence for the second time at follow-up. In this patient the systemic disease has continued in an aggressive form. Recurrence was more common in the interphalangeal joints than in the metacarpophalangeal joints, which showed a 14.1% recurrence in the 283 joints operated on.

I believe that careful measurements of preoperative and postoperative ranges of motion will usually show loss of motion after surgery. This is not necessarily bad, since the metacarpophalangeal joint frequently needs some additional fibrous support to resist the subluxation forces. In the series of Ellison, Kelly, and myself comprising 253 joints, the average postoperative loss for all digits was 20 degrees at the metacarpophalangeal joints and 14 degrees at the proximal interphalangeal joints not operated on (Table 7). The average loss of extension at the metacarpophalangeal joints operated on was 9 degrees, and the average loss of flexion, 11 degrees.

Transfer of the extensor indicis proprius tendon to the radial side of the index finger as a support against pinch activity is commonly done. In earlier studies we felt that this transfer tended to narrow the radial entrance to the hand by causing a flexion contracture of the metacarpophalangeal joint of the index finger. Therefore the 20 extensor indicis proprius transfers done in conjunction with index metacarpophalangeal joint synovectomy were reviewed separately. These metacarpophalangeal joints lost a total of 22 degrees (10 degrees of extension and 12 degrees of flexion). However, the unoperated proximal interphalangeal joints of the same fingers gained extension of 5.9 degrees, tending toward hyperextension, and lost 19 degrees of flexion (Table 8).

In addition to these unfortunate changes in joint motion, significant radial devi-

Table 7. Total postoperative motion in metacarpophalangeal synovectomies*

Digit	Preoperative range (degrees)	Early post-operative range (degrees)	Late post-operative range (degrees)	Average difference (degrees)	Number of joints†
Index					
Metacarpophalangeal	61	46	44	−17	
Proximal inter-					89
phalangeal	80	68	62	−18	
Long					
Metacarpophalangeal	66	57	44	−22	
Proximal inter-					78
phalangeal	76	83	69	− 7	
Ring					
Metacarpophalangeal	67	62	48	−19	
Proximal inter-					56
phalangeal	81	79	62	−19	
Small					
Metacarpophalangeal	70	56	48	−22	
Proximal inter-					30
phalangeal	66	65	53	−13	
Average loss in all metacarpophalangeal joints operated on				−20	
					253
Associated average loss in all joints not operated on				−14	

*From Ellison, M.R., Kelly, K.J., and Flatt, A.E.: The results of surgical synovectomy of the digital joints in rheumatoid disease, J. Bone Joint Surg. **53-A:**1041-1060, 1971.
†Totals for index and small metacarpophalangeal joints do not include those joints with extensor indicis proprius transfer or hypothenar release.

Table 8. Metacarpophalangeal synovectomy combined with extensor indicis proprius transfer and hypothenar release (postoperative difference in range of motion)*

	Average flexion (degrees)	Average extension (degrees)	Average total range difference (degrees)	Number of joints
Extensor indicis proprius transfer				
(index) metacarpophalangeal	−12	−10	−22	
				20
Proximal interphalangeal	−19	+5.9	−13.1	
Hypothenar release				
(small) metacarpophalangeal	−16	+10	−6	
				10
Proximal interphalangeal	−18	−10	−28	

*From Ellison, M.R., Kelly, K.J., and Flatt, A.E.: The results of surgical synovectomy of the digital joints in rheumatoid disease, J. Bone Joint Surg. **53-A:**1041-1060, 1971.

Table 9. Pinch strength*†

Surgical category	Lateral pinch (kg)	Precision pinch (kg)
Metacarpophalangeal synovectomy		
Preoperative	3.4	2.9
Postoperative	4.1	3.5
Average gain	0.7	0.7
Proximal interphalangeal synovectomy		
Preoperative	3.6	3.2
Postoperative	4.6	4.7
Average gain	0.7	1.5

*From Ellison, M.R., Kelly, K.J., and Flatt, A.E.: The results of surgical synovectomy of the digital joints in rheumatoid disease, J. Bone Joint Surg. **53-A:**1041-1060, 1971.
†Normal average (dominant) (tip pinch):
  Male—17.7 kg.
  Female—11.9 kg.

ation of the index finger also occasionally occurred. These facts and their adverse functional implications have caused me to abandon this transfer procedure.

Pinch strength is commonly used as a measure of success for synovectomy, but the measurements bear little or no relationship to the patient's overall spectrum of functional ability. However, improvement in pinch and grip strength do enhance the patients' ability to perform everyday tasks. The results in our series are shown in Table 9.

Lateral pinch and precision tip pinch strength were generally increased after synovectomy. Forty-seven of our patients (69.5%) had excellent (more than 2 kg gain) or good (less than 2 kg gain) results when strength alone was considered. In many instances this improvement occurred because of the elimination of pain. In others, it undoubtedly occurred because of greater postoperative stability at the metacarpophalangeal joints on the radial side of the hand. Despite this increased strength, power grip was frequently reduced postoperatively. This impairment resulted from the patients' inability to get the ulnar side of the hand into proper position. Thirty-four of our patients were unable to get the tips of the ring and small fingers to the palm postoperatively, as opposed to their ability to do so preoperatively.

Reprise

The results of controlled trials of digital joint synovectomy have not produced statistical blessings for the procedure. However, most hand surgeons have no doubt that synovectomy is useful, but there are differing degrees of optimism. Patients also have little doubt that the operation relieves their symptoms and frequently request that their opposite hand be operated on.

Gschwend, in examining this apparent schism, has shown that the controlled studies involved small numbers of patients derived from several different medical centers. Their results contrast unfavorably with those coming from the large medical centers in countries like Finland, Poland, Norway, and West Germany. His own extensive experience also confirms the value of joint synovectomy, particularly if it is performed early in the disease.

For my part I believe that in the majority of cases, a reasonable estimate of the results of surgery for any one patient can be provided. Results will always be indifferent unless there is a maximum of understanding and cooperation by the patient in the decision that an operation is necessary.

Long-term functional and symptomatic results are better in patients with mild systemic disease, with no lesions demonstrable by x-ray examination, and with an incipient rather than a late stage of mechanical derangement.

Synovectomy performed when the disease, both locally and systemically, is in a severe stage will result in less than optimum benefit to the patient. Surgery under these circumstances has merit but should be approached with the full understanding of patient and surgeon that results may be transitory and ultimately disappointing.

FUSION OF DIGITAL JOINTS

Many methods of fusing the digital joints have been published. All satisfactory procedures are based on the internal immobilization of the raw bony surfaces until union is complete, since adequate external immobilization is almost impossible to supply. Recent years have seen the introduction of joint compression techniques. For those skilled in these methods it is permissible to try their use. In the small digital joints, I have found the two most satisfactory means of supplying internal immobilization are Kirschner wires and bone grafting.

I have used Kirschner wire fixation for many years in both degenerative and rheumatoid arthritis. Both conditions have shown occasional failures, and in osteoporotic bones I often use the type of fusion advocated by Moberg. There is no doubt that solid union is obtained by this bone grafting and the risk of infection inherent in temporary Kirschner wire fixation is avoided. The technique can be used for the metacarpophalangeal or the interphalangeal joints. The procedure and its aftercare, as performed by Moberg, are as follows.

TECHNIQUE

The joint is approached by a curved incision approximately 3 cm long over the dorsolateral aspect of the joint. The skin is separated from the deep tissues by blunt dissection, and the joint is exposed. An attempt must be made to save the dorsal tendon mechanism by incising the tissue to the lateral side of the extensor tendon and dislocating the tendon to the opposite side. After the joint has been opened, the collateral ligaments are divided and the joint is dislocated. The joint surfaces are then nibbled away with rongeurs until apposition of the bone ends shows the digit to be in the right position (Fig. 8-6).

A small hole is drilled through the dorsal cortex of the proximal bone and centered approximately 1 cm proximal to the level of fusion. The direction of the drill must be slanted so that the drill point will enter the medullary canal of the distal component. When this small hole has been properly established, it is enlarged with a larger drill. The sizes of the drills must vary with the sizes of the bones being fused. The best guide to size that I have found is that the larger drill should completely fill the medullary canal of the distal bone. When the hole has been enlarged to the correct size, it should be converted, with a small file, to a square-sided opening.

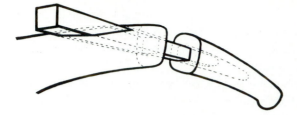

Fig. 8-6. Digital joint fusion. The Moberg technique of intramedullary pinning with a squared bone peg provides a sturdy fixation and encourages early union. (From Moberg, E., and Henrikson, B.: Acta Chir. Scand. **118**:331-338, 1959.)

The necessary bone graft is obtained from the ulna. A small, curved incision is made in the skin over the dorsal aspect of the ulnar and just distal to the olecranon. The length of graft required will be 1.5 to 3 cm and can be cut out with an electric saw. The most difficult part of the operation is shaping the bone so that it exactly fits the square hole. When the graft has been properly trimmed, it is driven home through the two bones and any excess bone is nibbled away, leaving the dorsal part of the proximal bone quite smooth. After the dislocation of the extensor tendon has been reduced, the tendon is sutured in place and the skin wound is closed with interrupted sutures. Moberg recommends that a well-molded plaster cast be applied, extending over the forearm and enclosing the whole of the finger that has been operated on. The cast can be removed after 4 to 6 weeks if a joint of the ring or small finger has been fused. Even in these fingers the period of immobilization should be lengthened if the joint is not stable on clinical examination. The index and long fingers are subjected to strong rotational forces when used in prehensile grips. The square hole and peg system is designed to resist this rotatory force, but it is probably wiser to add an additional 2 weeks' immobilization for these two radial digits.

This operation is time-consuming and demands a high degree of technical competence, but after some trials I have found the results so satisfactory that I believe it should be generally adopted for isolated fusions of digits in the rheumatoid hand.

If several joints are to be fused in one operative procedure, the Moberg technique becomes impractical because of the time involved; Kirschner wire fixation is then the method of choice for immobilization.

Carroll and Hill have published a useful technique for these fusions in which the bone ends are shaped to resemble a cone and spike. This technique provides large surfaces of raw bone for union but also allows a final fine adjustment of digital position that is not possible if the bone ends are fashioned into flat surfaces.

Fusion is also of value in stabilization of the flail "opera-glass hand." Froimson has reported satisfactory restoration of function in two severely crippled hands by a combination of digital joint fusions and phalangeal replacements using iliac bone grafts. I have little personal experience with this problem, but his operative plan is sound and the results are impressive.

RESULTS OF FUSION

The results of fusion are therefore largely judged on the basis of any improvement in function provided by the surgery since nonunion is uncommon. This improvement, in turn, is dependent on sound preoperative planning. The optimum position for fusion of flail, painful, or malaligned individual joints can usually be planned with precision. The positioning of multiple digital fusions often becomes a great problem. Experience with fusions in both thumb and fingers at the same time taught me that I could not always satisfactorily predict the functional end result. It is my practice to consider the hand in two phases. At one operation I complete the fusions within the fingers and postpone any similar work on the thumb until maximum finger function has been obtained. By this means I have been able to place the thumb in its optimum position at the second operation.

Although this means that my patient may need two operations, I believe that this more conservative approach will frequently yield a better long-term functional result in complicated reconstructive problems.

Metacarpophalangeal joint

Fusion of the metacarpophalangeal joint in the fingers is not commonly done because of the necessity of maintaining mobility at the key point of the longitudinal arch of each finger. If there is good mobility at both the interphalangeal joints in a "burned-out" hand, stabilization of the metacarpophalangeal joint of a finger can be of functional value.

In the past, arthrodesis of the metacarpophalangeal joint of the small finger was used in an attempt to prop up the ulnar side of the hand in ulnar drift. The results were bad because ulnar deviation of the more radial fingers was still possible on the dorsal or palmar surface of the small finger. In fact, the overlapping fingers were a greater functional handicap than even ulnar drift of all the fingers. This operation should be abandoned.

In some patients gross instability develops at the carpometacarpal joints, and some have advocated operative fusion to improve function. I am not aware of any extensive studies of this operation, and in the few that I have done there has been difficulty in obtaining fusion between some of the osteoporotic bones.

The problem with this concept is that although the palm may be improved, one's options at the metacarpophalangeal joint may be reduced. I have found that in patients whose disease has fused their metacarpals to the carpus, the palm is so rigid that an elective fusion of the metacarpophalangeal joints would almost reduce hand function to a primitive distal hook grip.

Proximal interphalangeal joint

The proximal interphalangeal joint of any of the fingers can be fused if there is good metacarpophalangeal motion. The index finger lends itself to this procedure because of the vital importance of stability for pinch. I largely follow the indications published by Vainio. He considers the main indications to be as follows:

1. Malposition of the finger—making grip and pinch impossible
2. Flail uncontrolled joint
3. Painful destruction of the joint

Vainio uses two crossed Kirschner wires for internal immobilization and does not use any form of external splinting. I have used both the crossed-Kirschner wires technique and the Moberg bone graft method. Both are satisfactory, but I believe that the Moberg method produces a firm fusion a little earlier than the crossed-wire technique. The most generally satisfactory angle of fusion is about 35 degrees of flexion.

Nonunion is uncommon, and Granowitz and Vainio report only 8 nonunions in 122 arthrodeses. The average duration of disease in these patients was 15 years, and the follow-up time averaged over 4 years. The functional results were pleasing in that 75% of the patients who could not oppose the thumb preoperatively could do so after fusion. Union, pinch, and a satisfactory functional position were more difficult to obtain in fingers with swan-neck deformity or flail joints than in those with a boutonniere deformity.

ARTHROPLASTY OF DIGITAL JOINTS

In the rheumatoid hand, arthroplasty is virtually confined to the metacarpophalangeal joints. Excisional arthroplasty of the proximal interphalangeal joint is uncommon and is confined to the long and ring fingers, since the index and small fingers lack lateral support on their outer sides.

As a late salvage procedure, arthroplasty is a very useful operation. Ideally the operation ought to provide a good range of painless motion over a period of many years. A careful assessment of the mechanical disturbance of the hand before surgery is essential. Operations aimed principally at cosmetic improvement can produce a hand that looks good but has less functional ability than before surgery.

The operation is designed to shorten the metacarpals and improve grasp by providing a palm that can be adequately cupped and fingers that can more readily adapt to different-shaped objects. Bony excision inevitably implies instability, and many techniques have been suggested to overcome this problem.

Metacarpophalangeal joint

Instability in this joint after excisional arthroplasty largely occurs in the dorsopalmar rather than the lateral plane. The basic problem is to hold the base of the proximal phalanx in proper relationship to the distal end of the shortened metacarpal. Two different approaches have distilled out of the many techniques suggested to overcome this problem. One approach is to use the dorsal extrinsic extensor tendon as a supporting mechanism. The operations devised by Fowler, Vainio, and Harrison are all variations on this theme. The other approach, favored by Tupper, is to provide a sling from the palmar surface of the phalanx by attaching the palmar plate to the dorsum of the shortened metacarpal.

GENERAL OPERATIVE TECHNIQUE

It is extremely rare for arthroplasty to be indicated for a single joint; when it is necessary, a satisfactory approach is a lazy-S-shaped, longitudinal midline dorsal incision, 5 cm long and centered over the joint. When several joints are to be operated on, they should be exposed through a transverse dorsal incision placed just proximal to the line of the joint when the fingers are extended. The longitudinal veins, which are usually found in the valleys between the metacarpal heads, must be preserved and protected throughout the operation. After the skin flaps have been mobilized and the veins retracted, the joints are opened. Each joint is opened through an incision on the radial side of the hood. The two sides of the hood are separated, by blunt dissection, from the underlying capsular and synovial tissues on both sides of the joint. The diseased capsular and synovial tissues must be carefully dissected away from the underlying bone and the articular surfaces inspected. An attempt should be made to identify and preserve the radial collateral ligament attached to the phalangeal base.

No matter which form of arthroplasty is to be used, the essential key to success is sufficient decompression of the joint, by bony excision, to allow adequate joint movement to occur after the base of the phalanx has been lifted up to the same plane as the metacarpal. To achieve this correct relationship it is usually necessary to detach the interosseous muscles' attachments to the sides of the phalanx. Occasionally the metacarpal neck attachment of the palmar plate may also have to be incised to obtain the correct alignment of the phalangeal base after removal of the metacarpal head. After completion of whatever arthroplasty procedure has been selected, closure of the joint follows the same basic pattern. The hood mechanism must be repaired. No attempt is made to reconstitute the ulnar side of the hood. The stretched radial side of the hood is passed under the extrinsic extensor tendon. Some prefer to use a double-breasting procedure. Others loop the hood back over the tendon and suture it to itself, thereby making a retinaculum that retains the extrinsic extensor tendon in the correct position. The skin wound is closed with interrupted sutures, and no drain is necessary. A large, fluffed-up gauze compression dressing is held in place by a self-adherent cotton bandage. The interphalangeal joints must not be included in the bandaging because gentle movement should be encouraged in the interphalangeal joints throughout the early postoperative period. No movement can be allowed in the metacarpophalangeal joints if Kirschner wires have been used. In recent years most surgeons have come to use some form of dynamic splinting such as the Swanson splint (Fig. 3-8, p. 52). The skin sutures are removed at about 2 weeks, and the dynamic splint is used to provide radial stabilization while motion develops. I believe it is helpful to maintain constant splinting for at least 6 weeks and night splinting for another 6 weeks.

SPECIFIC TECHNIQUES

Vainio arthroplasty. In the Vainio arthroplasty each joint is exposed by dissecting out the extensor tendon from the hood, dislocating the tendon sideways, and opening the two halves of the hood. In each joint the procedure is as follows. The metacarpal head is severed by a transverse cut with a slight radial inclination. The line of excision is dictated by the amount of bone that must be removed to provide good free joint movement. The site is usually in the distal portion of the metacarpal neck, but great care is always taken to dissect off the proximal attachments of the collateral ligaments from the sides of the metacarpal.

After the metacarpal head has been excised, an extensive synovectomy is performed. Every piece of synovium and adjacent diseased tissue is removed. It is

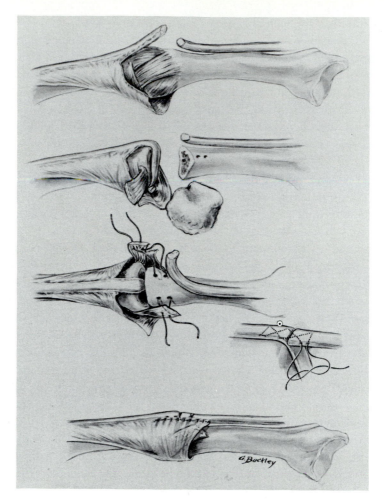

Fig. 8-7. Vainio arthroplasty. In this procedure the distal portion of the extrinsic extensor tendon is sewed down into the joint as an interposition layer between the two bone ends. The head of the metacarpal is excised and the neck squared. The collateral ligaments are tightened against the side of the metacarpal neck, and the extensor tendon is reconstituted.

unneccessary to trim the base of the proximal phalanx unless gross osteophytes are present that might interfere with free movement. After the new joint cavity has been created, the extrinsic extensor tendon is pushed down into the cavity until the distal portion touches the flexor aspect of the base of the phalanx when the joint is held flexed. The tendon is cut through at this point. The cut distal end of the extrinsic extensor tendon is sutured down to the base of the phalanx with fine nonabsorbable sutures. It is usually advisable to pass these sutures through the tissues of the palmar plate to anchor the cut end of the extensor tendon firmly.

A hole is now drilled in the dorsum of the neck of the metacarpal on each side. A suture is passed through each hole and into the proximal end of the collateral ligament, thereby tightening and lifting up the ligament (Fig. 8-7). An assistant then pulls distally the proximal part of the extrinsic extensor tendon until its cut end touches the distal extensor tendon where it bends downward over the dorsal edge of the base of the proximal phalanx. The two sides of the hood are stitched to the proximal tendon, and its cut end is then sewed to the distal tendon.

Tupper arthroplasty. After resection of the metacarpal head the palmar plate is incised transversely at the junction of the fibrous and membranous portions. This junction normally lies at about the level of the original metacarpal neck. The flexor sheath and retinacular fibers are then detached from each side of the plate distally to the base of the phalanx so that the proximal end of the plate can be gradually reflected up into the joint until it reaches the dorsal edge of the metacarpal stump (Fig. 8-8). Occasionally sesamoid bones are present and form a mechanical obstruction to good movement; they should be removed. It is easier to attach the proximal end of the palmar plate to the dorsal metacarpal edge if three or four holes are drilled first. All sutures are then passed, and each is tied individually.

The palmar plate is attached in this manner to:
1. Make a thick interpositional barrier equal in cross-sectional area to the metacarpal stump, which helps to make a good pseudarthrosis by completely preventing any bone-to-bone contact
2. Elevate the subluxated proximal phalanx
3. Stabilize the proximal phalanx and the flexor sheath by anchoring the palmar plate to the metacarpal, thereby preventing any palmar and ulnar deviating forces in the flexor tendons from acting directly on the base of the proximal phalanx

Reconstitution of joint stability by reattachment of the radial collateral ligament is important. With the joint held in 45 degrees of flexion, the ligament is reattached to the dorsoradial aspect of the metacarpal stump so that it produces slight radial deviation and mild supination. When all radial collateral ligaments have been attached, the fingers should be stable against gravity, without a tendency to drift or pronate. If they are not stable, the attachment site is wrong or the ligament is too loose. The error must be corrected before the hood fibers are closed over the joint.

RESULTS OF METACARPOPHALANGEAL EXCISIONAL ARTHROPLASTIES

The results obtained by the originating surgeon are always better than those obtained by others who attempt to copy the procedure. Equally, attempts at description of operative procedures usually omit subtle points of technique that are not easily described. I have tried to be faithful to the intent of the surgeons whose operations I have described and trust they will forgive any unintentional errors.

My personal experience with these two methods and laboratory investigations of each procedure make me believe that the most satisfactory plan is that of the Tupper arthroplasty. Long-term success of metacarpophalangeal arthroplasties depends on satisfactory resistance to palmar subluxation of the base of the proximal phalanx and successful maintenance of extension of the digital joints. I am concerned that methods that produce tenodesis of the extrinsic extensor tendon to the base of the phalanx must disturb this complex mechanism. Extension of the interphalangeal joints then

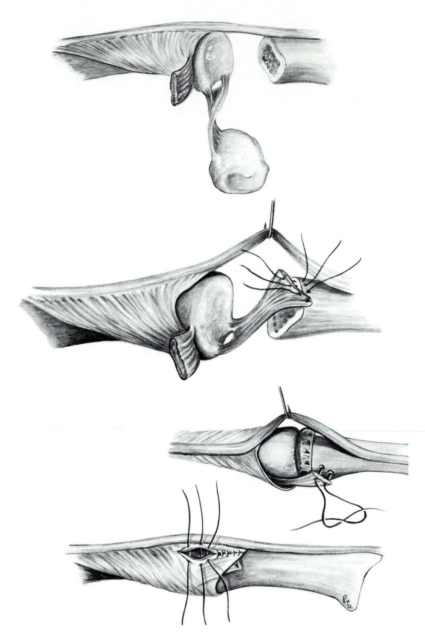

Fig. 8-8. Tupper arthroplasty. The metacarpal head is amputated at the level of the neck. The palmar plate is left attached to the phalanx but is cut proximally at the junction of its fibrous and membranous portions. Attachment of the proximal edge of the plate is made easier if three or four holes are drilled in the dorsal metacarpal neck and all sutures passed before each are tied individually. After the plate has been attached, the radial collateral ligament is reattached and the hood reconstituted.

becomes dependent on the intrinsic musculature, thus removing the option of intrinsic release should swan-neck deformity later develop.

The inclusion or exclusion of additional procedures—such as abductor digiti minimi release, crossed intrinsic transfer, and support of the first dorsal interosseous action by various transfers—varies with the state of the hand and the choice of the individual surgeon. Tupper, for instance, does not recommend adding the crossed intrinsic transfer procedure, whereas Vainio has recently reported a large series of excisional arthroplasties incorporating the crossed transfer.

I am not yet satisfied that the ideal excisional arthroplasty procedure has been devised for the metacarpophalangeal joint. The long-term follow-ups of my procedures and many of those I have seen performed by other surgeons are disappointing in the sense that the ideal balance between stability and movement has not yet been achieved. Most authors have commented that only about 30 to 60 degrees of simple hinge motion can be expected. Savill stated that useful motion is always sacrificed by this operation.

I have not done a large number of metacarpophalangeal arthroplasties, principally because of my deliberate testing of prosthetic replacement at this joint level. In those patients who have been followed up, there has been a very definite decrease in range of motion after surgery, and this decrease has been greater on the ulnar side of the hand.

The Fowler arthroplasty did not give a full range of movement at the metacarpophalangeal joint, but the combination of stability and limited movement usually yielded a useful functional result. If the movement of the proximal interphalangeal joint is normal, a 40-degree flexion of the metacarpophalangeal joints provides an excellent grip. A greater range of movement is essential only if there is gross limitation of movement of the interphalangeal joints.

In 1967 Vainio and colleagues reported a very thorough follow-up of the metacarpophalangeal arthroplasties performed at the Rheumatism Foundation Hospital in Heinola, Finland. Ninety-nine patients had arthroplasties of 283 joints in 111 hands. The age of the patients varied between 17 and 76 years, and the average follow-up time was 2.7 years. The average range of active motion was 43 degrees, and 78% of the joints showed a satisfactory range of motion. In 38 joints there was a flexion contracture of between 25 and 40 degrees; in the remaining joints the contracture was between 45 and 60 degrees.

Persistent postoperative pain was present in only 1.7% of patients. Palmar subluxation was a troublesome complication and occurred in 14% of patients. Ulnar deviation of the fingers was also a common sequel. Increase in the strength of grip was a common feature in all cases where the hand was really used. All patients in whom the Vainio type of arthroplasty had been combined with a transfer of the extensor indicis proprius tendon gained active and powerful abduction of the index finger.

This paper was followed in 1968 by a report of 159 arthroplasties in which crossed intrinsic transfers were also done. The recurrence of ulnar deviation was reduced to 6%, compared with 17% in the earlier series. All other results were comparable.

Jackson has reported that his experience with the Vainio procedure leads him to expect an improvement in the power of the hand and a range of movement of 60 degrees at the arthroplasty.

Weilby has reviewed his results with 75 Tupper arthroplasties followed for 2½ to 4½ years. The average passive range of motion was 63 degrees; the active range averaged two thirds of the passive range. He stresses that the palmar plate provides complete separation of the base of the proximal phalanx and the raw neck of the metacarpal. Fastening the plate to the metacarpal provides good resistance to palmar subluxation. Bone resorption rarely occurs and the operation can be used even in severely destroyed joints. A good detailed review of metacarpophalangeal arthroplasty is that reported by Robinson and colleagues from the University of British Columbia.

A carefully planned test situation was created in which a standard type of arthroplasty was performed after detailed preoperative functional testing. The tests were repeated 6 months and 1 year after the operation. The tests were applied to 14 consecutive hands in 12 patients. These authors point out that the operation should be regarded as a salvage procedure in a group of patients who had access to carefully applied physical and occupational therapy both before and after surgery.

In all patients except 2, some degree of flexion range was lost in the attempt to allow full metacarpophalangeal joint extension and an open grasp. The realignment of the fingers was maintained in 13 out of 14 hands. There is no comment on any recurrence of subluxation, and ulnar drift recurred in only 1 patient. The majority of patients showed an improvement in pinch strength, dexterity, applied strength and hook strength. These improvements were attributed to the realignment of the fingers and to a significant reduction in pain in the hands. Power grip was improved in only a small percentage of the patients because flexion of the joints had been deliberately sacrificed in favor of a more open grasp than was present before surgery.

I would stress that I do not believe there is such a thing as a universal arthroplasty procedure suitable for all the disturbances seen at the metacarpophalangeal joint of the fingers. The Tupper and Vainio procedures have stood the test of time, but more work is needed to define the precise indications of the various procedures that are now available.

Proximal interphalangeal joint

Arthroplasty of the proximal interphalangeal joint is rarely indicated in patients with degenerative or rheumatoid disease of the hand. Because of the postoperative instability of the joint, the procedure can be used successfully only in the long and ring fingers. Several acceptable methods of arthroplasty of the proximal interphalangeal joint have been published, and Curtis and Carroll and Taber have written on the subject. The operation I use employs features from a number of different procedures. The principles of the operation are the excision of sufficient bone to decompress the joint completely and the maintenance of joint traction during subsequent healing. No tissue need be interposed between the bone ends.

TECHNIQUE

The joint is approached through an incision in the neutral border of the finger. It makes no difference which side of the finger is opened. The neutral border is defined as a line joining the apices of the flexion creases of the finger when it is viewed from the side. The incision should extend from the middle of the proximal phalanx to the middle of the middle phalanx.

After the skin edges have been mobilized and retracted, the free edge of the intrinsic hood can be seen crossing the wound from the palmar surface to the dorsal surface in a distal direction. Next, the free edge is retracted so that the collateral ligament of the opposite side will be exposed. It should be detached from the neck of the proximal phalanx and the base of the middle phalanx rotated so that the ligament can be completely excised. The articular cartilage on the base of the middle phalanx is left intact unless gross joint disease has caused marked osteophyte formation. It is important that only minimal trimming be done, so that as much as possible of the articular cartilage and cortical bone will be left intact. Excessive trimming would leave a large, raw bone surface that would increase the chance of new bone formation occurring across the arthroplasty space.

The head of the proximal phalanx is trimmed back until a gap of at least 5 mm is made between the bone ends. The end of the proximal phalanx should be trimmed off square to the shaft. It is often necessary to detach the palmar plate from the base of the middle phalanx to obtain sufficient distraction.

After the bone ends have been satisfactorily prepared, the joint is reduced and the

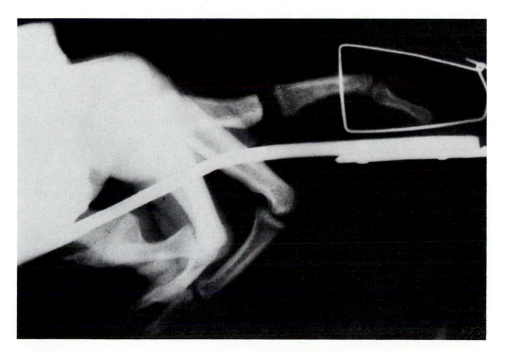

Fig. 8-9. Proximal interphalangeal joint arthroplasty. Excisional arthroplasty of this joint yields good results in the long and ring fingers. It is essential to maintain a distraction force after the operation. The force is supplied by passing a wire through the middle phalanx and connecting this wire to a hook on the distal end of the splint via an elastic band.

free edge of the hood is returned to its normal position. The skin wound is closed with interrupted sutures.

A Kirschner wire is then passed completely through the middle third of the middle phalanx from side to side. Each end is bent over, and excess wire is cut off. A padded aluminum splint with a hook on the distal end is bandaged to the forearm and hand and built into the dressing around the finger. Elastic band traction between the hook on the splint and the bent ends of the Kirschner wire supplies the necessary distracting force (Fig. 8-9).

Continuous traction must be applied for at least 2 weeks; at the end of this time the skin sutures are removed. Intermittent traction must continue for another 2 weeks but should be removed for increasing lengths of time while active movements of the joint are practiced. It is wise to apply the traction during sleeping hours for these 2 weeks.

Although this type of arthroplasty may seem a formidable operation for such a small joint, I believe that the method yields the most satisfactory results in what I consider a rather unsatisfactory procedure.

PROSTHETIC REPLACEMENT OF DIGITAL JOINTS

Over the last quarter of a century three generations of substitutes for finger joints have been developed (Fig. 8-10). The first generation of rigid stainless steel joints used in the 1950's are no longer available. The second generation, made of silicone rubber, are still in use. The third generation are, in effect, on clinical trial, since sufficient large-scale experience is not yet available to fully assess their value.

This multiplicity of choices creates a difficult problem in deciding which joint substitute to select. I have used examples of all that are available and have spent considerable time testing and reviewing these different devices.

I have no doubt that the simplest to use and the most forgiving is the Swanson implant. In no sense do I imply that the placing of these devices is easy. To get a good result demands meticulous attention to detail throughout the procedure and equally meticulous postoperative care. I confess to a theoretical liking for the Niebauer design concept over the Swanson "spacer," but I must stress that many thousands of the latter have been used throughout the world. Certainly Swanson's extensive field trial has shown that a large group of surgeons can use the spacer successfully with a low incidence of complications. I believe that it is slightly easier to insert than a Niebauer prosthesis, but the total operative plan is not significantly easier to carry out.

The third-generation devices are precisely designed and demand equal precision in their placement; particularly in regard to the orientation of their stems. Several follow-up studies have been published, but I am not as yet convinced that the results achieved are better than those obtained with the silicone rubber devices.

Operative procedures

Although these devices were originally developed for use in the rheumatoid hand the inevitable extension of their use for the degenerative joint has occurred. The operative procedure is essentially the same in both conditions.

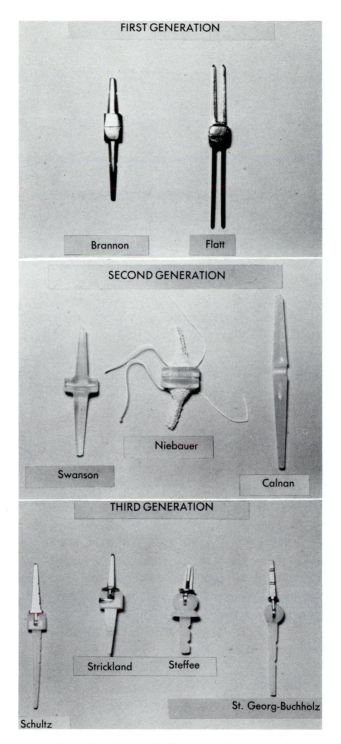

Fig. 8-10. The three generations of prostheses. The first generation were made of SS 316, the second of silicone rubber, and the third of a variety of metals and plastics.

Metacarpophalangeal joint

NIEBAUER PROSTHESIS

In the published description of his procedure, Niebauer prefers a transverse dorsal skin incision over the joints. However, if crossed intrinsic transfers are also to be done, he prefers a longitudinal incision centered over the midportion of each joint. Personally I have not found this necessary and believe that the crossed intrinsic transfer can also be done through the transverse incision, provided the separation of tissue planes is carried distally into the fingers.

After the dorsal veins have been retracted, the joint is approached by incising the hood on its ulnar side and reflecting it away from the capsule. In the small finger the tendon of the short abductor is resected. In each joint the collateral ligaments are cut free from their insertion into the metacarpal head and the neck of the metacarpal is transected so that the cut end angles about 10 degrees toward the radial side of the hand. One centimeter of clearance is mandatory between the cut surface and the base of the phalanx. If the proximal phalanx has been destroyed over the dorsal portion of its articular surface, it should be squared off. The intramedullary canals of the two bones are then broached or hollowed out and the appropriately sized prosthesis is inserted.

Before selecting and inserting the prosthesis it is important to relieve any palmar subluxation of the base of the proximal phalanx. The base of the phalanx must be released sufficiently for it to be easily brought up so that its dorsal surface is on the same plane as that of the metacarpal when the finger is extended. To obtain this release it may be necessary to detach the intrinsic insertions on the sides of the phalanx and to perform a wing tendon release. Sometimes it is necessary to free the palmar plate from the palmar edge of the phalanx to obtain full correction.

To ensure good placement of the prosthesis it is important to tie it in place, passing the sutures from the prosthesis through two small holes drilled in the dorsal cortex of each bone (Fig. 8-11).

Securing the stems in this manner allows much easier manipulation of the hand during the rest of the operation and is particularly important if crossed intrinsic transfers are to be done after placing the prostheses. It also allows early postoperative motion with the certain knowledge that stem dislocation will not occur.

Niebauer completes the operation by centralizing the extensor tendon. He comments that he has tried, not always successfully, to increase its extensor force by suturing a slip of the dorsal capsule arising from the proximal phalanx into a slit in the extensor tendon as suggested by Dr. Leonard Goldner.

I believe that the best results are obtained if early controlled motion is used. I try to apply a dynamic extensor splint to the dorsum of the forearm and hand on the third postoperative day. Active movement of the proximal interphalangeal joints is encouraged from the first postoperative day.

SWANSON IMPLANT

In his definitive paper published in 1972 Swanson recommends a transverse dorsal skin incision centered over the neck of the metacarpals. The dorsal veins are

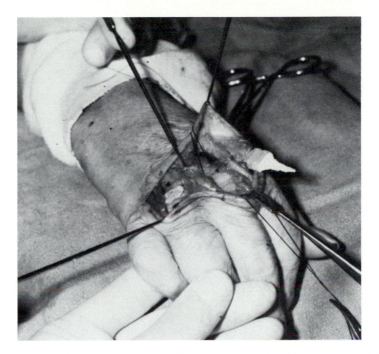

Fig. 8-11. Niebauer prosthesis. The index finger shows a prosthesis placed in the metacarpal. In the long finger black silk sutures have been passed through each prosthetic stem and through holes in the dorsum of each bone. The ring finger prosthesis is held firmly in place by the two tied-off sutures. Current models have tie-in sutures incorporated in the metacarpal stem.

carefully freed and retracted out of harm's way. The extensor hood is incised parallel to the extensor tendon on its radial side and separated from the underlying capsule. The neck of the metacarpal is exposed subperiosteally and cut across, leaving part of the flare of the metaphysis. After the collateral ligaments and capsule have been incised, the head, together with any attached hypertrophied synovial tissue, is removed en masse. Next a comprehensive soft-tissue release is done around the base of the proximal phalanx to allow full reduction of the subluxation of the joint. Release of tight ulnar intrinsic muscles is often necessary, and both the abductor and short flexor of the small finger are routinely released. None of the base of the proximal phalanx is resected except for marginal osteophytes that might interfere with the implant (Fig. 8-12).

On occasion it will be necessary to release the palmar plate to obtain full reduction of the subluxation, but on the index finger the palmar plate must be incised longitudinally and not transversely as in the other fingers. This longitudinal incision allows the radial half of the plate to be used later as a substitute for the radial collateral ligament.

The shaft of the metacarpal is cleaned out with a curette or broach. I use the efficient burr with a smooth leader point that Swanson has devised for this purpose. The joint surface of the proximal phalanx then has a rectangular hole cut into it with an osteotome or similar tool, and the medullary canal is reamed out through this hole.

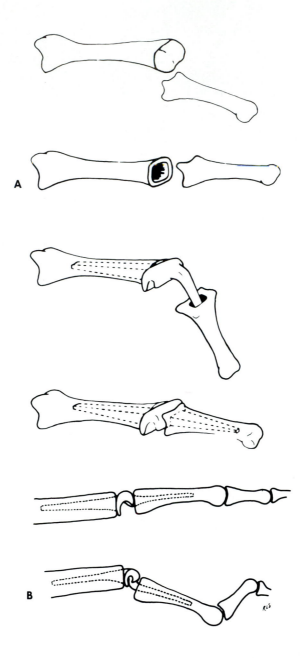

Fig. 8-12. Swanson implant technique. **A,** The head of the metacarpal is resected, leaving part of the flair of the metaphysis. No bony resection of the base of the proximal phalanx is usually performed unless there are marginal osteophytes, which might interfere with the implant. A comprehensive soft tissue release must be done so that the base of the proximal phalanx can be displaced dorsally above the metacarpal. The largest implant size that can be well seated should be used. **B,** Without appropriate soft tissue release and bone removal, there may be a dislocation tendency of the joint; subluxation may recur; and the implant may be impinged on by the bone. (From Swanson, A.B.: Flexible implant resection arthroplasty in the hand and extremities, St. Louis, 1973, The C.V. Mosby Co.)

The largest implant possible should be used, and the stem should fit well down into the canal so that the cross bar of the implant abuts against the metacarpal end, which should be smooth and free of any sharp points.

After all the fingers are tested, the appropriately sized implants are inserted with blunt instruments, by means of a no-touch technique. With the joint in extension, the metacarpal and the phalanx should not impinge on the implant. If there is impingement, either the soft-tissue release or bone resection has been inadequate.

To correct any tendency for the index finger to pronate, and to improve lateral stability for pinch, a flap consisting of the radial half of the palmar plate can be used to reconstruct the collateral ligament (Fig. 8-13). The flap, which should be 1.5 to 2 cm long and 5 to 8 mm wide, is attached to the radial aspect of the neck of the metacarpal with a nonabsorbable suture through a hole in the dorsal-radial cortex of the neck of the bone. Swanson does not recommend that this reconstruction be done routinely, but it is useful when the first dorsal interosseous is inadequate or there is a definite pronation deformity of the index finger.

After the extensor tendon has been centralized or even placed slightly to the radial side of the center of the joint, the stretched radial hood is passed beneath it, and the joint cavity is closed with a series of synthetic sutures. The skin wound is closed with interrupted nylon sutures. I frequently use a drain for 24 hours. A large compression dressing is placed on the dorsum of the hand, and a palmar plaster slab extending

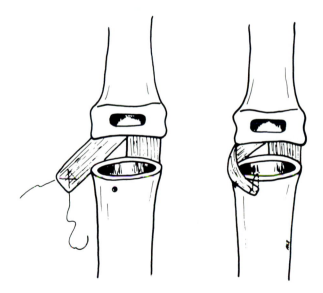

Fig. 8-13. Reconstruction of the radial collateral ligament of the metacarpophalangeal joint of the index finger. The palmar plate and its attachments are incised longitudinally in the midline. The sesamoid bone, if present, is resected. A distally based flap of 1.5 to 2 cm in length is made of the radial portion of the palmar plate and the radial collateral ligament, which are separated from the intrinsic muscle and flexor tendon. This flap is pulled around the radial aspect of the joint and attached to the neck of the metacarpal by a nonabsorbable suture through a hole in the dorsal radial cortex. (From Swanson, A.B.: J. Bone Joint Surg. **54-A:**435-455, 1972.)

beyond the metacarpophalangeal joints is incorporated in the bandages. The hand is elevated for at least 48 hours. Movement of the extensors and the proximal interphalangeal joints is encouraged as soon as the postoperative discomfort subsides.

Usually on the third postoperative day the palmar slab can be removed and a dynamic extensor splint placed in the dorsum of the forearm and hand. Intermittent elevation should be continued for several days. The metacarpophalangeal joints should be held in full extension and slight radial deviation (Fig. 3-8, p. 52). Swanson attaches great importance to the immediate postoperative positioning and control of joint movement during the first 6 to 8 weeks after surgery. He states that this postoperative program is just as important as the surgery itself. Swanson stresses that a carefully controlled follow-up and rehabilitation program should be provided for at least 3 months after surgery.

The brace may need constant readjustment so that 0 to 70 degrees of flexion is possible. The joints often stiffen during the second postoperative week, and sometimes a flexion cuff is useful as part-time passive assistance. The brace should be worn night and day for the first 3 weeks and then may usually be left off during the day for the second 3 weeks. Some patients do not progress satisfactorily because they flex largely at their proximal interphalangeal joints. By splinting these joints in extension during exercise periods, their full flexion force can be concentrated on the metacarpophalangeal joints. This temporary splinting can be done by taping on short padded aluminum strips or by using small plastic or cardboard cylinders placed over the fingers.

THIRD GENERATION IMPLANTS

The recommended technique for the insertion of third-generation devices varies with each model but a good general description has been published by Steffee. For his device, Steffee recommends a separate 4-cm straight dorsal incision centered over each metacarpophalangeal joint. I continue to use the transverse incision when I am inserting any type of these third-generation prostheses.

After the usual soft-tissue dissection with preservation of the veins and nerves, Steffee recommends cutting the neck of the metacarpal just proximal to the origins of the collateral ligaments. The base of the phalanx is squared off by removing about 1 to 3 mm of bone perpendicular to the long axis of the proximal phalanx. It may be necessary to remove more bone if the phalangeal base is sloped because of longstanding subluxation. As in all other types of prosthetic replacement, it is vital to reduce the subluxation sufficiently to obtain easy full extension. The palmar plate may have to be released and any ulnar deviation tendency relieved by sectioning the ulnar intrinsic tendon to each finger. The medullary canals of all eight bones are then lightly reamed to remove any soft cancellous bones, and the trial components are used to select the appropriate sizes.

I agree with Steffee's recommendation that only half a batch of cement be mixed at one time. It is inserted first into the proximal phalanges after it has become sticky. I prefer to hold all four fingers in my nondominant hand with the metacarpophalangeal joints flexed and distracted so that I can push the stem of the distal component into the cement with the dorsal border parallel to and just beneath the dorsal cortex. By holding all four fingers together, side by side, it is easier to ensure the transverse axis of the component is parallel to the nail bed. The proximal components are inserted in similar fashion by sighting down the line of the metacarpal and placing the stem up underneath the dorsal cortex of each bone.

The components are then articulated, and each finger is tested separately for proper orientation. All four fingers as a group are then flexed and extended. No overriding, lateral deviation, or rotational deformities can be allowed. These devices are unforgiving; if there is any abnormal orientation, the cement and the device must be removed from the affected finger and the whole process repeated.

I hold all four fingers fully extended while repairing the dorsal capsule and closing the skin wound. I usually drain the incision and use a large compression dressing with a palmar slab for immobilizing the metacarpophalangeal joints in full extension.

The postoperative course I use is similar to the course followed when Niebauer or Swanson prostheses have been implanted. However, Steffee maintains continuous elevation for 5 days and does not apply the dorsal splint until 5 to 7 days after the operation.

Proximal interphalangeal joint

METAL PROSTHESIS

Because it is made of a rigid material, this prosthesis can be made to block hyperextension, thereby preventing recurrent swan-neck deformity such as can occur if Silastic devices are used (Fig. 8-14). This prosthesis is now available only on special

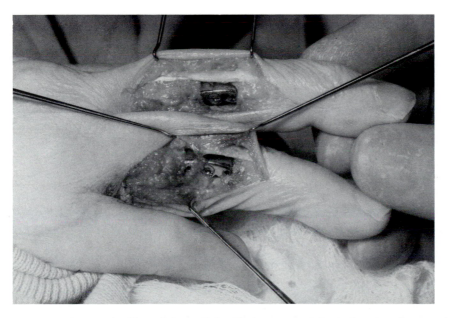

Fig. 8-14. Approach to proximal interphalangeal joint. The best approach for the insertion of an interphalangeal prosthesis is through the neutral border of the finger. (From Flatt, A.E.: J. Bone Joint Surg. **43-A:**753, 1961.)

order and requires specific tools for its insertion. The method of insertion has been described in earlier editions of this book.

NIEBAUER PROSTHESIS

Niebauer approaches this joint through a longitudinal incision over the dorsum of the joint, with wide reflection of the skin to either side. He stresses the importance of preserving the central extensor tendon during any preliminary synovectomy. After the collateral ligaments have been excised, the head of the proximal phalanx is removed piecemeal with rongeurs, and the necessary space for the prosthesis is created. Most of the bone should be removed from the proximal phalanx. The medullary canals are reamed out, and the correct size of prosthesis is selected. It is particularly important to ensure that buckling of the prosthesis does not occur. If it does occur, decompression of the joint has not been adequate, and swan-neck deformity is likely to occur later.

I have not found that the stems tend to dislocate so readily at this joint compared with the metacarpophalangeal joint, and I do not usually sew the stems into the bones. The problem of selecting the correct size of prosthesis has been greatly simplified by the introduction of a broad model that can be trimmed on its sides to the appropriate width without harm to the prosthesis.

The postoperative regime used by Niebauer consists of 4 or 5 days' splinting of the joints in extension, after which active motion is encouraged. The joints should be protected in extension on night splints for at least 3 weeks.

SWANSON IMPLANT

The operation is basically the same whether the implant is to be used in an osteoarthritic or a rheumatoid joint. The approach can be made through a dorsal gentle S- or C-shaped incision over the dorsum of the joint. In the index and small fingers the incision should be kept away from the outer borders of the digits. Swanson recommends the use of a midlateral incision when surgical treatment of the flexor tendon mechanism is also indicated.

If the joint has stiffened without collapse deformity, it is approached by incising the central tendon proximally from its insertion along the distal two thirds of the proximal phalanx. In swan-neck deformities the central tendon is divided by a step cut and dissected off the proximal phalanx. For boutonniere deformities the stretched central tendon is usually detached from the base of the middle phalanx and later reattached or replaced by the use of the lateral tendon on the radial side of the finger.

After the tendon mechanism has been retracted from the area of the joint, the collateral ligaments and the palmar plate are dissected from the head of the proximal phalanx. A transverse osteotomy through the neck of the phalanx will allow the head to be removed either in one piece or piecemeal. The base of the middle phalanx is not resected, but any osteophytes present should be trimmed away. Both medullary canals should be reamed and shaped to accept the rectangular stem of the implant.

The largest suitable implant should be used: Swanson records that sizes 0, 1, 2, or

3 are most frequently used for this joint. The cross bar must seat well against the adjacent surfaces of the phalanges, which should have been smoothly trimmed to prevent any bone spicules from puncturing the skin of the implant. The proximal stem of the implant is inserted first and the distal stem is inserted by bending it down to fit into the middle phalanx when the joint is held in flexion.

The joint must be tested when it is in extension; if the bone ends impinge too much on the cross bar of the implant, more bone must be removed or additional soft-tissue release must be done. This is the most difficult part of the operation because judgment, rather than technique, is involved. Too much decompression of the joint produces a floppy system liable to buckling, and inadequate soft-tissue release may lead to swan-neck deformity. The only advice I can give the inexperienced is to study Swanson's writings with the utmost care before operating, and after insertion of the implant to repeatedly test the joint in passive flexion, proceeding cautiously with additional bony excisions or soft-tissue releases.

The joint must also be tested for lateral stability. If instability or deviation is present, the distally based flap made of the collateral and accessory collateral ligaments must be reattached. Small holes should be drilled on the dorsolateral sides of the trimmed neck of the proximal phalanx and 3-0 synthetic sutures used to reattach the ligaments. Passive flexion must now be tested. If the ligaments are too tight, adjustments must be made before the central extensor mechanism is appropriately repaired. A small drain is placed in the wound; the skin is closed with interrupted 5-0 nylon sutures; and a voluminous compression dressing applied.

On the third postoperative day the drain is removed, the dressing changed, and exercises started. The patient should be encouraged to flex and extend the digits within the limits of discomfort while the proximal phalanges are supported with a brace cast or other exercise device. For the first 3 to 6 weeks small aluminum splints holding the joints in extension should be used at night.

The postoperative regimen for fixed swan-neck deformities should include fixing the joints in 20 degrees of flexion on aluminum splints for the first 10 days. Active exercises can then be started, but hyperextension must be avoided for the first 6 weeks. When an implant has been used in a boutonniere deformity the finger should be splinted in extension for 10 days before guarded flexion movements are permitted. It should then be held in extension part time for 3 to 6 weeks, depending on the degree of extensor lag.

RESULTS OF PROSTHETIC REPLACEMENTS

A significant number of papers of varying critical quality have been published assessing the value of prosthetic replacements. Even after 25 years of work in this field I find it impossible to present a scientific unbiased opinion of the situation. I cannot always justify my views by statistical evidence. I take comfort, however, in a quotation from Sir Herbert Seddon, who wrote, "Forthright dogmatism is better than conclusions propped up by shaky statistics."*

---

*From Seddon, H.: Surgical disorders of the peripheral nerves, Baltimore, 1972, The Williams & Wilkins Co., p. 310.

I started to use metal prostheses in 1957 with the narrow intention of investigating whether or not fixed swan-neck deformity could be helped by prosthetic replacement of the proximal interphalangeal joint. In a short time the large number of patients with dislocated metacarpophalangeal joints prompted me to expand the indications to include the metacarpophalangeal joints of the fingers and thumb. As time went on, I tried many of the other devices that became available and have tried to keep accurate preoperative and postoperative records of the state of the hand in order to form an unbiased assessment of the results. Virtually all patients report significant loss of pain in their joints after replacement. Replacement of the metacarpophalangeal joints often seems to precipitate discomfort and stiffness in the proximal interphalangeal joints, presumably because of the new demands made on the joints after stabilization of the metacarpophalangeal joints. Restoration of motion by prosthetic replacement in the proximal interphalangeal joints often has a salutary effect on metacarpophalangeal joint motion because of increased use of the hand.

The full range of motion that is built into a prosthesis is never obtained. The greater range is achieved at the proximal interphalangeal joint. At the metacarpophalangeal joint large cross sections of raw bone are exposed, there is considerable bleeding, and subsequent fibrosis occurs, which tends to limit both the active and passive range of motion.

Metacarpophalangeal joint

NIEBAUER PROSTHESES

Several authors have now reported their results with this silicone-Dacron prosthesis. In 1976 Goldner reported that after using 441 Niebauer prostheses he felt that they can be expected to relieve pain, improve function and appearance, and consistently provide a reasonably predictable result. He reported a 5.4% fracture rate for the series; however, 30% of those followed for 6 years were found to be fractured. He considered that the presence of a fracture did not preclude a good functional result. The average range of motion achieved for each joint was 54 degrees. Beckenbaugh, Dobyns, Linscheid, and Bryan reported an average range of motion of 35 degrees and a fracture rate of 38.2%. They commented that early implant types and some variations from the designer's recommended rehabilitation protocols were used.

SWANSON IMPLANTS

Many thousands of the Swanson implants have been used, and many surgeons have published their results in many languages. There is no question that the overall results are pleasing and that most patients are gratified at the functional and cosmetic improvement of their hands. I see little point in reproducing a battery of figures, because the standards used in measuring results vary so much that true comparison is impossible.

Results with the earlier Swanson model disclosed an unsatisfactory rate of fracture. The newer, high-performance silicone rubber implant has shown a significantly reduced rate of fracture. Most patients whose implants have fractured are not aware of it and suffer no functional loss.

The majority of the Swanson implants have been used at the metacarpophalangeal joint; some have been used at the proximal interphalangeal joint and relatively few at the terminal joint. There have been isolated reports of silicone lymph-adenopathy and synovitis with silicone particles being present in distant lymph nodes or in the synovium of the joint. I have also seen this associated with a fractured wrist implant. After removal of the broken pieces and the associated synovitis the painful symptoms subsided. Swanson has stated that "the presence of silicone particles in tissue causes one of the most benign reactions that one can see from foreign material and that there need not be fear or any implication that this can be a problem with patients who have silicone implants." One would not expect these Swanson implants to show any special affinity for postoperative infection. Millender and his colleagues reported only 10 instances in 2105 prosthetic implants. In the 7 patients whose Swanson implants were removed, nearly all had stable, somewhat stiff, but pain-free joints.

Swanson is currently conducting a multiclinic field trial of the new high-performance silicone rubber implants, and I believe the long-term results will prove satisfactory. Because of the large number of these implants that have been used with reasonable results, the Swanson implant has established a level against which the results of any other device should be measured. It is significant that those who have used two different versions of the third-generation devices both defer to the results obtained with the Swanson implant. I too frequently use these implants at the metacarpophalangeal level; however, I repeat my earlier comment that this implant appears deceptively easy to use, but in fact, good results can be obtained only by faithfully following Swanson's published directions.

THIRD GENERATION PROSTHESES

Steffee and his colleagues report that a sizable number of his Type I prostheses were inserted in 1973 and 1974, but the results were variable and disappointing. Recurrent ulnar drift and extensor lag were sufficient problems to stimulate the development of the Type II model. From 1974 to 1977, 577 of the Type II design were implanted. In a very frank report on the follow-up of the Type II prothesis, this group pointed out the problems encountered. Loosening of both components at the bone-cement interface has occurred, and the hoped-for improvement in grip strength and prevention of recurrent ulnar drift have not materialized. Despite these disappointments the average range of active flexion was 42 degrees, and pain was relieved in 96% of the patients. He concludes that these complications dictate the continued routine use of the Swanson implant as the treatment of choice, while limited clinical trials should continue in selected investigative centers.

The St. George prosthesis has been used in Europe since 1971. Karl Tillmann reported disappointing results at the First International Federation of Societies for Surgery of the Hand in 1980. Long-term follow-up showed less joint mobility when compared with resection arthroplasty or Swanson implants. The theoretical advantages of mechanical stability were outweighed by mechanical failure, there being an especially high rate of stem loosening.

I have used a number of the original Schultz prostheses and found a high rate of fracture of the narrow neck of the metal component. I have not yet used sufficient numbers of the redesigned and stronger model to be able to pass judgment.

MY OWN SERIES

In the early 1970's I reviewed 242 metal prostheses that I had placed in the hands of 84 patients during the years 1957 to 1971. In an attempt to avoid the influence of personality and patients' loyalty, all the postoperative assessments were done by another surgeon in my absence. One hundred and sixty-seven prostheses were inserted into the metacarpophalangeal joints, the principal indication being gross subluxation or even frank dislocation associated with ulnar drift. Fifteen of these prostheses were later removed. The results of these metal prostheses were examined at three different times after implantation. Preoperatively the average range of motion was 24 degrees, and the average arc was from 47 to 71 degrees of flexion. Postoperatively the measurements for the average range of motion and the average arc were as follows: up to 7 months, a range of 16 degrees and an arc from 45 to 61 degrees; at 8 months to 5 years, a range of 25 degrees and an arc from 37 to 62 degrees; and at 5 to 14 years, a range of 16 degrees and an arc from 15 to 31 degrees. Thus there was an initial decrease, then an increase, and finally another decrease in motion (Fig. 8-15). The average ranges of motion for the metacarpophalangeal joints of all four fingers decreased postoperatively. But the average axes of motion were in a more functional position, since they moved toward extension as time passed. Motion of the associated proximal interphalangeal joints that were not operated on tended to increase because of the reciprocal interaction of the metacarpophalangeal and proximal interphalangeal joints.

The gradual decrease in range of motion as time went by proved to forecast the results we found in a similar survey in the early 1980's. In this review we studied the results of postoperative therapy and subsequent hand function in 125 patients with 5 different types of implants. This group included all patients available for interview and examination who were under my care between 1957 and 1978. The follow-up period ranged from 1 year to 21 years with an average of 8.5 years. Implants evaluated included 191 Swanson, 88 Flatt, 35 Niebauer, 32 Schultz, and 16 Steffee prostheses. Follow-up interviews and examinations were always performed by investigators other than the patient's surgeon. Evaluation of active range of motion and strength and functional testing, as well as interview assessment of function, and the patient's subjective evaluation of their results were recorded. X-ray films were taken to assess any structural causes of change demonstrated by physical examination.

The results with all five types of implants had several common features. In each type of implant, evaluation of the patient's function shortly after surgery demonstrated improved range of finger joint motion, decreased ulnar drift with improved prehension, and relief of pain, except for a single patient who had persistent discomfort. Long-term evaluation showed a progressive loss of finger motion, a decrease in strength, and a recurrence of deformity. Ulnar drift, broken prostheses, bone resorption, and increasing periarticular thickening were the most common complications identified.

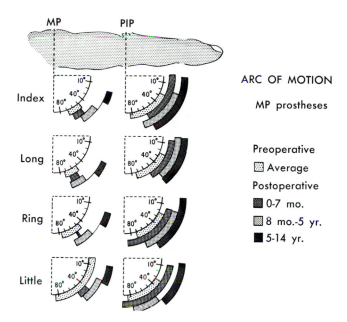

Fig. 8-15. Metacarpophalangeal prostheses: arcs of motion. Average arcs of metacarpophalangeal and proximal interphalangeal motion before and after insertion of a metacarpophalangeal prosthesis in the index, long, ring, and little finger. Although, after 14 years, metacarpophalangeal motion has decreased, the arc of available motion has moved toward extension and the reciprocal interaction of the metacarpophalangeal and proximal phalangeal joints has maintained the arc of motion in the latter joint. (From Flatt, A.E., and Ellison, M.R.: J. Bone Joint Surg. **54-A:**1317-1322, 1972.)

Although comparison of the types of implants was difficult because of differences in the numbers of each type and the average lengths of follow-up, we did identify differences in the frequency and types of complications. Fingers with the metal prostheses had the highest incidence of skin breakdown, and they tended to develop fatigue fractures after about their fifth year. In the entire series, the index finger had the highest incidence of prosthetic fracture, accounting for 78% of all Niebauer prostheses implanted in the index metacarpophalangeal joint, 40% of the Schultz implants, 10% of the Swanson implants, 7% of the metal prostheses and none of the Steffee implants. The Swanson implant was the only type with a higher fracture incidence in a finger other than the index finger (12% in the long finger). The Niebauer prosthesis had a 50% fracture rate, and the Schultz a 20% fracture rate in the small finger metacarpophalangeal joint. For the Schultz prosthesis, patients with a grip strength greater than 14 pounds fractured their prostheses, as did patients with greater than 12 pounds lateral pinch. Average active metacarpophalangeal ranges of motion by type were 28 degrees for the Flatt, 44 degrees for the Swanson, 39 degrees for the Niebauer, and 22 degrees for the Schultz implants.

These complications have occurred in prostheses implanted up to 21 years ago. There have been many design changes in the prostheses, and current models should be much less prone to problems than their forebearers. However, I believe it is significant that in time all five types of implants show steadily decreasing hand func-

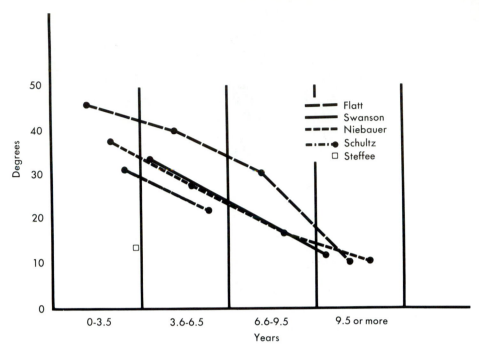

Fig. 8-16. Comparison of active range of motion of five MCP joint substitutes. All showed decreasing range of motion as time went by.

tion (Fig. 8-16). I do not believe current designs have yet solved the problems of decreasing finger motion and strength, recurrence of deformity, and bone resorption around the implant.

The pronated index finger

Because of its vital importance in many precision activities, the index finger is subjected to forces that the other fingers and their implants do not have to endure. Pronation of the index finger has proved to be a significant complication for many patients.

In the normal pinch mechanism the index finger is held in slight supination, thereby presenting the working palmar surface of the fingertip. When the finger pronates, it is the radial border of the finger that meets the thumb. This rotation takes place at the metacarpophalangeal joint and is largely the result of soft tissue laxity and force imbalance. The articular surfaces of the joint are so shallow that even in the normal joint they do not present any mechanical restraint against rotation.

After an implant arthroplasty has been done the index metacarpophalangeal joint must be carefully protected against ulnar deviation and pronation for many weeks. Even despite such care, pronation deformities do occur; I have seen such deformities a number of times in my patients. Fatigue fractures were particularly prone to occur in the prongs of the metal prostheses, either in the proximal phalanx or within the metacarpal (Fig. 7-12, p. 172). I have also seen loosening of the stems in the third-generation implants in the index finger. The separation usually occurs at the bone-cement interface in the proximal phalanx. Control of the axial torque to the digit is therefore not provided by a rigid, constrained implant and clearly cannot be supplied by a flexible implant, which has been known to rotate with the medullary canals. Meticulous soft-tissue surgery is the best that can be offered against the natural tendency to pinch pronation. Biddulph has suggested splitting the extensor indicis proprius into two longitudinal strands with each slip being passed downwards into the base of the proximal phalanx just dorsal to the radial collateral ligament. He reports that this transfer produces supination of the index and long fingers and also strengthens radial deviation of these two digits. He believes that this use of an actively contracting musculotendinous unit is better than a local tissue rearrangement that runs the risk of stretching.

Certainly the use of such a transfer would be a useful supplement to local tissue repair, but I believe the latter is still an essential part of an arthroplasty of the two radial fingers. I believe an important factor in the pronation deformity is the subluxation of the first dorsal interosseus tendon below and under the axis of the index metacarpophalangeal joint. I agree with Swanson that it is essential to relocate this tendon in its proper anatomical position on the side of the joint. One must be careful not to place it too far above the axis of the joint because this produces a grotesque abduction deformity of the joint.

The best protection that can be supplied is to leave the radial collateral ligament attached to the base of the phalanx and to reinsert the proximal end on the dorsoradial side of the neck of the metacarpal. The ligament should be firmly attached with 3-0 nonabsorbable sutures passed through small drill holes. If, as frequently occurs in late disease, there is no real ligament left to reattach, then the radial part of the palmar plate can be brought up and sewn to the neck of the metacarpal. This will certainly rotate the digit out of its pronated posture. Careful capsular repair and centralization of the extensor tendon are also essential.

Pronation deformity tends to be greatest when the metacarpophalangeal joint is flexed to about 45 degrees. Postoperative therapy should be directed to training the patient to pinch with the joint in greater extension. It is also helpful to teach three-point pinch activities because the buttress effect on the long finger aids in preventing pronation.

POSTOPERATIVE MANAGEMENT

Whatever may be the merits of any one particular device, it is clear that a significant factor in obtaining a satisfactory result is the postoperative management program. It has been gradually accepted that early motion and a prolonged splinting program yield the best results.

The paper by Madden, DeVore, and Arem is a major contribution to an understanding of the value of rational postoperative management. They have developed a postsurgical program for metacarpophalangeal joint arthroplasty based on the biology of scar tissue. Although developed specifically for arthroplasties using the Swanson device, I agree with them that the biological principles on which their program was developed seem applicable to all current arthroplastic techniques.

All alloplastic material becomes encapsulated by scar tissue. This scar capsule remains metabolically active for months after implantation. The major factor influencing the architectural arrangement and the size and shape of the capsular scar tissue is controlled tension. Thus controlled movement should produce tension in some planes and static stability in others. The scar tissue on the palmar and dorsal aspects of the capsule must remain long enough to allow extension and flexion whereas tissue on the sides of the implant must remain short and compact to provide stability.

Madden waits until the fifth postoperative day to apply a dorsal splint with 15 to 20 degrees of extension for the wrist. An outrigger holds the rubber bands and finger loops for the index, long, and ring fingers, keeping the metacarpophalangeal joints in extension and in slight radial deviation. The rubber band tension is adjusted to hold these joints in approximately minus 10 degrees of extension. Note that the small finger is not supported by a rubber band sling but is taped to the ring finger. The small finger is notorious for its obstinacy in gaining flexion and usually does better if it is not splinted.

I agree with this group that the use of individually fitted splints is preferable to routine use of universal splints. Custom-made splints can be more easily fitted to fixed deformities in the wrist, thumb, and elbow and can be readily modified as treatment progresses.

Madden, DeVore, and Arem's program differs from many others, because instead of encouraging early maximum passive motion, they *insist* on it. They also insist on a prolonged dynamic splinting program. By using a minimum of 14 weeks of dynamic night splinting, gains achieved during the first 2 months are maintained. They have been able to show that if this program is carried out fully, the gains in active motion are maintained through at least 2 years. Their paper should be read in its entirety by all those implanting prostheses, because it demonstrates so clearly the vital importance of responsible and detailed postoperative care in obtaining good results. I do not believe surgeons should implant joint replacements if they are not able to provide comparable complete and proper postoperative care.

Proximal interphalangeal joint

The anatomical features of the proximal interphalangeal joint are such that prosthetic replacement should not be a major design problem, since little, if any, rotation or lateral motion is expected in a normal proximal interphalangeal joint. Unfortunately, we have an inadequate number of preoperative and postoperative follow-up studies on patients in whom we have placed two-pronged metal prostheses. Seventy-five prostheses were inserted, and 11 were later removed. The majority of these proximal interphalangeal joints were replaced because of persistent swan-neck deformity or ankylosis of the joint. In no case was prosthetic replacement done for joints showing a boutonniere or severe flexion deformity. The longest follow-up study we have among these patients is of a 63-year-old housewife who has had rheumatoid disease for 27 years. Her left hand was severely involved, with fixed swan-neck deformities that were not improved by intrinsic release. Over 19 years ago prostheses were placed in her index, long, and ring fingers. A prosthesis was placed in the small finger 1 year later (Fig. 8-17). The hand was changed from a flipper to a useful prehensile organ and has continued to be of great use to her. Her general disease has continued to worsen, and the metacarpophalangeal joints of the index and long fingers have remained useful, but the ring and small fingers show almost no motion in their prostheses.

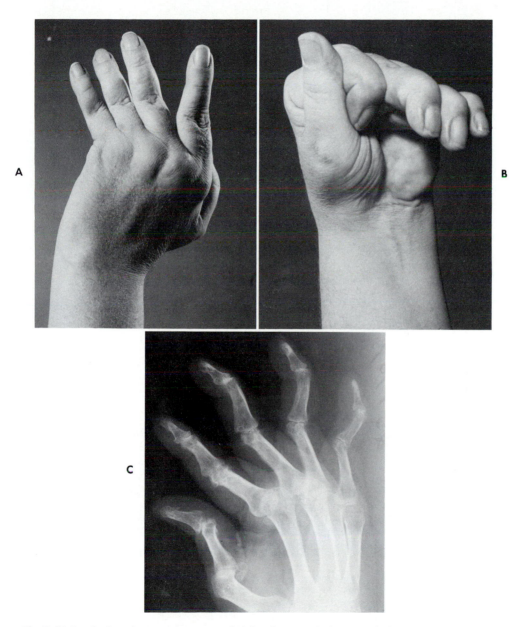

Fig. 8-17. Prosthetic replacement in swan-neck deformity. **A,** Typical swan-neck deformity in the left hand of a patient who had rheumatoid disease for 9 years and hand symptoms for 6 years. **B,** Patient attempting to make a fist after an intrinsic release operation. **C,** Because of the joint destruction, the operation failed.   *Continued.*

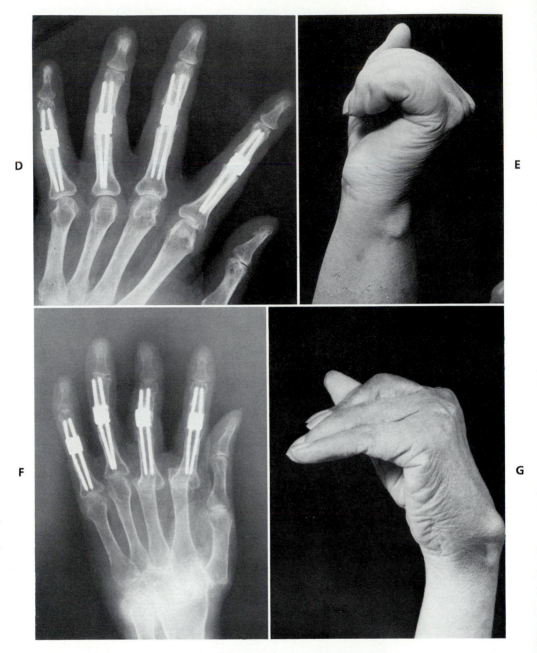

Fig. 8-17, cont'd. D, Middle phalanx of the long finger shows signs of bone absorption around the prongs of the prosthesis. **E,** Flexion possible 9 months after a fourth prosthesis had been placed in the small finger. **F,** This x-ray film shows the state of the hand 7 years after prosthetic replacement; note the dislocation of the metacarpophalangeal joints of the index and long fingers. **G,** Hand still remains useful 12 years after surgery; motion is acceptable in the index and long fingers, but there is little motion in the prostheses in the ring and small fingers. It is now nearly 20 years after the original surgery and the hand still functions. (From Flatt, A.E.: J. Bone Joint Surg. **43-A:**753, 1961.)

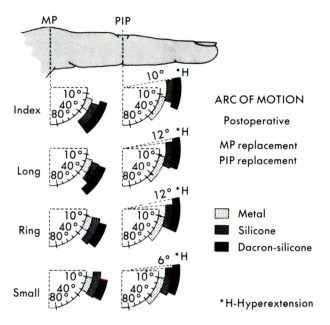

Fig. 8-18. Prosthetic replacement: arcs of motion. These arcs of motion summarize my results using three different joint substitutes at the metacarpophalangeal and proximal interphalangeal levels. There is a disproportion in the total number of the types used because of my longer experience with metal prostheses. The figures show that at the metacarpophalangeal joint the silicone rubber substitutes yield more motion than the metal prosthesis. At the proximal interphalangeal joint hyperextension can occur in the silicone varieties but not in the metal ones, which provide a good range of motion.

This result is included in this edition not to prove the longevity of the two-pronged prosthesis at this joint level, but to stress that with a mechanical block to hyperextension, swan-neck deformity does not recur. My results using either the Niebauer prosthesis or the Swanson implant have not been as pleasing, and recurrence of joint imbalance has frequently occurred (Fig. 8-18). I have not been able to find any large series of implants with several years of follow-up for either device. In 1972 Goldner and Urbaniak reported that the 27 proximal interphalangeal prostheses they had used provided an average range of motion of 63 degrees. They commented that the prosthesis gave a better range of motion in the degenerative arthritic joint than in joints of a rheumatoid patient.

At about the same time, Swanson reported only 85 implants in the proximal interphalangeal joint in his large personal series. These patients showed an average range of motion from 4 degrees of extension lag to 70 degrees of flexion. Patients with an implant in the index finger preferred to use pulp pinch, and when using lateral pinch they supported the index finger by using the lateral fingers to increase stability.

Since the metal prostheses are no longer available, I do occasionally use a Swanson implant at this joint level. I far prefer to place them in the long or ring fingers, since lateral support is available to these fingers. I have had considerable trouble developing lateral stability in the two border fingers.

CURRENT STATUS OF PROSTHETIC REPLACEMENT

There is no longer any need to publish pictorial justifications of prosthetic replacement of destroyed finger joints; it is an accomplished fact and has been proven to be a useful procedure. Any prosthetic device within the human body is an inferior substitute for the normal organ. A prosthesis becomes of value only when the limited function it can supply is better than that provided by the natural, but diseased, tissue. All prosthetic devices have a limited useful life, and it becomes a difficult matter of judgment to decide whether to employ a prosthesis, and, if so, which one to use. Because of the drawbacks of the current devices and because there is still a large number of patients who would benefit from prosthetic replacement of their destroyed digital joints, several new prostheses are currently being developed. Use of the new prostheses should be confined to major medical centers where strict control over development can be exercised.

The use of current prostheses is gradually expanding into replacement of single joints destroyed by degenerative arthritis. The strong normal forces within the hand place great strains on the artificial joint, and, because of this, fractures must be anticipated.

The argument as to whether prosthetic stems should or should not be fixed is still not settled, nor has the ideal material from which to construct these prostheses yet been found. In the meantime I repeat my earlier hope that all hands meriting surgical rehabilitation will be referred to the hand surgeon in the early stages of the disease and will therefore never arrive at the stage of needing prostheses. This is, of course, the counsel of perfection, and it will be many years before such a state is reached.

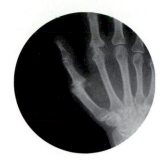

CHAPTER 9

The thumb

The thumb is the single most important digit of the hand. In effect it endures half of the work load of the prehensile hand and is therefore subject to all forms of arthritic changes.

Although there are large variations in the movement of the three joints of the thumb, the carpometacarpal joint has the greatest range of motion. Each joint contributes specific motions to the articular chain, and each can be affected by the imbalance of its neighbors. This integration of activities implies that destructive changes in one joint will inevitably affect the posture and function of the others.

Osteoarthritic disease occurs most commonly at the carpometacarpal joint, but rheumatoid disease of the thumb involves all its joints. Brewerton showed that in the rheumatoid outpatient clinic about 68% of the patients have deformities of their thumbs that have a significant effect on function. Pulkki found virtually the same incidence (67%) in a study of 500 rheumatoid patients. Thirty-five percent of these patients showed limited opposition because of restricted rotation of the thumb. One third of Brewerton's patients showed a loss of at least 30 degrees of internal rotation of the thumb, making normal opposition impossible. Forty-five percent of Pulkki's patients showed instability of the metacarpophalangeal joint, and 10% had instability of their interphalangeal joint.

ANATOMICAL PROBLEMS
Carpometacarpal joint

The carpometacarpal is the key joint of the thumb. The fundamental movements of opposition, rotation, flexion, extension, abduction, and adduction all take place at this joint (Fig. 9-1).

To accommodate all these various movements, the joint is saddle shaped, with two principal axes: (1) a dorsopalmar axis for abduction and adduction and (2) a radioulnar axis for flexion and extension. When the thumb is fully abducted or adducted, the joint surfaces are congruous and are held in close contact by tense capsular and ligamentous structures. These two postures should be regarded as the

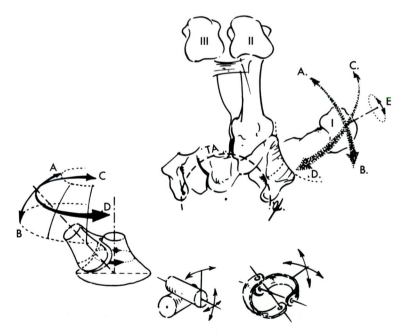

Fig. 9-1. Carpometacarpal joint of the thumb. **Top,** Three basic motions are possible; *A* to *B,* palmar adduction to palmar abduction; *C* to *D,* extension abduction to· flexion adduction; and *E,* rotation that occurs on the long axis of the metacarpal. **Bottom,** The geometry of this joint is represented by a tapered cone with a curved surface on which rests the saddle-shaped base of the metacarpal. (After Bausenhardt; from Littler, J.W.: Clin. Orthop. **13:**182-192, 1959.)

stable "positions of function" of the joint. The third, and vital, motion of longitudinal rotation takes place in the midposition of the joint when the capsular structures are sufficiently slack to allow rotation. Rotation of the thumb is essential for opposition, and in full opposition, tightening of the ligaments provides stability even though the joint surfaces are no longer congruous. When the metacarpal also moves into flexion and adduction, as in pinch activities, the forces on the dorsal ligament and the dorsal joint facet increase significantly. Thus even in the normal hand, usage produces severe demands on this joint, and the wear and tear of aging is inevitable. If the joint is already weakened by rheumatoid synovitis, significant loss of function must occur.

Since this joint is the most proximal of the three thumb joints, laxness of its restraints from either ligament destruction or joint collapse sets the stage for zigzag collapse in the more distal joints.

Metacarpophalangeal joint

Although the anatomical relationships of the metacarpophalangeal joints of the thumb and fingers are basically similar, there are certain differences that have an important bearing on the development of deformities of the metacarpophalangeal joint of the thumb. The dorsal fibrous capsule of the joint contains the terminal portion of the extensor pollicis brevis tendon. In this area the tendon gives fibers to the hood as well as inserting into the proximal phalanx. On the ulnar side of this tendon lies the strong tendon of the extensor pollicis longus muscle, passing to its attachment on the base of the distal phalanx. These two tendons are usually joined together by a considerable number of cross fibers, which also blend into the fibrous capsule.

Rupture of the extensor pollicis longus will deprive the interphalangeal joint of its major source of extension. Also lost, however, will be some extension of the metacarpophalangeal joint and a major contribution to adduction of the thumb.

The two wings of the hood on the sides of the joint are formed by contributions from the intrinsic muscles of the thumb. On the ulnar side of the joint the adductor pollicis muscle supplies both transverse and oblique fibers to the hood as well as fibers of insertion into the proximal phalanx. On the radial side transverse and oblique fibers of the hood are contributed by the abductor pollicis brevis and the flexor pollicis brevis muscles, which also insert into the proximal phalanx.

Extension of the distal phalanx of the thumb can therefore be accomplished not only by the long extensor tendon but also by the short extensor tendon via its insertion into the hood and by the intrinsic muscles through their insertions into either side of the hood. This integrated group of extensor tendons plays an important part in the production of deformities at the metacarpophalangeal and interphalangeal joints of the thumb.

As in the other digital joints, rheumatoid synovitis of the metacarpophalangeal joint will cause a distention of the structures surrounding the joint. Particularly affected are the fibers of the hood over the joint and the insertion of the extensor pollicis brevis tendon into the base of the proximal phalanx.

In established rheumatoid disease of the joint the fibers of the bony insertion of the extensor pollicis brevis muscle disappear, leaving the weak extensor action of this muscle to act solely on the hood mechanism. The lateral hood attachments of the intrinsic muscles stretch the hood fibers transversely, and the tendon of the extensor pollicis longus muscle displaces to the ulnar side. This displacement is particularly noticeable when the thumb is in adduction.

These distortions of the normal anatomy will cause a zigzag collapse. Controlled extension of the metacarpophalangeal joint is lost, and all the various components of extension act on the more distal interphalangeal joint, thereby producing a hyperextension deformity. (Fig. 9-2, A). Because the line of pull of the extrinsic muscles has been altered by the hyperextension deformity, these muscles become strong flexors of the metacarpophalangeal joint and ultimately produce what can best be described as an intrinsic-plus deformity of the thumb. Nalebuff has stressed that the initiating factor in this chain of collapse is the weakening and effective lengthening of the terminal part of the extensor pollicis brevis tendon. At this stage it is better to consider this deformity an extrinsic-minus thumb rather than an intrinsic-plus thumb, since the contribution of the intrinsic muscles becomes significant only as the extrinsic extensor muscles become weaker. As the metacarpophalangeal joint passes into permanent flexion, the hood slips distally over the joint and thereby contributes an additional deforming factor that increases the flexion deformity.

Interphalangeal joint

Throughout the time that the deformity of the metacarpophalangeal joint is developing, the thumb is being used. Normal use of the thumb tends to accentuate the deformity, because the most common position for most prehensile activities is palmar pinch. The pressure is exerted between the pulp surfaces of the distal phalanges of the thumb and index finger. This form of pinch is most efficient when the metacarpophalangeal joint is held straight or in very few degrees of flexion (Fig. 2-9, p. 26). To retain efficiency of pinch, the interphalangeal joint will respond to flexion of the metacarpophalangeal joint by a compensatory, and roughly equal, degree of hyperextension.

Hyperextension of the interphalangeal joint is not necessarily a pathological state. The range of movement of the three joints of the thumb shows an astonishing variation among normal individuals. The variation in the range of movement at the carpometacarpal joint is not great, but at the other two joints it is considerable.

I used to believe that lack of range of movement at the metacarpophalangeal joint was compensated for by an increased range at the interphalangeal joint and that the reverse situation was also true. Measurements of the range of movement of the thumbs in a group of normal young adults have now convinced me that there is no direct correlation between the ranges of movement of these two joints. Nor can I find any correlation between functional ability and variations in total joint range. Many of the people studied were quite unaware that the range of movement of their thumbs was different from that of other people. The variations in range were extreme. Some double-jointed individuals showed a total range of movement in the two joints of over

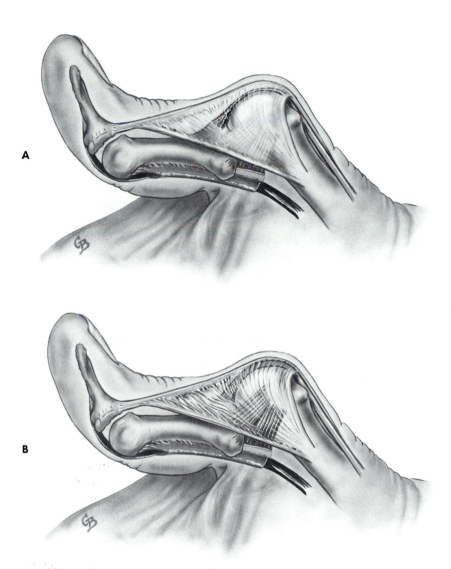

Fig. 9-2. Metacarpophalangeal joint of the thumb. **A,** Extrinsic-minus deformity; the terminal part of the extensor pollicis brevis has attenuated, the proximal phalanx has slipped into flexion, and a secondary hyperextension of the interphalangeal joint has occurred. **B,** Intrinsic-plus deformity; a postural deformity similar to **A** could be produced by overaction of the intrinsic muscles even in the presence of an intact extensor pollicis brevis tendon.

300 degrees, whereas others showed a total range of between 120 and 130 degrees.

Lateral instability of the interphalangeal joint is a severe handicap. Instability is made even worse when other joints in the thumb and index finger are also abnormal (Fig. 9-11).

CLINICAL PROBLEMS

The carpometacarpal joint of the thumb carries such a heavy workload that it is frequently subject to osteoarthritic changes. In rheumatoid disease the synovitis produces capsular distortion that leads to laxity, subsequent joint deformity, and collapse.

In both forms of arthritis, the trapeziometacarpal joint is always involved; in osteo-arthritis, there may be pantrapezial changes with involvement of the base of the second metacarpal, the scaphoid, and the trapezoid (Fig. 9-3). Osteoarthritic changes are probably most common in postmenopausal women, but they can also occur following Bennett's fracture or after severe soft-tissue injuries to the joint.

Arthritic changes, either from degenerative or rheumatoid disease, may produce an adduction contracture of the thumb metacarpal and a collapse into the swan-neck posture. The basic mechanical reasons for postural collapse of the thumb into various recognizable patterns are similar in all diseases. No operative treatment should be undertaken without a clear understanding of the causes of the postural deformity. It is profitless to consider the treatment of disease of an individual joint of the thumb. The plan for restoration of function must be based on both the preoperative range of movement in each joint and the state of the extrinsic and intrinsic muscles controlling these joints.

Etiology of collapse deformities

Nalebuff has been a major contributor in developing a workable classification of the collapse deformities of the thumb. Anatomically the thumb, compared with a finger, lacks one joint in which synovitis can precipitate joint laxity, but the pattern of deformities is analogous to that which occurs in the fingers. Nalebuff has shown that thumbs deformed by rheumatoid disease can be categorized into four basic types according to which joint was initially or most seriously affected.

TYPE I

The most common deformity of the thumb in established rheumatoid disease is fixed flexion of the metacarpophalangeal joint and hyperextension of the interphalangeal joint.

The chain of events leading to this collapse starts with a synovitis of the metacarpophalangeal joint. This joint is frequently the first to show signs of rheumatoid disease of the hand. Probably synovitis is also present in other digital joints, but the work demands on the thumb metacarpophalangeal joint are so great that functional deterioration first shows up at this site.

As the synovitis progresses, the dorsal joint capsule stretches and the long extrin-

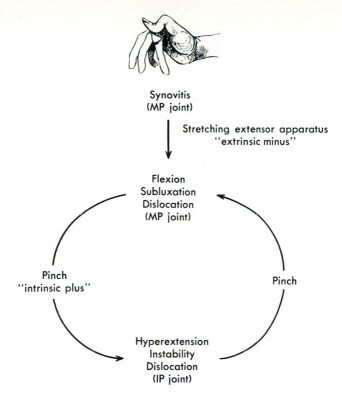

Synovitis
(MP joint)

Stretching extensor apparatus
"extrinsic minus"

Flexion
Subluxation
Dislocation
(MP joint)

Pinch
"intrinsic plus"

Pinch

Hyperextension
Instability
Dislocation
(IP joint)

Fig. 9-4. Type I deformities of the thumb. The chart indicates the steps leading to fully developed Type I deformity. (From Nalebuff, E.A.: Bull. Hosp. Joint Dis. **29:**119-137, 1968.)

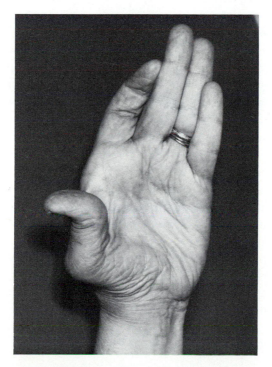

Fig. 9-5. 90-90 degree thumb. A typical late deformity of the thumb with the metacarpophalangeal and interphalangeal joints each at 90 degrees.

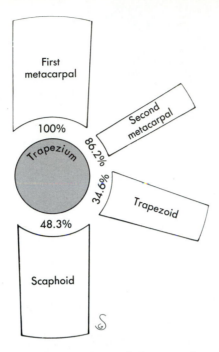

Fig. 9-3. Pantrapezial arthritis. The trapezium is frequently the center of a generalized arthritic process. The trapezio-first-metacarpal joint is most frequently involved; the least involvement occurs between the trapezium and trapezoid. (Courtesy A.B. Swanson, M.D.)

sic extensor tendon displaces ulnarward just as it does in a finger. The bony insertion of the extensor pollicis brevis is intimately related to the dorsal joint capsule and stretches as the synovitis expands (Fig. 9-4).

Concurrent with this synovial expansion is a slackening of the collateral ligaments of the joints, and palmar subluxation of the base of the proximal phalanx commences. Thus both extrinsic extensor tendons acting over the joint are now at a severe mechanical disadvantage. At this stage of deformity the posture of the interphalangeal joint is unchanged and the thumb is in an extrinsic-minus state (Fig. 9-2, A).

As subluxation of the base of the phalanx continues, both of the extrinsic thumb extensors and the intrinsic muscles all extend the interphalangeal joint. In the early stages of this posture both joints can be passively corrected, but a vicious cycle is soon created in which metacarpophalangeal flexion and interphalangeal extension accentuate each other with every pinch action, and the thumb soon becomes fixed in the 90-90–degree position (Fig. 9-5). This posture closely resembles the fully developed boutonniere deformity of a finger.

Although the great majority of thumbs in this posture are created by such a combined action of extrinsic and intrinsic muscles, one can still identify occasional patients in whom it seems that pure intrinsic tightness is the major factor. Tightness of the thumb intrinsics is tested for in the same basic manner as finger intrinsic tightness (Fig. 9-6). The interphalangeal joint must first be tested for passive flexion, and then the metacarpophalangeal joint is hyperextended and an attempt made to

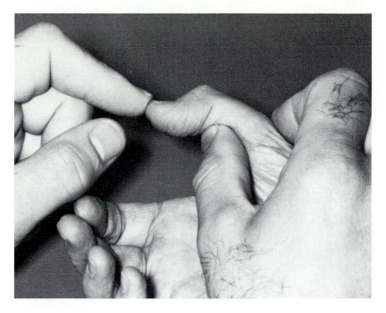

Fig. 9-6. Intrinsic-plus thumb. Tightness of the intrinsic muscles of the thumb is tested by holding the metacarpophalangeal joint in extension and attempting passive flexion of the interphalangeal joint. This thumb's test result is negative in the sense that there is no great resistance to passive flexion.

passively flex the interphalangeal joint while the patient is consciously relaxing the extrinsic extensors.

TYPE II

Type II deformity is not common, and its end result superficially resembles that of a Type I deformity in that there is hyperextension of the interphalangeal joint and flexion of the metacarpophalangeal joint. However, the precipitating factor in this collapse is synovitis of the carpometacarpal joint (Fig. 9-7).

The synovitis of this joint causes a stretching of the joint capsule followed by subluxation or dislocation. The head of the metacarpal tends to tilt as its proximal end becomes loose, resulting in a secondary adduction contracture. When the metacarpal is fixed in adduction, either the interphalangeal or the metacarpophalangeal joint will hyperextend as the patient tries to bring the thumb away from the palm. Which of the joints hyperextends depends on individual variations in joint laxity. More commonly it is the interphalangeal joint that hyperextends, whereas the metacarpophalangeal joint falls into compensatory flexion with every pinch action.

TYPE III

Type III deformity is the opposite of Types I and II in the sense that the interphalangeal joint is in flexion and the metacarpophalangeal is in extension (Fig. 9-7). As in Type II the original precipitating factor is a synovitis of the carpometacarpal joint, which leads to an adduction/flexion deformity of the metacarpal. Since the proximal thumb joint is now in flexion, it naturally follows that zigzag collapse will

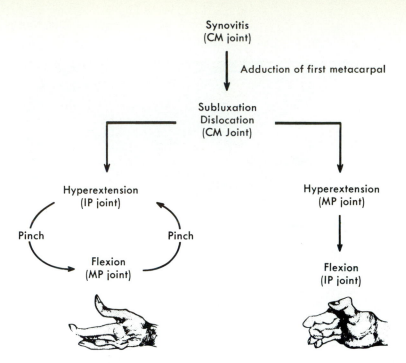

Fig. 9-7. Types II and III deformities of the thumb. This chart indicates the two courses of deformity the thumb may take after synovitis is established in the carpometacarpal joint. On the left is the less common Type II and on the right the more common Type III. (From Nalebuff, E.A.: Bull. Hosp. Joint Dis. **29:**119-137, 1968.)

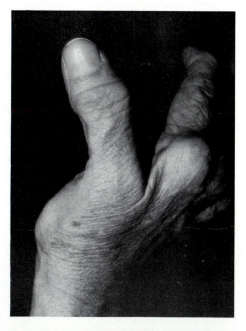

Fig. 9-8. Type IV thumb deformity. In this deformity the posture is one of adduction of the metacarpal and radial abduction of the proximal phalanx. (Courtesy Dr. E.A. Nalebuff, Brookline, Mass.)

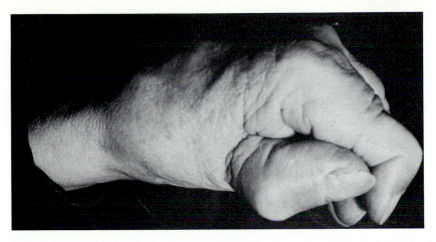

Fig. 9-9. Instability of the thumb. Absorption and instability of the metacarpophalangeal joint of this thumb allowed lateral instability, which totally destroyed the power of controlled pinch.

produce extension of the metacarpophalangeal and flexion of the interphalangeal joint. This self-perpetuating deformity is similar to the swan-neck collapse deformity seen in the finger.

TYPE IV

There is one other deformity of the rheumatoid thumb that Nalebuff considers can be usefully classified. Probably the precipitating synovitis occurs at the carpometa-carpal joint, but it must be closely associated with a synovitis of the metacarpophalan-geal joint, since the posture is one of adduction of the metacarpal and radial abduction of the proximal phalanx (Fig. 9-8). This deformity is known in nonrheumatoid hands as game-keeper's thumb because it is produced by specific occupational patterns.

Noncollapse deformities

An unstable single joint of the thumb will produce a deformity that is not neces-sarily associated with a collapse of the whole thumb posture. Occasionally more than one joint can be involved without concomitant collapse of the whole articular chain. The classic example of this type of deformity is seen in arthritis mutilans. This rela-tively uncommon variety of rheumatoid disease is characterized by gross bone absorption in the region of the joint, causing instability of the digit. Vainio notes that this deformity was first given the name "la main en lorgnette," or opera-glass hand, because the transverse folds of the skin of the fingers resembled a folded telescope. Mutilans deformities of the hand are especially crippling in the thumb. Instability of the interphalangeal joint shortens the functional length of the thumb and thereby destroys the single-handed power of grasp used for large objects. Patients are forced to use both hands to hold such objects as a drinking glass. A similar functional short-ening of the thumb is produced by absorption and instability of the metacarpophalan-geal joint (Fig. 9-9). Any lateral instability of this joint totally destroys the power of pinch prehension. When the metacarpophalangeal joint retains lateral stability, the destruction of prehension is not severe unless the interphalangeal joint is also unstable.

CLINICAL TREATMENT

Stability is more important for useful function of the thumb than movement, particularly at the metacarpophalangeal and interphalangeal joints. If a good range of motion is present in these joints, the vital carpometacarpal joint can even be fused for localized destruction, provided there is no pantrapezial involvement. The best position is about 35 degrees of abduction and 10 degrees of extension of the joint.

Although fusion has been used for many years, particularly in younger patients, excision of the trapezium with or without prosthetic replacement can provide stability and acceptable motion. Each operation and each implant device have their supporters, and the indications for the various combinations appear to overlap. A recent study of trapeziectomy by Amadio, Millender, and Smith in a comparable series of 45 patients did not show any significant difference between the results obtained by an "anchovy" tendon implant and a Silastic replacement. No matter what type of procedure is used for retaining motion at the basal thumb joint, meticulous restoration of the ligamentous supports of the joint is essential. In early degrees of joint instability, ligamentous reconstruction may well be sufficient.

Although local arthritic changes in the metacarpophalangeal joint can be treated by prosthetic substitution, the joint is more often fused. The same provision of stability by fusion is usually indicated for the interphalangeal joint with prosthetic replacement being rarely, if ever, indicated.

The osteoarthritic thumb

Osteoarthritic or posttraumatic degenerative changes can occur in any of the three joints of the thumb, particularly after direct violence to the articular surface. Because a painfree thumb is essential for normal functional use, some form of corrective surgery is usually necessary. The joint most commonly painful is the carpometacarpal joint.

CARPOMETACARPAL JOINT

In many instances the onset of pain in the carpometacarpal joint is associated with hypermobility of the joint. This idiopathic hypermobility is more common in women and is probably a major factor in producing the common arthrosis of this joint. Persistent hypermobility predisposes the joint to trauma and increasing damage to the articular surface. Restoration of ligament stability will not only relieve the pain and stabilize the joint but, when done prior to the onset of articular damage, may prevent or at least retard subsequent joint degeneration.

Eaton and Littler have discussed this condition in great detail in their paper; they stress that there is a large group of patients, predominantly postmenopausal women, in whom painful, progressively unstable carpometacarpal joints develop. Symptoms usually begin with a painful synovitis in the dominant thumb during the fifth decade of life. These authors have described four states of carpometacarpal arthrosis as follows.

Stage I. In the synovitis phase, before significant capsular laxity has developed, x-ray examination may show slight widening of the joint space (joint capsule distention caused by effusion), normal articular contours, and less than one third subluxation in any projection.

Stage II. Significant capsular laxity is present in this stage. There may be at least one third subluxation of the joint. The instability is particularly apparent in stress x-ray examinations. Small bone or calcific fragments less than 2mm in diameter are present, usually adjacent to the palmar or dorsal facets of the trapezium.

Stage III. Greater than one third subluxation is present. Fragments greater than 2mm are present dorsally or palmarly, usually in both locations. There is slight joint-space narrowing.

Stage IV. Advanced degenerative changes are now present. This stage is generally applicable to rheumatoid arthritis, although this process will produce more joint collapse than sclerosis and osteophyte formation. Major subluxation is apparent, and the joint space is narrow with cystic and sclerotic subchondral bone changes. The margins of the trapezium show lipping and osteophyte formation, and there is significant erosion of the dorsoradial facet of the trapezium.

CAPSULAR RECONSTRUCTION

In the synovitis stage, splinting and antiinflammatory medication may temporarily relieve the pain; but splinting the thumb severely compromises hand function, and most patients remove the splint. Weakness, persistent unrelieved pain, and demonstrable instability show the presence of articular surface deterioration. For these early cases capsular reconstruction is indicated rather than prosthetic replacement or joint fusion. Several ligament reconstruction procedures have been described, but I use these authors' methods to reinforce the existing palmar ligament that inserts on the basal beak of the metacarpal and create a new radial ligament perpendicular to it.

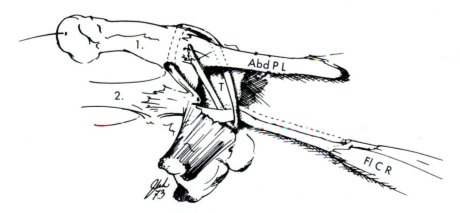

Fig. 9-10. Carpometacarpal joint capsule reconstruction. A new ligament is made from a strip half the width of the flexor carpi radialis tendon. This "ligament" is passed through a hole made in the first metacarpal and secured in place. (From Eaton, R.G., and Littler, J.W.: Ligamentous reconstruction for the painful thumb carpometacarpal joint, J. Bone Joint Surg. **55-A:**1655-66, 1973.)

The detailed description of the operative technique should be read in Eaton and Littler's paper before attempting this procedure because many details essential to the success of the operation are carefully described. The new "ligament" is made from a strip half the width of the flexor carpi radialis tendon. It is made from the radial half of the tendon, 6 cm long, and left attached distally. This ligament is then passed through a tunnel created in the metacarpal from the apex of the palmar beak to the dorsum of the metacarpal. It is stitched to the periosteum where it emerges on the dorsum, passed beneath the abductor pollicis longus and the extensor pollicis brevis, looped around the intact flexor carpi radialis, and finally stitched to the radial margin of the joint (Fig. 9-10). The joint must be completely reduced before the new ligament is sewn in place. Postoperative immobilization for at least a month is mandatory.

This is an excellent operation for patients with the minimal articular damage of Stages I and II. Patients with the moderately advanced Stage III changes sometimes do well, but those with the Stage IV changes would probably do better with prosthetic replacement or arthrodesis.

PROSTHETIC REPLACEMENT

Replacement of one or the other side of the trapeziometacarpal joint or even the whole joint is now possible. A variety of devices are currently available, such as those designed by Ashworth-Blatt, Braun, de la Caffiniére, Eaton, Kessler, Mayo, Niebauer, and Swanson; no doubt others will be forthcoming. Silastic implants are most commonly used. Some physicians resurface either the trapezial or metacarpal articular surface, and others replace the trapezium. Articulated devices that are held in place by methyl methacrylate are also available. I have not used all of these devices. I would strongly advise a careful study of the available literature before placing one of these implants for the first time. When both sides of the joint need replacement, I have a personal preference for the Niebauer device, because its tie strings provide a secure resistance to dislocation of the prosthesis.

There are several operative approaches to the basal joint of the thumb. Most surgeons use the straight radial approach paralleling the extensor pollicis brevis described by Gervis in 1949; others use Wagner's J-shaped radiopalmar approach. In recent years I have come to prefer a C-shaped modification of the Wagner J in which the incision passes around the base of the thumb with the concavity facing distally. Immediately beneath the skin lie important veins and branches of the superficial radial nerve that must be gently retracted toward the dorsal and palmar ends of the incision.

The capsule is incised transversely and carefully dissected back toward the metacarpal shaft and scaphoid for later replacement. The trapezium is usually removed more easily by cutting it up into major fragments. It is important to remove the spur of bone that is frequently found between the first and second metacarpal bases. The base of the metacarpal is squared off and the medullary canal reamed out to receive the stem of the prosthesis. If the Niebauer prosthesis is used, the two strong ties are passed through and tied into the flexor carpi radialis tendon lying in the depths of the wound. I have always found this satisfactory, but it should be noted that Niebauer now recommends that the ties be passed up through the base of the index metacarpal and tied off at holes drilled at the midpoint of the metacarpal shaft. Two additional holes are needed at the base of the thumb metacarpal through which two thinner ties are passed and tied. These ties retain the prosthetic stem in its correct place while fibrous tissue is growing into the Dacron cover of the stem.

Whatever form of replacement is used, I believe it vital to reconstruct and reinforce the capsule over the joint. The two portions of the capsule should be overlapped if possible, and then portions of the abductor pollicis longus tendon should be used as a superficial reinforcement for the capsular repair. The use of a slip of the flexor carpi radialis tendon for additional reinforcement, as described by Swanson, is also useful.

I close the skin with 5-0 nylon sutures and do not use a drain. The thumb is immobilized in the position of opposition using a split, below-the-elbow cast. Skin sutures are removed 2 weeks later, and a complete below-the-elbow cast that incorporates the thumb metacarpophalangeal joint is kept on for another 6 weeks.

Immobilization for this length of time is not needed for total joint replacement devices, nor is it probably needed for Niebauer's "tie-in" trapezium prosthesis. However, I have seen no long-term ill effects from this immobilization time, and I believe it gives proper protection to the capsular repair.

The rheumatoid thumb

The fundamental objective in the treatment of the rheumatoid thumb is the restoration and maintenance of stable motion.

It must be accepted that splinting the thumb accomplishes little. Splinting cannot affect the progress of soft-tissue disease, and there is no form of splinting that can effectively prevent the development of an intrinsic-plus contracture. In the late stages of an intrinsic-plus deformity, there is no form of splinting that will correct the position or restore function to the thumb.

Splinting can be useful as a temporary measure to demonstrate to a patient the increase in function that would result from a proposed fusion. The basic problem with external splinting is the impossibility of obtaining an adequate grip on the unstable thumb without covering a large part of its tactile, palmar surface and depriving its joints of essential motion.

GENERAL OPERATIVE INDICATIONS

Surgical correction of thumb deformities still tends to be one of the most neglected areas in treatment of the rheumatoid hand. Great improvements can be made by surgery, but procedures must be carefully planned because rheumatoid disease is a continuing process, and the state of function of the hand will change; therefore the functional effects of any particular operation may also change. Synovectomy has a definite place in the treatment of early disease, but most patients show such a combination of deformities that synovectomy alone is inadequate. Pure intrinsic-plus deformity of the thumb can be relieved by an operation that is basically similar to that used for intrinsic-plus deformity of the finger. There are, however, certain technical differences in the procedure for the thumb.

In established adduction contracture, the thumb can be mobilized by operative release of the adductor muscle or its overlying fascia. Additional work is often necessary on the carpometacarpal joint, since primary disease or secondary contractures of this joint may prevent full mobilization of the thumb.

Tendon function of the thumb is often compromised, and careful examination is necessary to establish the loss of function and site of rupture. Loss of flexion of the interphalangeal joint is almost invariably caused by attrition rupture of the flexor pollicis longus on a spur of the scaphoid. Control can best be established by transferring the superficialis tendon of the ring finger. I have not had good results using cable grafts. Even if fusion of the interphalangeal joint is used instead of a tendon transfer, exploration of the wrist, particularly on the floor of the flexor canal, is necessary to remove bony spicules that might later cause rupture of the index profundus tendon.

Extensor power is usually lost by attenuation or rupture of the extensor pollicis longus at the level of the metacarpophalangeal joint. Power is easily restored by transferring the extensor indicis proprius and sewing it in tightly. The repair should be splinted for at least a month and protected against strong pull for another 2 weeks. If the interphalangeal joint lies in hyperextension, but retains both flexor and extensor power, it can be secured into flexion through tenodesis by splitting the terminal portion of the flexor tendon and attaching it to the neck of the proximal phalanx with unabsorbable sutures. I transfix the joint in about 30 degrees of flexion with a Kirschner wire before completing the tenodesis and leave the wire in place for 3 weeks.

Particular care must be taken when fusion is considered. When a joint is fused, the increased stability that results often puts undue strain on an adjacent joint, which may develop troublesome symptoms.

The patient illustrated in Fig. 9-11 became progressively more handicapped as the interphalangeal joint of her thumb became less stable. The situation was aggravated by a previously performed fusion of the proximal interphalangeal joint of the index finger. In addition, there was marked disease in the metacarpophalangeal joints of both the thumb and the index finger. Stability and movement were restored to the index finger by prosthetic replacement, but fusion of the interphalangeal joint was the only possible means of supplying stability to the thumb. This stability was achieved at the expense of some function, leaving the patient with a very rigid form of tip pinch.

The problem of fusion is more often not how to obtain a firm fusion but deciding whether one or two joints should be fused. Fusion of the interphalangeal joint and/or the metacarpophalangeal joint must not be undertaken unless there is adequate stability of the carpometacarpal joint.

In the normal hand of a patient with isolated degenerative arthritis of the carpometacarpal joint, fusion of the base of the metacarpal to the trapezium is sometimes advised. This operation is not advisable for the rheumatoid hand because it imposes appreciable functional limitations on even a normal hand. In the normal hand degenerative changes in the carpal joints cause decreasing movement only with increasing

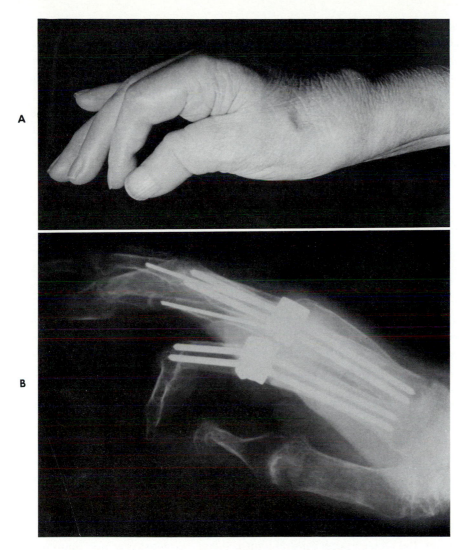

Fig. 9-11. Instability of interphalangeal joint of thumb. Rheumatoid disease of the interphalangeal joint of the thumb, leading to lateral instability, is a gross handicap to pinch. **A,** Lateral deviation occurring at this joint in the hand of a patient who previously had a surgical fusion of the proximal interphalangeal joint of the index finger. **B,** Prosthetic replacement of the metacarpophalangeal joint of the index finger, which was necessary to stabilize this finger so that lateral pinch could be used. The interphalangeal joint of the thumb is completely destroyed. Fusion of this joint supplied stability to the thumb but at the expense of function.

age. In the rheumatoid hand these changes occur very early and are often already present at the time of the proposed fusion. Thus fusion of the carpometacarpal joint results in a thumb that sticks out as a rigid pillar from the palm of the hand. The thumb is an obstruction when the patient attempts to place the hand in a confined space or lift any large, flat object with the palm of the hand.

In the rheumatoid hand it is essential to maintain movement at the carpometacarpal joint, and this movement must be provided before any more distal joints are fused. It is usually necessary to carry out some form of excisional arthroplasty to provide the necessary mobility. Several different procedures including prosthetic replacements have been developed for this joint. I believe that when this operation is necessary, it should be performed as a first, and separate, procedure. In many patients an adduction contracture of the thumb will also be present and should be relieved at the same operation. A short postoperative period of immobilization is necessary, but it must be followed by active exercises planned to produce controlled movement of the metacarpal.

After a satisfactory arc of movement has been regained at the carpometacarpal joint, fusion of one or both of the other thumb joints can be carried out. Dual joint fusion has the functional disadvantage of producing a completely rigid pillar of bone that can be moved only at the basal carpometacarpal joint. Although the two joints can be placed in a functional position, the long arch of bone cannot adapt to variously shaped objects. The functional limitations of this type of thumb are great, but patients are grateful after the operation, since it affords them a limited degree of function that they previously did not possess. I consider gross lateral instability of both joints to be an indication for fusion of both joints or for fusion of one joint and prosthetic replacement of the other. The thumb prosthesis has been designed for this problem. The hinge replaces the metacarpophalangeal joint, and the phalangeal prongs are sufficiently long to be used as internal fixation in fusion of the interphalangeal joint (Fig. 9-16).

If there is reasonable lateral stability in either joint, I do not believe that there is an absolute indication for fusion of one joint in preference to the other. Clayton believes that the metacarpophalangeal joint is of less functional importance than the interphalangeal joint and is therefore the joint of choice for fusion. I believe that this view is correct for normal hands but is not of great importance in thumbs with greatly reduced functional capacity. The factors of greatest importance are the degree of lateral instability of the joint in which movement is to be retained and the posture of the fingers against which the thumb will work.

When the metacarpophalangeal joint is fused, the most common optimum position is about 20 degrees of flexion and 15 degrees of both internal rotation and abduction. Fusion of the interphalangeal joint in the straight position usually provides excellent function. It is probably wise to use some form of internal splinting with a bone graft in both joints to encourage union. For those patients in whom bone absorption has caused gross shortening of the thumb, additional length can be provided by a bone graft of appropriate size.

SPECIFIC OPERATIVE INDICATIONS

Synovectomy. In early disease before postural deformity has developed, excision of synovium from the distal two joints of the thumb is an excellent operation. Synovectomy of the carpometacarpal joint is apparently not often done. I have done few myself and found no report of any series in the literature. Synovectomy of the metacarpophalangeal joint is rarely done so early in the disease that a "pure" synovectomy is performed. More often some form of extensor hood reconstruction and realignment of the tendons are also necessary. Inglis and colleagues, in reviewing their cases, commented that reconstruction, in contrast to fusion, should be used when the joint has a normal passive arc of motion without subluxation and good lateral stability when the thumb is extended. In the 21 patients they followed, half were free of pain, 6 had pain with extreme activity and 2 with mild activity, and 2 had pain at rest. Late lateral instability developed in the latter 4 patients. Those who had recurrence of deformity after synovectomy and dorsal hood reconstruction proved on review to have been unsuitable for reconstruction in the first place because ligamentous support was marginal or the thumb could not be extended to a neutral position, indicating a subluxation. Synovitis did not recur during the follow-up period, which varied between 8 years and 12 months.

I completely agree with these authors in their support of the concept that "a little joint motion when painless and stable is better than no motion." My only reservation is that my own follow-up on synovectomy has not been so pleasing. Eleven percent have shown a recurrent synovitis in the metacarpophalangeal joint, and a depressing 50% in the interphalangeal joint.

Intrinsic release operation. Intrinsic contracture over the metacarpophalangeal joint of the thumb can occur in isolation but more commonly is a secondary or later result of an extrinsic-minus deformity. When it does occur in isolation it resembles a Type I deformity but is distinguished from it by demonstrating the presence of an active pull in the extensor pollicis brevis. In addition, it is necessary to demonstrate a tightening of resistance to passive flexion of the interphalangeal joint while the metacarpophalangeal joint is held in hyperextension. In early cases excellent relief is obtained, and even in well-established cases the restoration of function can be significant (Fig. 9-12).

Type I deformity. In early stages of Type I collapse, before either the flexion deformity or the palmar subluxation of the metacarpophalangeal joint has become fixed, synovectomy with or without restoration of extensor power is the operation of choice (Fig. 9-13). It is usually impossible to satisfactorily reattach the attenuated tendon of the extensor pollicis brevis, and Nalebuff has therefore introduced an operation rerouting the extensor pollicis longus tendon.

Two prerequisites determine the feasibility of this operation:

1. The surgeon must be able to passively correct any flexion deformity or palmar subluxation of the joint.

2. Clinical and x-ray examination should establish that little if any degenerative change has occured in this joint.

If these requirements can be met, an excellent powerful extensor of the metacarpophalangeal joint can be provided by rerouting the proximal end of the tendon through a hole in the dorsal capsule and suturing the cut end back on itself. Extension of the interphalangeal joint is provided by the intrinsic muscles.

In late fixed stages of this deformity the basic treatment is arthrodesis of either or both of the metacarpophalangeal and interphalangeal joints (Fig. 9-13). This procedure will restore stability and relieve pain. The choice of which joint to fuse can be

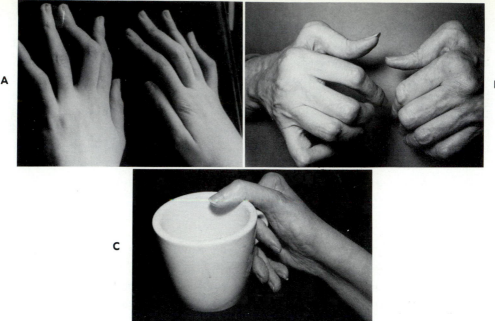

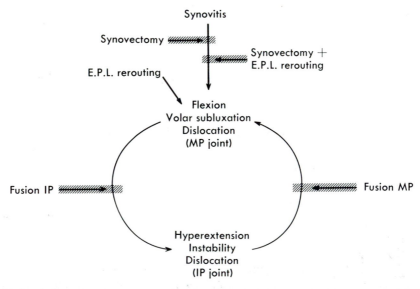

Fig. 9-12. Intrinsic contracture of thumb. **A,** The patient whose hands are shown had rheumatoid disease of the hand, but the thumbs were not affected at this time. **B,** Eight years later typical deformity of contracture of the thumb intrinsic muscles can be seen. The metacarpophalangeal joint could not be extended, and the hyperextension of the interphalangeal joint became steadily greater as the intrinsic contracture increased. **C,** After operative release of the intrinsic muscles the normal functional arch of the thumb was restored.

Synovitis

Synovectomy

Synovectomy +
E.P.L. rerouting

E.P.L. rerouting

Flexion
Volar subluxation
Dislocation
(MP joint)

Fusion IP

Fusion MP

Hyperextension
Instability
Dislocation
(IP joint)

Fig. 9-13. Surgical treatment of Type I deformities. This chart correlates the various appropriate surgical procedures with the different stages of Type I deformity. (From Nalebuff, E.A.: Bull. Hosp. Joint Dis. **29:**119-137, 1968.)

made only after a thorough review of the state of the thumb. In some patients the major functional loss is at the interphalangeal joint, where gross instability causes collapse with every pinch motion. Fusion in a straight position gives good function even though the metacarpophalangeal joint may be in flexion. When fusion of the metacarpophalangeal joint is the choice, I usually fix it in about 15 to 20 degrees of flexion and about 15 degrees of internal rotation; the degree of abduction needed, if any, is dictated by the posture of the fingers against which the thumb will be working. As long as there is satisfactory carpometacarpal joint motion, both joints can be fused, although I believe that this entails a significant loss of function. It is for this sort of problem that I occasionally use a prosthesis (Fig. 9-16).

Type II deformity. Patients with the uncommon Type II deformity have great difficulty grasping large objects because of the hyperextension of the interphalangeal joint and adduction of the metacarpal. The first objective of surgery is to bring the adducted metacarpal out into abduction. Although this can be done by fusion of the carpometacarpal joint, an arthroplasty of the joint is a better alternative. The distal phalanx can be brought down into a straight line with the proximal phalanx either by tenotomy of the terminal extensor tendon or by fusion of the interphalangeal joint. I regard the latter as the better choice.

Type III deformity. Type III deformity is the most difficult to treat, since it combines hyperextension of the metacarpophalangeal joint with flexion of the distal joint. Two types can be distinguished: one in which the metacarpophalangeal joint can be passively corrected and the other in which it cannot.

If the metacarpophalangeal joint retains a reasonable degree of lateral stability after it is passively corrected, it is best to fuse the carpometacarpal joint so that the metacarpal is held in abduction. This realignment of the metacarpal is helpful in maintaining the corrected position of the metacarpophalangeal joint. An additional useful way of maintaining this correction is to fix the joint in about 20 degrees of flexion by Kessler's method, using the tendon the extensor pollicis brevis.

When the metacarpophalangeal joint cannot be passively corrected or when it is grossly unstable, it seems reasonable to fuse it. But this type of problem must be carefully evaluated since a combination of fusion of the metacarpophalangeal and the carpometacarpal joint would leave a virtually useless rigid thumb. If there is any possibility that fusion of the metacarpophalangeal joint can be postponed, the first metacarpal should be brought out into abduction first by such procedures as arthroplasty of the carpometacarpal joint, excision of the trapezium, or even osteotomy of the metacarpal. Fusion of the interphalangeal joint should be postponed until the position of the metacarpophalangeal joint is determined, since its position will influence the selection of the best angle for interphalangeal fusion.

Type IV deformity. The prime factor in maintaining Type IV deformities appears to be the fascial aponeurosis covering the adductor muscle. Kessler advised that the aponeurosis should be incised over the entire length of the first web space parallel to the first metacarpal. Occasionally a Z-plasty of the thumb web skin is necessary, and surgical decompression of the carpometacarpal joint is almost invariably necessary. Excisional arthroplasty is usually best, and Kessler has devised a silicone spacer to replace the excised base of the metacarpal; its use must be associated with careful reconstruction of the joint capsule.

Once the metacarpal has been fully mobilized into abduction, the metacarpophalangeal joint is stabilized either by arthrodesis or by tightening of its ulnar and palmar supporting tissues. It is important to replace the extensor pollicis longus tendon, which is displaced radially.

OPERATIONS
Synovectomy

Excision of the synovium from the distal two joints of the thumb is usually carried out at the same operation. The interphalangeal joint is commonly approached by a dorsal curvilinear incision. After the skin flaps have been developed and mobilized, the thin capsule tissue on either side of the central extensor tendon is identified. The joint can be successfully cleared of virtually all synovium by entering the cavity on each side of the extensor tendon between its lateral edge and the dorsal edge of the adjacent collateral ligament. Occasionally the major portion of the synovial disease lies on the palmar aspect of the joint. In these patients it is better to approach the joint through a lateral neutral border incision, clearing both dorsal and palmar aspects of the joint. If the joint is very lax after synovectomy, temporary splinting by Kirschner wire fixation, with the joint held straight or in a few degrees of flexion, is useful.

The metacarpophalangeal joint is readily approached through a dorsal longitudinal curvilinear incision stretching from about the middle of the metacarpal to the middle of the proximal phalanx. An incision of this length gives adequate exposure to the sides of the joint and allows additional procedures such as intrinsic release, extensor tendon surgery, or hood reconstruction to be done.

If the synovectomy is done relatively early in the disease and no additional work is to be done, I usually approach the joint cavity by incising between the two extrinsic extensor tendons. If the extensor pollicis brevis is badly attenuated and a rerouting of the extensor pollicis longus is necessary, this tendon is divided just distal to the metacarpophalangeal joint and dissected proximally. The synovium can then be excised, with particular attention being paid to the tongue of synovium lying between the metacarpal head and the collateral ligaments. Removal of any palmar synovium under the metacarpal neck is made easier by flexion of the joint.

If no other reconstruction is necessary, the two extensor tendons should be approximated, but sutures must not be passed through the tendons themselves. A thorough synovectomy often leaves significant joint laxity, and temporary Kirschner wire splinting in almost full extension for about 10 days is helpful. After removal of the skin stitches active motion should be encouraged; if there is significant extensor lag, a small dorsal night splint can be tried for a month or 6 weeks. Such a splint is difficult to apply, and about the only effective way is to strap it directly to the whole length of the thumb with adhesive tape.

Extensor pollicis longus rerouting

After the metacarpophalangeal joint has been approached through a dorsal skin incision, the extensor pollicis longus tendon is divided just distal to the line of the

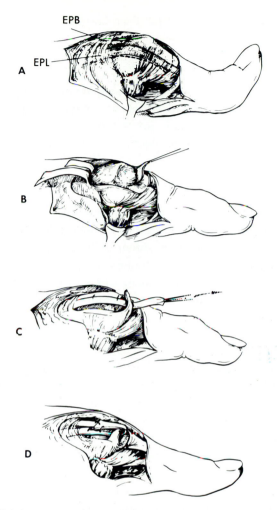

Fig. 9-14. Extensor pollicis longus rerouting. **A,** The incision in the extensor apparatus. (*EPB,* Extensor pollicis brevis tendon; *EPL,* extensor pollicis longus tendon.) **B,** The two extensor tendons have been separated and turned proximally. **C,** The extensor pollicis longus has been passed through a cuff of tissue at the base of the proximal phalanx. **D,** The tendon has been resutured back to itself and the extensor pollicis brevis tendon. Note that the intrinsic muscles are shown reattached to the extensor apparatus to restore interphalangeal joint extension. (From Nalebuff, E.A.: Bull. Hosp. Joint Dis. **29:**119-137, 1968.)

joint and dissected out from the hood. The attenuated extensor pollicis brevis tendon is also dissected from the base of the proximal phalanx and detached from the hood (Fig. 9-14).

The dorsal capsule of the joint is dissected up and left firmly attached to the base of the proximal phalanx. A hole is then made in the midline position and the proximal cut end of the extensor pollicis longus passed through. The tendon is pulled back over itself until the tension is adequate to hold the joint in extension. After the folded-back end has been sutured to the underlying tendon, the extensor pollicis brevis is pulled distally and sutured into the side of the extensor pollicis longus.

In this procedure the intrinsic tendons on either side of the joint are left intact and through their cross attachments to the distal portion of the extensor pollicis longus provide interphalangeal joint extension. It is often helpful to tighten or imbricate the transverse and interlacing fibers to ensure direct action on the stump of the extensor pollicis longus.

Postoperatively the thumb can be held in a splint or plaster-of-paris cast with both distal joints in extension. The skin sutures are removed at about 10 to 14 days, at which time the immobilization can be altered to allow active motion of the interphalangeal joint. The metacarpophalangeal joint should be supported in extension for 4 to 6 weeks.

Intrinsic release of the thumb

Deformity of the thumb resulting from intrinsic contracture can be relieved in its early stages by surgery. In the late stages of the deformity some increase in function can be obtained, but full restoration cannot be expected.

If a synovectomy is unnecessary, the joint is approached through two incisions, one on either side of the metacarpophalangeal joint along the side of the joint to the midpoint of the proximal phalanx. A synovectomy is usually a necessary part of the operation, and the usual dorsal longitudinal curvilinear skin incision should be used.

The wings of the intrinsic hood of the metacarpophalangeal joint lie immediately beneath the subcutaneous tissues. Retraction of the skin edges of either limb of the incision will show the hood fibers in the depth of the wound. A blunt hook is passed beneath the free edge of the hood on either side of the joint. Sliding the hook backward and forward will free the undersurface of the hood from any adhesions. When the hood has been completely mobilized, it is released on both sides. The tendon of the long extensor of the thumb passes over the dorsum of the proximal phalanx and is the division between the two wings of the hood. An incision is made on each side of the extensor tendon, extending from a point just distal to the metacarpophalangeal joint to the point where the two free borders of the hood join the long extensor tendon. The free edges are cut through and the wing tissues turned proximally. It will be found that the hyperextension of the interphalangeal joint is considerably relieved after both free edges are cut through, but the flexion deformity of the metacarpophalangeal joint is not usually corrected at this stage.

The two incisions releasing the wings of the hood will have to be extended proximally for a varying distance through the transverse fibers until the flexion deformity of the metacarpophalangeal joint is overcome. When this joint can be fully extended, the tissues around the neck of the metacarpal should be exposed. The origins of the capsule, the periosteum, and the muscle fibers in this region are the sites to which the two detached wings of the hood should be attached. The wings are trimmed of excessive length and sewed securely to the tissues on both sides of the neck of the metacarpal. It does not matter to which soft tissues the wings are attached, provided the site of attachment is far distal on the metacarpal but is proximal to the metacarpophalangeal joint.

If a synovectomy is necessary, the joint is opened after the intrinsic release has been completed. If the flexion contracture of the joint cannot be fully corrected after the synovectomy, the joint must be fully flexed and a knife blade must be passed between the two bones to detach the palmar plate from the base of the proximal phalanx.

After completion of the synovectomy, the collateral ligaments are tested for stability. If an appreciable degree of instability is present, or if the ligaments have dislocated to a position low on the side of the joint, the ligaments must be tightened. Holes are drilled through the cortex of the bone and sutures are passed through these holes, anchoring the ligaments to the neck of the metacarpal (Fig. 8-7, p. 198). Although this procedure may partially restrict flexion of the joint, the added stability is of greater importance than the lack of a few degrees of flexion.

The wound in the capsule of the joint is closed with a few fine catgut sutures, and the skin incision is closed with interrupted fine nylon sutures. A fluffed-up compression dressing is applied and held in place with a self-adherent cotton bandage.

I use a complete plaster-of-paris cast up to the tip of the thumb for patients with severe deformity and particularly for those in whom the thumb did not readily correct after the release operation. The normal arch of the thumb is maintained by the cast, which should be left in place for 3 weeks. I do not use plaster-of-paris immobilization for patients with mild deformity; instead, I encourage early movement after removal of the skin sutures.

Release of thumb web contracture

Release of thumb web contracture is usually combined with an arthroplasty of the carpometacarpal joint but can be used as a solitary procedure when the joint is normal. The principle of the operation is to release the fascial covering of the muscle and, if this is not sufficient, to also strip the first metacarpal of all muscular attachments on the dorsoulnar surfaces. This releases the bone to the full power of the muscles of the thenar eminence that produce rotation and opposition.

The approach is along the same line used for arthroplasty of the carpometacarpal joint. The incision extends along the dorsoulnar border of the first metacarpal from the carpometacarpal joint to a point just distal to the metacarpophalangeal joint. Since there is no primary loss of skin, there is no need for skin grafting to supply extra skin to the web space. It is often helpful, however, to incorporate a Z-plasty into the incision, thereby allowing an increase in abduction of the thumb without a great increase in the tension on the edges of the incision. The Z is planned with its central third lying along the edge of the web and the two other limbs arising at an angle of 60 degrees from each end of the central limb (Fig. 9-15). The dorsal flap is planned to be based on the thumb, thereby allowing the proximal portion of the incision to be developed naturally from this flap.

As the skin incision is developed, it may be necessary to tie off a few dorsal veins crossing the field. It is wise to preserve these veins if their presence does not interfere with the operation. The dorsal branches of the radial nerve fanning out to supply the dorsum of the hand must be sought and preserved. The tendon of the extensor pollicis longus muscle crosses the operative field obliquely and should be released from its tendon sheath and retracted toward the second metacarpal.

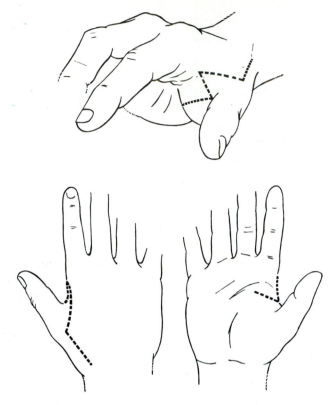

Fig. 9-15. Thumb web contracture. If a Z-plasty is incorporated into the skin incision, an increase in abduction of the thumb can be obtained without an increase in the tension on the edges of the skin incision. The central limb of the Z should lie along the edge of the thumb web.

The most superficial muscle encountered is the first dorsal interosseous. It arises by two heads from the adjacent sides of the first and second metacarpals. Beneath this muscle lies the conjoined tendon of the heads of the adductor pollicis muscle. Immediately on the palmar side of this tendon lies the neurovascular bundle to the ulnar side of the thumb. This bundle must be protected before the aponeurosis covering the muscle is fully exposed. The aponeurosis is frequently fibrosed and is a major factor in the development of the adduction contracture. It should be incised longitudinally over the entire length of the web parallel near the first metacarpal. If the adductor also has to be released, it is my practice to excise a small portion of the conjoined adductor tendon and to tuck the muscular end toward the ulnar side of the cleft beneath the first dorsal interosseous muscle to prevent its adherence to the original site of attachment.

After the fascia and muscles have been released, passive abduction, rotation, and opposition should be tried. It is often necessary to release the tissues on the ulnar side of the carpometacarpal joint to obtain full correction, but before doing so it is wise to identify and protect the radial artery, which lies deep in the wound at this site.

Before the incision is closed with interruped fine sutures, the skin over the dorsum of the second and third metacarpals should be loosened by a subcutaneous spreading of blunt scissor ends. This maneuver mobilizes the skin, thereby reducing tension on the edges of the wound. If a Z-plasty has been used, the flaps must be rotated and the incisions closed with interrupted sutures. The skin sutures should be placed at close intervals (at least every 5 mm), because there may be considerable tension on the wound edges after the the thumb is placed in the fully corrected position. No drain is necessary if a compression dressing is properly applied. The thumb is brought into full abduction and rotated to lie in a plane opposite the third metacarpal. Fluffed-up dressings must be packed against both palmar and dorsal sides of the thumb web and between the fingers and thumb at the distal edge of the web. The dressings are held in place by a self-adherent cotton bandage, and one or two plaster-of-paris bandages are used to protect the position of immobilization. The bandages are kept in place for approximately 16 to 18 days. The skin sutures are then removed and active exercises started.

Arthroplasty of carpometacarpal joint

Arthroplasty can be used alone or in combination with other procedures planned to restore mobility to the metacarpal of the thumb. The operation is commonly combined with a release of the web space between the first and second metacarpals. Prosthetic replacement for this joint is described earlier in this chapter under the osteoarthritic thumb. When web space release is also done, the postoperative immobilization period must last 6 weeks.

Fusion of thumb joints

CARPOMETACARPAL JOINT

I believe that fusion of the carpometacarpal joint is rarely indicated in the rheumatoid hand. If a sound indication has been established, then the method described by Carroll and Hill is probably the most satisfactory. Their operative approach has evolved from the method they have used in other small joints of the hand and does not require bone grafting. The proximal end of the metacarpal is made into a smoothly rounded blunt point, and the trapezium is carved into a cup-shaped receptacle for the metacarpal. The two bones are held together by Kirschner wire fixation.

METACARPOPHALANGEAL AND INTERPHALANGEAL JOINTS

Fusion of the metacarpophalangeal joint of the thumb is a good operation and is quite commonly practiced; Vainio reports a series of 102 cases. Nonunion did not occur in his series, in which the position of choice for fusion was slight flexion and abduction, with sufficient rotation for good pinch to be possible. Fusion of an unstable interphalangeal joint of the thumb is often helpful if there is reasonable controlled motion at the more proximal joints. It is often necessary to add a bone graft to maintain length of the thumb because of the destruction that usually occurs to the head of the proximal phalanx. It is uncommon for nonunion to occur.

I usually fuse these joints by following the principles of the Moberg fusion (p. 193). When fusion of the grossly unstable mutilans joints is being attempted, it is usually necessary to reinforce the intramedullary bone graft with Kirschner wire fixation.

The metacarpophalangeal joint should be fused in 20 degrees of flexion and 15 degrees of both internal rotation and abduction. The interphalangeal joint should be fused straight. Either joint is approached through a curvilinear, dorsal skin incision. The cutaneous nerves beneath these incisions must be carefully protected because, as Milford has stressed, they may supply the sensibility to the terminal pulp of the thumb.

In the metacarpophalangeal joint, care must be taken to preserve the extensor mechanism where it crosses the joint. The joint is opened and all granulation tissue and remains of synovial tissue are removed. Any remnants of articular cartilage and subchondral cortical bone are also removed. It is probably wise to use a bone graft at either joint, since even at the metacarpophalangeal joint there is rarely sufficient bone present for fusion to be obtained by simple immobilization. The graft should be taken from the tibia and shaped to fit the medullary canals of the bones on either side of the joint. If the thumb must be lengthened because of absorption around the joint, the graft is trimmed to provide the appropriate length in its middle section. Cancellous chips are obtained from the tibia and are packed around the joint area before the soft tissues are closed. If the bones are not stable on the graft, a Kirschner wire should be used for additional stability.

After the skin wound has been closed, the thumb is immobilized in plaster of paris. If the interphalangeal joint has been fused, the cast must extend to the tip of the thumb; if only the metacarpophalangeal joint has been fused, the interphalangeal joint can be left free. In the early postoperative weeks the cast must include the proximal part of the forearm. It is usually necessary to retain a cast for at least 2 months, but during the latter part of this time the cast can be changed to a smaller size. The smaller cast should start just distal to the wrist, include the thumb, and extend over the palm to the level of the metacarpophalangeal joints of the fingers. This smaller cast allows a good grip to be made and permits free movement of the wrist.

Prosthetic replacement of metacarpophalangeal joint

The ideal indication for prosthetic replacement of the metacarpophalangeal joint in the rheumatoid thumb is destruction without accompanying distortion of the proximal or distal joints. Such a situation rarely occurs. More common indications include joint destruction associated with stiffness of the basal and distal joints or hyperextension and instability of the distal joint.

Whatever device is used, it is essential that a careful reconstruction of the extensor apparatus be done and that this repair be protected by splinting for at least a month. If possible, the two components of each collateral ligament and the palmar plate should be left attached to the base of the proximal phalanx for later reattachment to the metacarpal neck.

Over 20 years ago, I introduced a two-pronged metal prosthesis for this joint. The distal prongs were made sufficiently long to be used as intramedullary pins for fusion of the interphalangeal joint when necessary (Fig. 9-16). A number of these devices

Flatt, AE.   Care of the Arthritic Hand
1983.

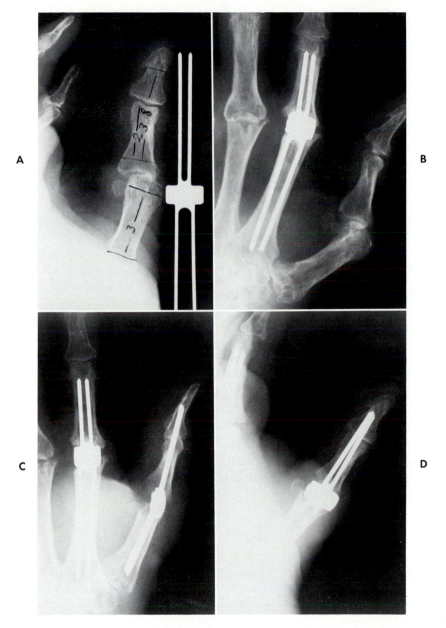

Fig. 9-16. Prosthetic replacement within the thumb. **A** and **B,** X-ray films of a thumb in which dislocation had occurred in two planes. Instability was also present at the interphalangeal joint. The figures in the x-ray film shown in **A** represent the measurements of the bones before prosthetic replacement. **C** and **D,** X-ray films of the prosthesis in place. Movement and stability have been supplied at the metacarpophalangeal joint, and the prosthetic prongs have been left long enough to aid in fusion of the interphalangeal joint.

have been used. Ferlich has reported his experience with nine of these prostheses followed-up for 3 months to 15 years. Bony resorption occurred around the prongs in every case, and fracture of the junctional screw happened in one case. Even with these problems, all interphalangeal joints fused, and the patients obtained 20 degrees of motion, which they found to be functional. All of the patients claimed to be satisfied with their results.

Despite this encouraging report, I believe this device has rightly been generally abandoned in favor of flexible implant and fusion of the interphalangeal joint as needed.

Swanson has reviewed 44 of these implants. All cases were not strictly comparable, and not all received the current high-performance elastomer implants. In general, however, the results were pleasing and stability of the joint was much improved postoperatively. The performance of activities of daily living improved in all but one patient whose implant fractured 7 months after arthroplasty.

When placing a flexible silicone implant in this joint, it is important to decompress the joint sufficiently to allow it to be easily brought up into full extension with the implant in place. This may require total release of the collateral ligaments and the palmar plate with significant resection of the metacarpal head and neck.

Careful reconstruction of the structures surrounding the joint is essential, since it is subject to significant forces during use. The ulnar collateral ligament must always be tested for lateral stability and may have to be attached using holes drilled in the metacarpal neck.

Swanson recommends that the extensor pollicis brevis be detached early in the procedure and later reattached by passing the sutures through two small holes drilled in the dorsum of the base of the proximal phalanx. The two intrinsic extensor expansions should then be brought up and sewn over the top of the pollicis brevis insertion. The extensor pollicis longus can either be joined to the brevis or sewn into the midportion of the phalanx in the midline.

The joint must be protected by a dorsal splint applied directly after postoperative swelling has subsided. Active motion can be started at a month, but night splinting is advisable for another month.

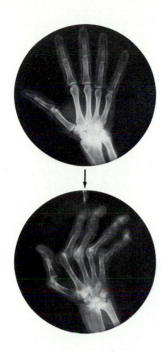

CHAPTER 10

Ulnar drift

Etiology
Intrinsic forces
    Wrist
    Extrinsic tendons
        Extensor tendons
        Flexor tendons
    Intrinsic muscles
    Force nucleus of Zancolli
    Extrinsic forces

Early ulnar drift

Treatment
Mild ulnar drift
Severe ulnar drift

Ulnar drift is not solely the prerogative of rheumatoid disease; it occurs in many other conditions. It has been shown to be present in congenital deformities, poliomyelitis, arthrogryposis, parkinsonism, and various occupations. The posture of ulnar drift is the end position produced by dynamic imbalance of forces within the hand. The problem is to identify any common factors that either from within or without the hand could produce this deformity in so many different conditions.

The term *ulnar drift* was originally coined by the late Dr. Sterling Bunnell nearly 30 years ago. It is a useful phrase for describing the result of a combination of two abnormalities of the metacarpophalangeal joint: ulnar deviation and ulnar shift (Fig. 10-1). *Ulnar deviation* is a deformity produced by the ulnar rotation of the proximal phalanx with respect to the metacarpal head. *Ulnar shift* is a deformity produced by the ulnar translation of the proximal phalanx base with respect to the metacarpal head.

ETIOLOGY

Ulnar deviation is present in the normal hand; at rest there is an ulnar inclination of the phalanges in relation to the line of the metacarpals that is greatest in the index finger (Fig. 10-2). This deviation becomes a threat to function only after it cannot be corrected. Ulnar shift is always a pathological state. I believe that this distinction into component parts is valid, since there are abnormal hands in which one or the other type can be distinguished and in which full ulnar drift ultimately develops.

The key to this problem must be in the alterations produced in the functional anatomy of the metacarpophalangeal joint and its surrounding structures. In recent years several detailed studies of this joint have been published, and prominent in this

255

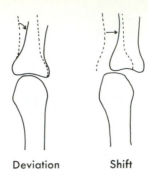

Deviation   Shift

Fig. 10-1. Ulnar drift. Ulnar drift is the product of ulnar deviation and ulnar shift. Deviation is a deformity produced by ulnar rotation of the proximal phalanx with respect to the metacarpal head. Shift is the deformity produced by ulnar translation of the proximal phalanx base with respect to the metacarpal head.

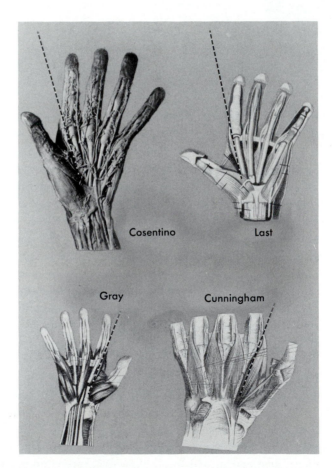

Fig. 10-2. Ulnar deviation of the index finger. Four standard texts of anatomy show that the index finger lies in deviation in relation to its metacarpal. The total index ray is only straight when the first dorsal interosseous muscle is acting strongly as an abductor. (From Flatt, A.E.: Plast. Reconstr. Surg. **37:**295-303, 1966.)

field are the works of Landsmeer, Backhouse, Straub, Hakstian and Tubiana, and Smith and Kaplan. Although there are areas of disagreement, or at least differences of emphasis in these papers, there is a general agreement on several important aspects of the anatomy. In many hand activities the metacarpophalangeal joints are used not in pure flexion but with ulnar deviation and rotation. On the radial side of the hand, the index and long finger metacarpals show a small sloping ulnar condyle and asymmetrical attachments of the collateral ligaments, so that rotation and deviation are an inevitable result of either passive or active flexion in these joints. During such motion the radial collateral ligament of the index finger acts as an anchor resisting the imposed forces, and any laxity in this ligament must have a profound influence on the integrity of this system.

The metacarpophalangeal joints, unlike the interphalangeal joints, normally have lateral mobility when in extension. The integrity and stability of this lateral movement are controlled by the intrinsic muscles and supported by the capsular and ligamentous structures. Acting on, and against, this joint are two force systems. One is the system of intrinsic forces generated within the hand by the actions of the extrinsic and intrinsic muscles, and the other is the system of extrinsic forces created by pressures of usage.

Intrinsic forces

WRIST

It is now well accepted that the posture of the wrist has a profound effect on the function of the digits. Shapiro was the first to document the relationship between wrist posture and the pathodynamics of ulnar drift. His study of the serial x-ray films of 100 rheumatoid hands showed a relationship between radial deviation of the metacarpus and carpus and the development of ulnar drift. He demonstrated that Landsmeer's concept of the "intercalcated bone" applies to the carpometacarpal bones as a unit; thus, when they deviate radially, there is a tendency for the fingers to pass into ulnar deviation, creating a zigzag deformity. Some physicians believe that much of the radial carpal deviation seen on the x-ray films is positional. However, the evidence would seem to be overwhelming that there is true merit in the concept of the intercalcated bone.

Pahle and Raunio's investigation of wrist-hand alignment following wrist fusions supported Shapiro's views invoking the intercalcated bone system. They showed that a radial tilt of the carpometacarpal unit greater than 5 degrees is associated with ulnar drift of the fingers. If the theory of zigzag collapse had merit, then it would be logical to expect occasional examples of radial drift. Fig. 10-3 shows ulnar destruction of the wrist joint to a greater extent than the radial. Radial drift of the index finger has resulted. Pahle and Raunio have shown similar examples in wrists fused in ulnar deviation. The importance of the study by Pahle and Raunio is in showing that it is the posture of the carpometacarpal unit and not the activity of the wrist motors that determines the digital deviation. Taleisnik has pointed out that patients with a normal wrist and paralysis of the extensor carpi ulnaris do not develop carpometacarpal deviation if all other supportive wrist structures are intact.

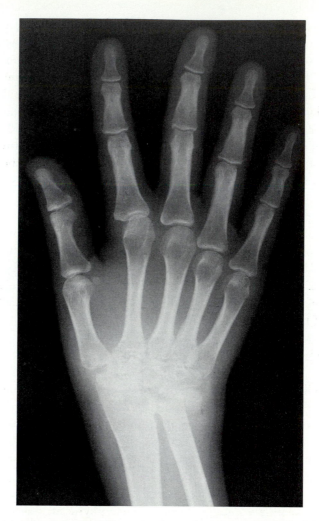

Fig. 10-3. The wrist and radial drift. With greater destruction of the ulnar half of the wrist joint, the carpometacarpal unit has tilted ulnarward and a radial drift of the index finger has occurred.

The wrist joint is only one link in the longitudinal chain over which pass the powerful extrinsic flexor and extensor tendons. When these tendons act over a weakened metacarpophalangeal joint, it is reasonable for this proximally acting force to induce a collapse of the system. Certainly as Linschied and Dobyns have pointed out the deformity increases during active use of the flexor muscles.

The basic movement in the zigzag collapse is an ulnar translation of the carpus along the inclined plane of the radial articular surface (Fig. 10-4). Taleisnik points out that this can occur as a result of the disorganization initiated by intraarticular synovitis and the consequent loss of ligament support. This then leads to changes in carpal function, particularly of the scaphoid. There is a widening of the scapholunate joint and palmar flexion of the scaphoid. Hastings and Evans have shown, by measurement, a proximal migration of the capitate into the space provided by destruction of the scapholunate ligament together with a palmar flexion of the scaphoid.

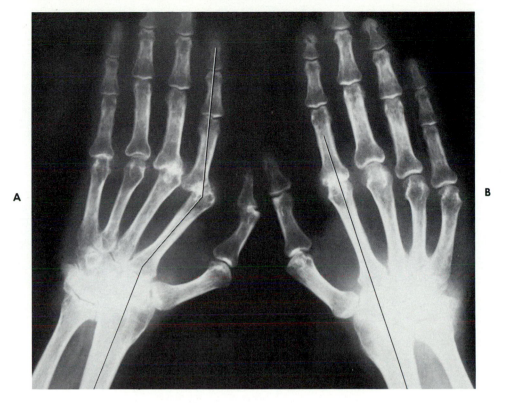

Fig. 10-4. The wrist and ulnar drift. **A,** With radial carpal collapse the unbalanced tendon forces produce the zigzag deformity of ulnar drift. **B,** If the carpal disease is even, tendon equilibrium is not disturbed and ulnar shift does not occur.

Collapse of the carpus does not inevitably initiate ulnar deviation of the fingers, but it certainly can do so. It will certainly aggravate a preexisting tendency to ulnar deviation and must adversely influence any surgical correction at the metacarpophalangeal joint level—particularly if the wrist imbalance is not corrected at the same operation.

Correction of the radial metacarpocarpal tilt is commonly done by extrinsic transfer. We analyzed the results of transferring extensor carpi radialis longus to extensor carpi ulnaris in 20 patients and showed that 13 had significant correction of their wrist deformity. However, the transferred tendon did not contract during active ulnar deviation of the wrist. In a concurrent laboratory study we demonstrated that the transferred tendon acts as a dynamic checkrein in helping rebalance the forces around the destroyed distal radioulnar joint.

EXTRINSIC TENDONS

In 1951 Snorrason commented on the ulnar deviating tendency of dislocated extensor tendons and also on the potential for a similar tendency in the flexor tendons. There is no general agreement among anatomists or clinicians about whether one or the other group is of more importance. The extensor tendons invite attention because they can be readily examined and deviations from their line of pull are easily

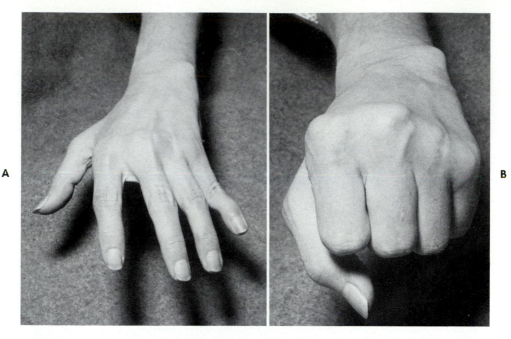

Fig. 10-5. Dislocation of extensor tendons. **A,** In early stages of ulnar drift the extensor tendons may appear to be in a normal position when the fingers are in extension. **B,** When a fist is made, the extensor tendons will slip from the top toward the ulnar side of each joint.

detected. It is a matter of fact that ulnar shift of the extensor tendons may occur late in drift and is not a consistent primary etiological factor. In the early 1960's experimental and clinical work, particularly by Smith, Juvinall, Bender, and Pearson, drew attention to the vital role played by the flexor tendons. It serves no purpose to promote the cause of one group versus the other, and it must be accepted that either, according to the pathological circumstances, could be the prime factor.

Extensor tendons. As ulnar deviation of the fingers increases, a fundamental change occurs in the relationship between the extrinsic extensor tendons and the metacarpophalangeal joints. Each extrinsic extensor tendon gradually slides off the dorsum of its joint and lies on the ulnar side. This shift of tendon position steadily increases the aberrant pull on the joint, and the condition becomes self-perpetuating (Fig. 10-5). Eventually the extensor tendons will dislocate completely and come to lie on the ulnar side of their metacarpals deep in the valley between the metacarpal heads. In this position the tendons have crossed the flexion-extension axis of the joint and lie on its palmar aspect, thereby adding a flexor-deforming force to the joint. The flexion deformity produced by this dislocation of the tendons is seen in late stages of ulnar drift.

Backhouse has stressed that because of the difference in the anatomy of the dorsal hood area over the joint, synovial swelling can show selective bulging into the thin radial triangle and hence precipitate an ulnar shift of the long extensor tendons. This unilateral herniation of synovium has been commented on by several observers and has been extensively studied by Professor Tsuge of Hiroshima, who published his views in 1966. He agreed with Backhouse that thickening of the synovium causes distention of the dorsal joint capsule and that herniation of this swelling tends to occur differentially on the radial side, particularly in the index finger.

This weakening of the radial hood is coupled with the pressure that is applied to the radial side of the index finger during pinch, and that, Tsuge feels, plays a major role in the gradual displacement of the extensor tendons into the ulnar grooves and consequent ulnar drift of fingers. In this connection it is interesting that Vainio has observed a similar occurrence in the ring and small fingers. In a personal communication in 1968 he wrote: "One more cause seems to be sure in the etiology of ulnar drift starting from the ring and little fingers. In several cases a big mass consisting of hypertrophic synovial tissue and rheumatoid nodules can be found between the bases of the first phalanges. The lump pushes the little finger ulnarward and causes its luxation. Later on the ring may follow. This seems to be one additional important cause of ulnar drift of the ulnar fingers, which are not subjected to the distorting forces of the daily life and in which the direction of the flexor and extensor tendons does not pull the tendon sheaths ulnarward."

These observations are accurate and in the circumstances described may create a mechanical situation in which ulnar shift of the extensor tendons can occur.

Flexor tendons. The influence of the extrinsic flexor tendons as a factor in the production of ulnar drift is no longer a matter for debate. The work of Smith, Juvinall, Bender, and Pearson shows how, on the radial side of the palm, significant forces exist within the flexor tendons that tend to produce an ulnar torque. My experimental work confirmed the vital role that the flexor tendons play in the onset of ulnar drift in the radial half of the hand.

Although this discussion is concerned with the influence of the flexor tendons on the initiation of ulnar drift, I must repeat that they also contribute major palmar dislocating forces to the metacarpophalangeal joint. During any fingertip grip activity there is a considerably greater force acting on the base of the proximal phalanx than the resultant output at the fingertip (Fig. 10-6, A).

The flexor tendons do not exert traction in the line of the metacarpal; like the extensors, they converge toward the base of the fourth metacarpal. They are kept in the line of each finger by the digital fibrous sheaths, which only begin at the level of the metacarpophalangeal joints, and considerable forces are exerted during prehension on the entrance to the fibrous tunnel. These forces, in the case of the index and long fingers, act both in a palmar and an ulnar direction. The ulnar border of the inlet to the sheath acts as a reflexion pulley. Normally in rheumatoid disease the thick palmar plate acts as a barrier between the expanding synovium of the joint and the pulleys. It is not the fibrous flexor sheath that is weakened first but the joint structures from which it is suspended. Both the metacarpophalangeal and the metacarpo-glenoidal portions of the collateral ligaments are affected; the latter initially take most of the strain. After the ligaments are loosened or stretched, the entrance of the pulley will be displaced palmarward and ulnarward. Such a displacement will have a double effect on the weakened joint (Fig. 10-6). First, the base of the phalanx will tend

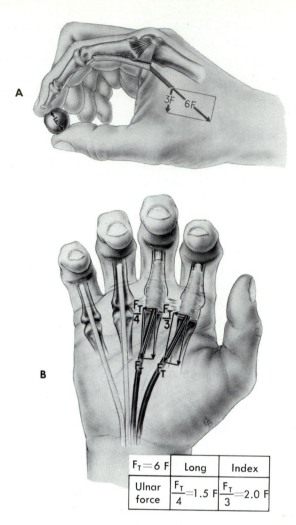

$F_T = 6\,F$	Long	Index
Ulnar force	$\dfrac{F_T}{4} = 1.5\,F$	$\dfrac{F_T}{3} = 2.0\,F$

Fig. 10-6. Flexor tendon forces. **A,** The forces developed in the flexor tendons of the index during pinch. Palmar subluxation must result if the metacarpophalangeal ligaments are destroyed. **B,** The forces pulling on the radial side of the flexor tendon sheath of the index and long fingers. Ulnar displacement of the tendons will result if the restraints are diseased.

toward subluxation in a palmar direction, and second, the ulnar displacement of the line of the flexor tendons as they enter the sheath will result in ulnar shift of the base of the phalanx.

If the synovium around the flexor tendons is also diseased, the fibrous flexor sheath will expand and the flexor tendons will displace in an ulnar direction and contribute an ulnar deviation force to the fingers.

Combinations of this shift, both of the base of the phalanx and the flexor tendon, can also occur and are illustrated in Fig. 10-7.

An operation known as the flexor sheath release procedure is designed to increase the flexor power over the metacarpophalangeal joints by cutting the proximal portion

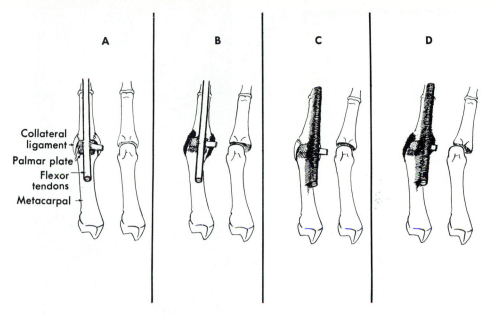

Fig. 10-7. Synovial disease around the metacarpophalangeal joint. **A,** Normal anatomy. **B,** Ulnar shift of the phalangeal base when the collateral ligaments are slackened. **C,** Flexor sheath slackening, producing tendon displacement and finger deviation. **D,** Ulnar drift produced by a combination of **B** and **C.** (From Flatt, A.E.: Plast. Reconstr. Surg. **37:**295-303, 1966.)

of the flexor sheath. Putting the entrance of the flexor sheath, and therefore the pulley around which the tendon works, more distally into the finger might seem an easy way of increasing the power of grasp. However, when considered in terms of more than one plane, this method can be seen to have an inherent disadvantage (Fig. 10-8, *A*). Advancing the site of the pulley into the finger also releases the flexor tendons from a restraint that had previously kept them in the longitudinal line of the finger. Ulnar deviation should result (Fig. 10-8, *B*). If this operation, or the similar trigger finger release operation, is done on all four fingers, ulnar drift can be expected to develop (Fig. 10-8, *C*). Several rheumatoid patients I have seen have had flexor tendon sheath release procedures done in both hands to improve weakness of grip. They all reported that after this operation the ulnar drift increased "very rapidly."

INTRINSIC MUSCLES

Although the actual force generated by the intrinsic muscles is significantly less than that of the extrinsic extensor and flexor tendons, intrinsic muscle activity can undoubtedly contribute to the production of ulnar drift by both the flexion and the deviating components of their action.

The contribution of their flexion activity to subluxation of the metacarpophalangeal joints has been concisely illustrated by a patient reported by Hueston. He records a "natural experiment" in which a man who suffered a midforearm ulnar nerve lesion in World War I developed rheumatoid disease 10 years later. Despite his

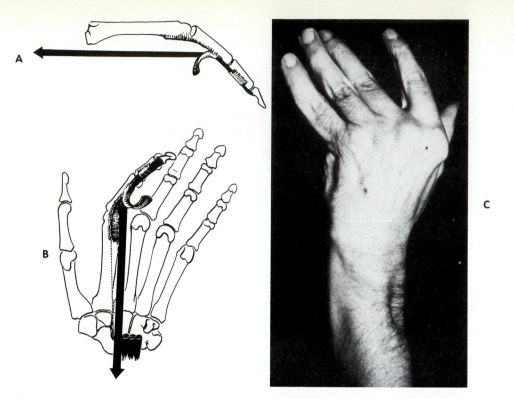

Fig. 10-8. Flexor sheath release operation. **A,** In the lateral plane release of the flexor sheath can be seen to place the entrance to the sheath within the finger. **B,** However, this release also allows a significant increase in the ulnar deviating tendency. **C,** A clinical example; this deformity resulted many years after trigger finger release had been done on all four fingers. (**C** courtesy Dr. Daniel C. Riordan, New Orleans.)

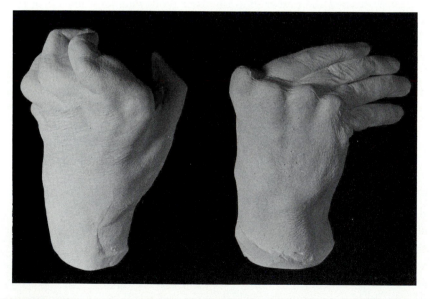

Fig. 10-9. Influence of intrinsic muscles. These plaster casts illustrate the two hands of a man who has had rheumatoid disease of both hands for many years but who suffered a complete ulnar nerve lesion to his left hand before contracting rheumatoid disease. Symmetrical ulnar drift is present, but palmar metacarpo-phalangeal subluxation is present only in the right hand, in which the intrinsic musculature is still working. (Courtesy Dr. J.T. Hueston, Melbourne, Australia.)

disease he stoically continued his heavy laboring occupation. His hands now show symmetrical ulnar drift, but palmar subluxation of the metacarpophalangeal joints is present only in the right hand, in which the intrinsic muscles are still working (Fig. 10-9). In the left hand, in which the intrinsic muscles are paralyzed, the typical claw deformity has developed, together with the usual ulnar deviation secondary to unopposed extrinsic extensor activity over the metacarpophalangeal joints.

When the deviating actions of the intrinsics are considered, I agree with Backhouse that it is useful to abandon the old concept of strict anatomical descriptions of these muscles. I believe it to be of clinical value to accept his suggestion that they be thought of in the functional grouping of ulnar and radial muscles. In the majority of hands each ulnar insertion of the muscles is stronger, more transverse, and more intimately related to the extensor tendon than its radial counterpart. These anatomical differences imply that there is a significant difference between the patterns of activity on the two sides. Backhouse has shown that the ulnar interossei are either stronger or work to a better mechanical advantage than their radial counterparts. Tubiana and Valentin have also remarked on the mechanical advantage of ulnar over radial interossei when they are acting in flexion, deviation, or rotation.

Boyes has also stressed the importance of the link between the wing insertions of the interossei and the extrinsic extensor tendons and makes the important observation that ulnar deviation does not seem to occur in fingers with ruptured extrinsic extensor tendons. This predominance of the ulnar-sided intrinsics is probably related to their activity in all forms of firm grasp.

Power grip is particularly associated with the ulnar border of the hand and flexor-ulnar deviating activity of the fingers. Completion of the tightening of power grip results in flexion of the ring and small finger carpometacarpal and metacarpophalangeal joints. This "descent" of the fourth and fifth metacarpals is considered of prime importance by Zancolli, who points out in his stimulating and original book, *Structural and Dynamic Bases of Hand Surgery*, that there is a consequent marked ulnarward pull on the extensor tendons and their juncturae tendinum (Fig. 10-10). During such activity the radial collateral ligament of the index finger acts as the ultimate vital anchor resisting the imposed forces.

Dynamic support for the radial side of the index finger metacarpophalangeal joint is supplied by the first dorsal interosseous muscle. In detailed dissections of this area Straub has pointed out that the first dorsal interosseous muscle has a broad area of attachment to the capsule of the metacarpophalangeal joint at the base of the proximal phalanx of the index finger and that it also attaches indirectly to the palmar plate of the joint. If the capsule is distended by disease and the joint becomes unstable, the insertion of the first dorsal interosseous muscle slides forward, the muscle loses its ability to abduct, and it becomes a flexor of the joint. His anatomical studies have also confirmed Backhouse's view that the ulnar-sided interosseous muscles, including the hypothenar muscles of the small finger, show a significant power dominance over their radial counterpart. Straub is particularly impressed by the abductor digiti minimi, which he regards as a surprisingly strong muscle (Fig 10-11). He has also stressed the importance of the transverse intermetacarpal ligament, to which the abductor

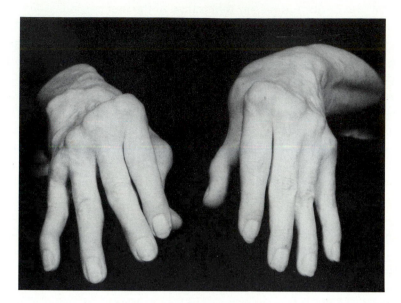

Fig. 10-10. ''Descent'' of the ring and small fingers. Established palmar descent or collapse of the ulnar sides of both hands. Synovitis of the carpometacarpal joints of the ring and small fingers coupled with deforming forces within the hand leads to this significant deformity.

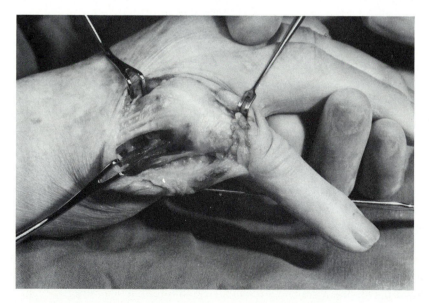

Fig. 10-11. Hypothenar muscles. The phalangeal insertions of these muscles in the small finger extend a surprising distance distally and thereby obtain a great mechanical advantage in the production of ulnar deviation.

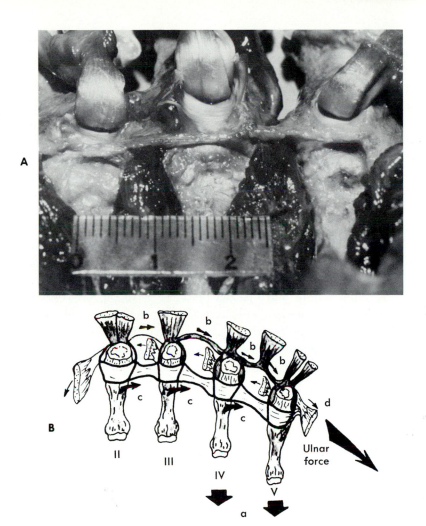

Fig. 10-12. The transverse intermetacarpal ligament. **A,** Dissection of the palm showing the transverse intermetacarpal ligament lying across the center of the picture parallel with the ruler. Note that the flexor tendons have been turned upward to reveal the palmar plates on which they normally lie. Each palmar plate is connected to its neighbor via the intermetacarpal ligament. **B,** Zancolli's illustration showing how the intermetacarpal ligament *(c)* and the juncturae of the extensor tendons *(b)* transmit the ulnar pull of the abductor digiti minimi *(d)*. (**B** from Zancolli, E.: Structural and dynamic bases of hand surgery, Philadelphia, 1968, J.B. Lippincott Co.)

digiti minimi muscle shows a strong attachment. This ligament has no bony attachment and is a strong link between all the palmar plates of the metacarpophalangeal joints (Fig. 10-12).

Straub is supported by Zancolli in the concept that the possibility exists that a strong pull by the abductor digiti minimi muscle will be transmitted to all palmar plates and through their attachments to the bases of the proximal phalanges of all the fingers. Zancolli has pointed out that "the anatomical characteristics of this ligament favor metacarpal descent because its ulnar part becomes progressively longer transversally and short longitudinally."*

Force nucleus of Zancolli

A variety of potentially deforming forces, generated by both extrinsic and intrinsic muscles, are concentrated in the area of the metacarpophalangeal joint. Zancolli has echoed Backhouse's plea for the combining of different descriptive anatomical parts into functional units by describing a "force nucleus" in the ligamentous and retinacular tissues around the metacarpophalangeal joint. The core of his thesis is that there is in space a point, or nucleus, at which all the forces exerted on the constituent anatomical structures balance each other. Damage to any one anatomical component will produce imbalance, and permanent deformity can result.

He states that "all of the components that form the metacarpophalangeal nucleus integrate into a closed apparatus, or circuit, which is formed by the ligamentous structures located on both sides of each joint. Each metacarpophalangeal circuit is formed by a dorsal, a middle, and a palmar bridge [Fig. 10-13]. Between the dorsal and middle bridges is the metacarpophalangeal joint, and between the middle and palmar bridges run the long flexor tendons. . . . The transverse intermetacarpal ligament unites all the metacarpophalangeal force nuclei and metacarpophalangeal encircling structures, thus contributing to a total transverse integration of the metacarpal arch of the hand."

Zancolli considers that the main forces transmitted through the nucleus are represented by (1) longitudinal gliding of the extensor tendon, both in a distal and a proximal direction during digital flexion and extension respectively; (2) traction transmitted in a palmar direction by tension of the flexor tendons during gripping and pinching; and (3) a force ("ulnar force of the hand") that originates from the ulnar side of the hand and pulls along the line of the transverse intermetacarpal ligament and the palmar plates, and that is accentuated by the "descent" of the last segment of the intermetacarpal ligament.

Zancolli's concept of the "descent" of the ring and small finger metacarpals is an important contribution to our understanding of ulnar drift. He points out that in rheumatoid ulnar drift one usually observes persistent palmar descent of the ulnar two metacarpals "due to synovitis of the carpometacarpal joints with stretching of their dorsal ligaments, and unresisted action of some of the contractured hypothenar muscles and the long flexor tendons of the fingers. This is aggravated with the permanent dislocation of the extensor tendons of the last fingers, which can no longer extend the last metacarpals when the fingers are completely flexed."*

I am largely in agreement with Zancolli's position that ulnar drift of the fingers "is the result of the imbalance created between the failure of the dorsal and radial stabilizing mechanisms of the extensor tendons and the proximal phalanges—synovitis consequence—against the strong palmar and ulnar forces of the hand."*

---

*From Zancolli, E.: Structural and dynamic bases of hand surgery, ed. 2, Philadelphia, 1979, J.B. Lippincott Co.

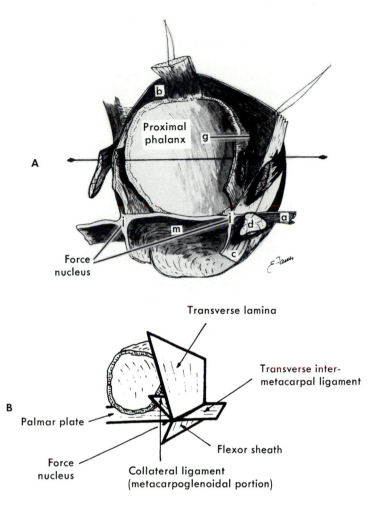

Fig. 10-13. Force nucleus concept of Zancolli. **A,** Anatomical constituents: *a,* transverse intermetacarpal ligament; *b,* transverse lamina; *c,* flexor sheath; *d,* lumbrical; *g,* aponeurotic sleeve; *m,* palmar plate; *j,* force nucleus. **B,** Schematic drawing relating the anatomical parts to the location of the "force nucleus." (From Zancolli, E.: Structural and dynamic bases of hand surgery, ed. 2, Philadelphia, 1979, J.B. Lippincott Co.)

Extrinsic forces

The extrinsic, or external, forces associated with the development of ulnar drift are largely those of use, and several clinical conditions demonstrate this association. The French have recognized the importance of the forces of usage by aptly naming the condition "coup de vent." It is significant that ulnar drift is twice as common in women as in men. Vainio and Oka found an incidence of 14.6% in men and 28.6% in women in 292 unselected cases. This greater incidence in women probably occurs for the same basic reason that young mothers are usually severely affected by poliomyelitis. When men are afflicted by any condition severe enough to demand rest, they rest completely. Women, however, tend to carry on their housework and family duties with great perseverance. From the very beginning of rheumatoid disease the constant activities of daily living and domestic chores will force these women's hands into ulnar drift.

Children suffering from juvenile rheumatoid disease have no domestic obligations whatsoever and are usually kept at complete rest. Ulnar drift could therefore be expected to be uncommon, and Vainio and Oka recorded an incidence of ulnar drift of only 3.3% in 30 patients with juvenile rheumatoid arthritis.

That use of the hand is of fundamental importance in the production of this deformity is shown by the occasional occurrence of radial drift. I have seen two patients with this deformity, and both had unusual occupations involving radialward pressures on the ulnar border of the hand.

Billich has stressed the importance of usage as a factor in ulnar drift. He examined the hands of nearly 200 carpenters who were known to be free of injury or disease to their hands. In those who had been working at the trade several years he found 40% had a mild and 20% a severe ulnar drift of the fingers. The drift could be easily corrected to the normal plane by passive pressure. He stressed that he felt this drift was caused by mechanical stretching of the radial tissues "by sidewards pressure of the tool which aggravates the normal ulnar position which is normally present to a very small degree." This emphasis on radial pressure from hand use is also reinforced by the common clinical observation that osteoarthritis of the hand is far more common on the radial than the ulnar side of the hand.

Vainio and Oka have recorded that in numerous cases of war injuries causing ulnar and/or median nerve paralysis, there was no ulnar drift when the metacarpophalangeal joints were undamaged. Although I concur with this observation, particularly in relation to adult hands, I have seen ulnar drift develop in the hands of children after poliomyelitic involvement of the intrinsic hand muscles when the children were infants (Fig. 10-14). I believe the differentiating factor in these two types of cases is that in the children's hands, the pressure of usage toward the ulnar border is unremitting over a long period of years, whereas in the adult's wounded hands, treatment is started before any drift can develop.

Ulnar drift frequently occurs if the collateral ligaments are totally resected during the correction of claw hands (Fig. 10-15). The drift does not appear immediately. It gradually develops as increasing use is made of the hand. Vainio and Oka recorded a case in which the patient obtained good flexion of the metacarpophalangeal joints by operation but developed ulnar drift during a subsequent course of occupational therapy. My own experience has been comparable, and I have modified my operative procedure for claw hand so as to lengthen, rather than excise, the collateral ligaments.

Ulnar drift, from whatever cause, cannot occur in the presence of normal anatomy; there must be aberrations of structure or function to initiate the deformity. In rheumatoid disease the critical precipitating factor is an expanding synovitis affecting the digital joints, the carpal and wrist joints, and the synovium around the extrinsic flexor and extensor tendons. This disease leads to slackening of normal restraints, a redistribution of forces normally present within the hand, and the development of

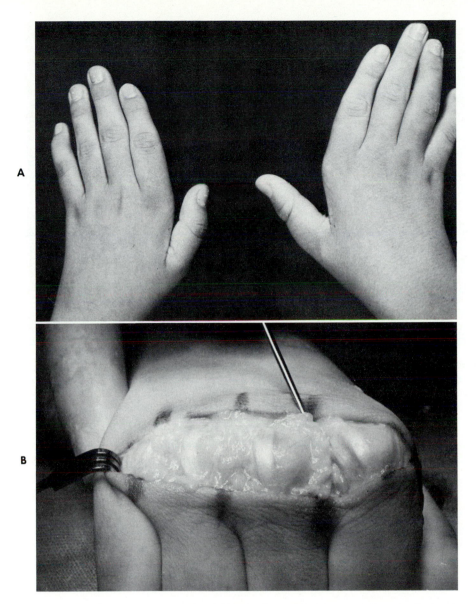

Fig. 10-14. Ulnar drift and poliomyelitis. This child had poliomyelitis at the age of 6 months. Her hands were photographed at the age of 7 years. **A,** Ulnar drift can clearly be seen. **B,** Dislocation of the extrinsic extensor tendons toward the ulnar side of each joint as seen at surgery.

unbalanced forces that lead to progressive deformity. Similar imbalance of forces can be created by traumatic incidents, selective paralyses, or iatrogenically by ill-conceived surgical procedures.

The relative importance of each and every one of these factors within the hand will vary in any given clinical situation, and all can be influenced by the placing of the hand in relation to the axis of the forearm. Disease of both inferior radioulnar and the

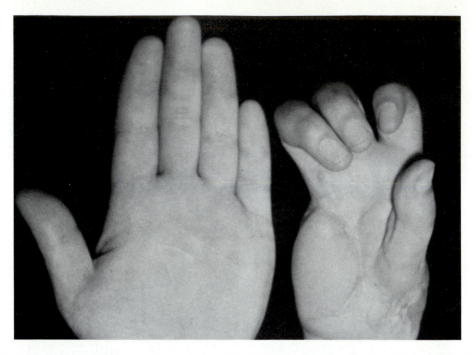

Fig. 10-15. Collateral ligament excision and ulnar drift. Major trauma to this patient's right hand resulted in total stiffness of the metacarpophalangeal and proximal interphalangeal joints. Excision of the collateral ligaments of the metacarpophalangeal joints was among the procedures carried out. The fingers subsequently passed into ulnar drift.

radiocarpal joints affects the function of the normal hand and will have a profound efect on the diseased hand. Loosening of the normal restraints of the inferior radioulnar joint leads to dorsal dislocation of the distal end of the ulna, displacement of the extensor carpi ulnaris tendon into the position of a wrist flexor, and disturbance of the posture of the ring and small finger metacarpals. Radiocarpal disease accompanied by radial carpal collapse will hold the carpometacarpal unit in radial deviation, making it mechanically inevitable that the phalanges will go into ulnar deviation.

Thus there are many causes for ulnar drift, and effective therapy cannot be prescribed unless the many possible aberrant factors are identified by a thorough clinical examination.

EARLY ULNAR DRIFT

Ulnar drift is insidious in its onset, and early stages of the condition are difficult to diagnose. Synovitis and swelling of the metacarpophalangeal joints must be considered the warning signs. Patients with rheumatoid disease frequently bear unduly on the radial border of their hands in everyday activites, and they must be taught to overcome this tendency.

In the late stages of the disease, weakness, wasting, and contracture of the interosseous muscles are easily recognized; in the early stages of the condition. however, careful clinical and radiological examination is necessary to elicit the early features of

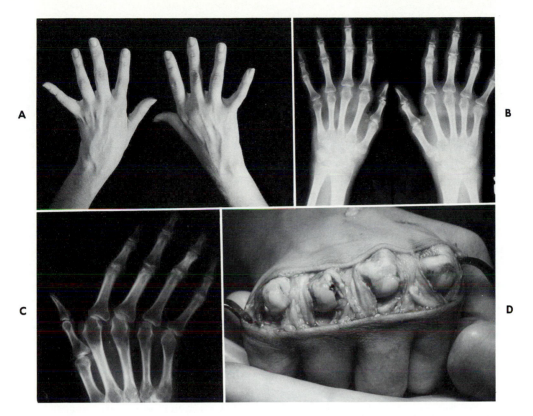

Fig. 10-16. Early ulnar drift. **A,** These hands might be regarded as normal, but there is wasting of the first dorsal interosseous muscle on either side. **B,** Shift of the base of the index finger proximal phalanx in an ulnar direction in each hand. **C** and **D,** State of the hand 11 months later with advanced destruction of the metacarpal heads. (**A** and **B** from Flatt, A.E.: Salvage of the rheumatoid hand. In DePalma, A.F., editor: Clinical orthopaedics, vol. 23, Philadelphia, 1962, J.B. Lippincott Co.)

the deformity. Commencing weakness of the first dorsal interosseous muscle is shown by an instability of lateral pinch as well as a weakness of the index finger in pure abduction against passive resistance. At this stage x-ray films may show an unequal balance of the base of the proximal phalanx on the head of the second metacarpal (Fig. 10-16). It is probable that the ulnar deviation torque described by Smith, Juvinall, Bender, and Pearson is largely responsible for this shift of the base of the phalanx. This displacement is not invariably present, but when it occurs, it is a definite warning that ulnar drift has begun and that treatment must be started immediately. The patient whose hands are illustrated in Fig. 10-16 is a 19-year-old college student with known rheumatoid disease. It can be seen that there is evidence of intrinsic muscle wasting and a definite displacement of the base of the proximal phalanx of the index finger. Consent for surgical treatment was not obtained at that time, and she did not return until 11 months later. By this time ulnar drift was well established, and an extensive operation was performed in an attempt to overcome the results of the disease. Unfortunately the disease was found to be far advanced, and gross destruction of the articular surface of the metacarpophalangeal joints had already occurred.

Another early sign of impending ulnar drift that can be detected on the radial side of the hand is ulnar displacement of the flexor tendons. Clinically this shift of the flexor tendons in an ulnar direction can be readily detected in the index and long fingers by palpation on the flexor aspect of the palm or on the ulnar side of the finger in its most proximal portion.

The examining digit must push on the ulnar side of the flexor tendon in a radial direction. If the finger in question is then flexed against resistance, the flexor tendon will displace ulnarward if its retaining sheath has been widened by synovitis (Fig. 10-17). If the tendon does move significantly in an ulnar direction, the prognosis is poor; the stage is set for steadily increasing ulnar deviation.

On several occasions I have been able to insert a wire marker in the profundus tendon and show on x-ray film the ulnar shift of the tendon during application of flexor power. Smith and Kaplan have shown similar illustrations in their paper. In some patients the sesamoid bone of the index finger provides a useful marker for such a shift; Fig. 10-18 illustrates the shift in the sesamoid bone of an index finger over a period of nearly 5 years. The index sesamoid lies within the angle between the palmar aspect of the palmar plate and the radial side of the flexor tendon sheath. It is intimately attached to the flexor sheath, and if there is a loosening of the attachments of the flexor sheath and the palmar plate, these structures could be pulled ulnarward by the flexor tendons if an ulnarward force existed. This shift of the sesamoid can be detected in some patients with early ulnar drift.

Contracture of the hypothenar muscles on the ulnar side of the hand is probably a powerful initiating factor in ulnar drift but it is hard to detect in its early stages. The tightness of the muscles can be detected only after the small finger has been passively placed into a straight line with its metacarpal. Early contracture is usually evidenced by resistance to radially correcting forces applied after any flexion and subluxation of the joint has been corrected.

Ulnar deviation of the fingers in rheumatoid disease can begin on the radial side of the hand or on the ulnar side. The patients illustrated in Figs. 10-20 and 10-21 are examples of such unilateral onsets. I find it hard to believe that gravity can make any significant contribution to the etiology of the deviation, and I believe that laxity of the tissues secondary to disease and the anatomical configurations combine to allow production of the deformity by the forces involved in the use of the hand. On the radial side of the hand these forces are largely supplied by prehensile activities and the flexor tendons, and on the ulnar side of the hand the strong forces of power grip and the hypothenar muscles with their relative distal insertion (Fig. 10-11) must be largely responsible for the deviation of the small finger.

The ring finger is probably least affected by either anatomical or aberrant force factors. The shape of its metacarpal head is almost symmetrical, and the flexor tendons do not tend to pull it ulnarward. I agree with Hakstian and Tubiana that it is probably most affected by external forces and either is pushed into ulnar deviation by the index and long fingers or falls into this position if the splinting effect of the small finger has been removed.

In the early stages of the deformity, ulnar deviation of the fingers occurs in the

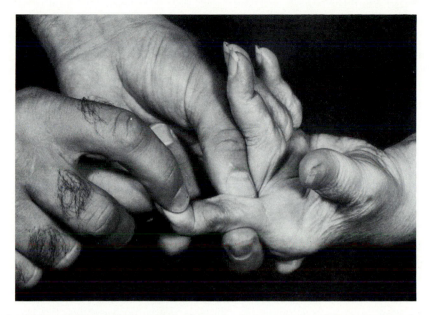

Fig. 10-17. Ulnar dislocating flexor tendons. When the flexor profundus of the index finger is pushed radially by the examiner's thumb, the tendon will move ulnarward when the finger is flexed against resistance if the flexor sheath has been enlarged by disease.

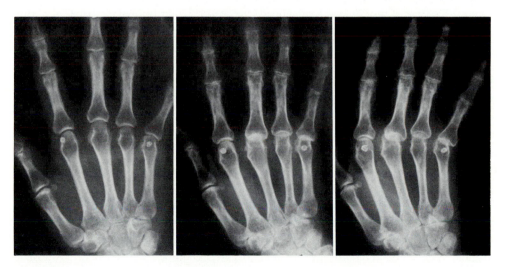

Fig. 10-18. Sesamoid shift in ulnar drift. Successive x-ray films show how the index sesamoid bone has moved in an ulnar direction as ulnar drift of the fingers increases. (From Flatt, A.E.: Plast. Reconstr. Surg. **37:**295-303, 1966.)

plane of full extension of the metacarpophalangeal joints. The fingers can still be fully extended by the tendons of the extrinsic extensor muscles, even though these tendons are beginning to slide to the ulnar side of the midline of their joints. As the deformity increases, the power to completely extend the metacarpophalangeal joints decreases. A true flexion contracture eventually develops in the joint, so that it cannot be fully extended even passively. This flexion contracture has been reported by several writers, and I believe that it plays a fundamental part in the development of later stages of the drift.

On the radial side of the hand the first dorsal interosseous muscle is quite unable to resist the ulnarward pressures of grip. On the ulnar border of the hand the unbalanced hypothenar group of muscles frequently pulls the proximal phalanx of the small finger into 90 degrees of lateral drift and complete palmar dislocation.

The destruction of stability of the index finger has a profound effect on the power of grasp. As the deformity becomes worse, the important precision handling of pinch is increasingly hampered. The contact area of the pulp of the thumb against the index finger moves progressively to a more proximal position. Eventually, tip grip is totally destroyed, and prehension is reduced to a form of proximal lateral pinch in which the thumb presses against the side of the middle phalanx or even of the proximal phalanx of the index finger.

The small finger is used mainly in relatively coarse power grips, and even total dislocation at the metacarpophalangeal joint may not completely destroy the ability to grasp objects along the ulnar border of the hand.

The fully developed state of late ulnar drift will therefore show partial or complete dislocation of the metacarpophalangeal joints in the compound planes of flexion and ulnar deviation. If the disease is advanced, there may be additional destruction of the joint surfaces and their underlying bone. The extrinsic extensor tendons will be dislocated into the valley on the ulnar side of their joints and will be unable to extend the joint. The pull of the intrinsic muscles will have become aberrant and contributes to the deformity.

TREATMENT

The ideal treatment would be to provide sufficient lateral stability for the fingers to counterbalance the radial pressure of pinch and all other forms of precision handling. It should also reconstitute the metacarpophalangeal joints of the ring and small fingers so that a good power grip may be developed.

Any form of surgery designed to restore the normal functional arch of the skeleton of the hand must eliminate the abnormal pull of the various muscle groups producing the original dislocation. Muscle power, which is required to support the restored arches, is reduced by both surgery and disease, making some form of additional splinting necessary to help maintain the correction. This splinting can be supplied either externally by some device or internally by surgery.

External splinting may be of help in the early phase of ulnar drift, but it cannot correct the multiple deformities of the late stages of the condition. Many ingenious, and often heavy, devices have been produced in an attempt to overcome the deformity, but I have yet to see a splint that efficiently corrects both planes of dislocation of the metacarpophalangeal joints. The basic function of most splints is to stabilize the position of the proximal phalanx by some form of radialward pull, forcing grasp to take place at the level of the interphalangeal joints. In effect, these splints move the grip of the hand distally and considerably reduce the possible range of grasp. Splints can be helpful in augmenting the results of surgery, but I do not believe that they are an efficient substitute for surgery in fully developed ulnar drift.

In the late stages of ulnar drift it is unlikely that surgery on the soft tissues alone can provide adequate function and stability. Excisional arthroplasty of the metacarpophalangeal joints of all the fingers is occasionally successful, but I believe that in neglected deformities additional internal splinting by prosthetic replacement is needed to supply the necessary stability.

Fusion of the metacarpophalangeal joint of the small and/or ring fingers is to be condemned, because this operation splints the two ulnar fingers in only the single position in which they are fused. Patients on whom I performed this operation tended to hold the radial fingers in the same position as the fused fingers, thereby nullifying the purpose of the operation, which is to supply stable mobility for these fingers. Several authors report similar experiences with their patients, commenting that this restriction of mobility is especially detrimental to patients with rheumatoid disease.

Mild ulnar drift

In the early phase of ulnar drift, rheumatoid disease affects the soft tissues sufficiently to alter the kinesiology of the hand. The articular cartilage and bone are usually only slightly involved, and surgical correction confined to the soft tissues yields excellent results.

The aim of these operations is to remove the diseased synovium, relocate the dislocated tendons, and correct any aberrant pull present in the muscles. Technically it is possible to reposition the extrinsic extensor tendons, but I am not aware of any operation that can successfully retain the flexor tendons in their normal anatomical pathways. During clinical examination of the hand it may be found that a significant degree of intrinsic contracture is present, and often there is a differential tightness of the ulnar intrinsic muscles. Should this be so, then a crossed intrinsic transfer must also be done. In recent years I have routinely done this procedure in mild ulnar drift even when I could not demonstrate differential tightness of the ulnar intrinsic muscles.

Synovectomy should always be combined with soft-tissue procedures that help maintain joint alignment. Harrison has pointed out that it is wise to correct moderate deformity at a stage when there is relatively minor joint destruction in an attempt to halt an ongoing chain reaction and thus improve hand function. Crossed intrinsic transfers and plication or reattachment of the radial collateral ligaments are consistently of value. Additional, more complex soft-tissue reconstructive procedures on the radial side of the joint are now being tried, and early results have been reported by Harrison and by Nicholle.

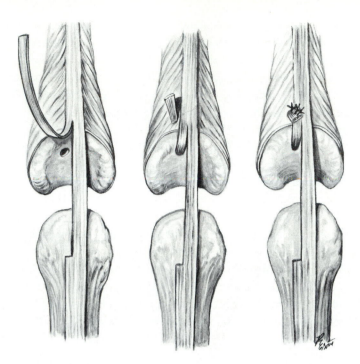

Fig. 10-19. Harrison arthroplasty. The extent of excision of the metacarpal head varies. (The site is not shown.) The stages in the extensor loop procedure are shown from left to right.

Harrison uses a hole drilled into the radial side of the base of the proximal phalanx for the crossed intrinsic transfer and, in addition, attempts to hold up the base of the phalanx by an "extensor loop" operation (Fig. 10-19). The slip of the extensor tendon used for the loop is passed through a midline dorsal hole drilled in the base of the phalanx. In a series of 103 joints he reported adequate maintenance of correction without serious loss of flexion and extension. Only those patients whose ulnar drift was not correctible before surgery failed to benefit.

Nicholle uses a 5- to 6-cm long slip dissected from the center of the extensor tendon, leaving it attached distally at the level of the metacarpophalangeal joint. The proximal end is passed through the phalangeal attachment of the radial collateral ligament. After repairing the central defect in the extensor tendon, the slip is brought proximally in an oblique direction and woven through the proximal portion of the extensor tendon. A variant on this operation is to use a radial slip from the extensor tendon and pass it around the bony insertion of the radial interosseous muscle. The effect of tightening the radial-side joint tissues would appear to be the same in both methods. Nicholle reports that in 32 joints, his method reduced the mean preoperative deviation from 45 degrees to 10 degrees and that flexion of the metacarpophalangeal joint exceeded 45 degrees in all patients.

All these procedures can be done through a transverse dorsal incision placed just proximal to the line of the metacarpophalangeal joint when the joint is in extension. This incision provides a good approach to the joints, but great care must be taken to preserve the longitudinal veins running from the fingers to the venous drainage network on the dorsum of the hand. These veins must be protected because their destruction will allow considerable venous congestion to occur distal to the incision. The ends of the incision should extend beyond the border joints just onto the lateral borders of the hand. At each end of the incision a relatively large but unnamed vein will be found in the subcutaneous tissues. These veins should also be preserved.

Synovectomy of the metacarpophalangeal joints is an essential part of the operation for correction of ulnar drift. As much synovium as possible must be carefully excised from all four metacarpophalangeal joints of the fingers. Each joint is approached on the radial side of the hood through an incision based about 5 mm below the level of, and parallel with, the extrinsic extensor tendon. The hood fibers are reflected both above and below the incision to expose the capsule and its diseased contents. Even when extensive synovial disease is present, it is usually possible to find a plane of cleavage between the deep surface of the hood and the underlying tissues. When the synovium is removed, particular care must be taken to excise completely the tongue of synovium that lies between the side of each collateral ligament and the side of the metacarpal head. The collateral ligament and the site of its bony attachment will be destroyed by this tongue of diseased synovium if it is left undisturbed. When adequate tissue is present, I often do a proximal recession or reattachment of the radial collateral ligament as suggested by Curtis. He has pointed out that if the radial tubercle, to which the collateral ligament is attached, is cut off in the long line of the bone, an excellent exposure of the joint is provided. Synovectomy can easily be done, and a firm, more proximal reattachment of the ligament can be accomplished when its origin from the bony tubercle has been left undisturbed.

When the synovectomy has been completed, the shortened ulnar side of the intrinsic wing insertion is released at a point well distal into each finger. The crossed intrinsic transfer illustrated in Fig. 6-18, *B* (p. 139) is then carried out.

The metacarpophalangeal joints of the long, ring, and small fingers can be corrected in this manner, but the index finger joint cannot. I abandoned transfer of the extensor indicis proprius muscle because it so often added an unwanted element of flexion to the metacarpophalangeal joint of the index finger. I now dissect the tendon of the first dorsal interosseous muscle from its insertion and transfer it to a more dorsal portion of the lateral joint capsule, where it attaches to the base of the proximal phalanx. This transfer has proved to be satisfactory in the long term. The extrinsic extensors must be repositioned on top of their metacarpophalangeal joints either by a double-breasting procedure of the hood fibers or by the creation of new retinacular fibers from local tissue (Fig. 10-20).

All skin incisions are closed with interrupted fine sutures; no drains are necessary. An ample compression dressing of Dacron batting is placed on both surfaces of the hand and held in place by a self-adherent cotton bandage. The position of the fingers is important. Because the extensor tendons have now been relocated, some weeks are necessary for the extrinsic extensor muscles to take up their slack. The fingers must therefore be kept in extension at all joints for 7 to 10 days. This grossly abnormal position might seem unacceptable because of the risk that stiffness will develop in the

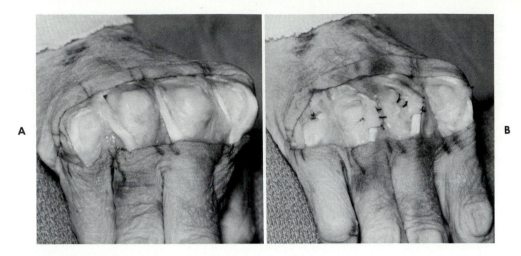

Fig. 10-20. Repositioning of extensor tendons. **A,** Gross ulnar dislocation of the extrinsic extensor tendons. **B,** Repositioning by use of local tissue to create retinacular ligaments.

fingers. Any stiffness caused by splinting in extension can always be overcome by the two extrinsic flexor muscles during subsequent active use of the hand.

After the sutures have been removed the crossed intrinsic transfers must still be protected from ulnarward strains for another week. A palmar plaster splint can be used to hold the metacarpophalangeal joints in extension, but it will need an ulnar flange on which the small finger can rest. The plaster splint should be removed for exercise during the third week, but the patient should be encouraged to wear the plaster splint during sleep.

Severe ulnar drift

Marked ulnar drift is not necessarily an indication for surgical intervention. Although cosmetic deformity may be significant even with gross ulnar drift, it may be possible for the patient to close the fist with grasp power by the ulnar three fingers. It was Savill's opinion that arthroplasty was not necessary so long as three-point pinch had been maintained.

However, when function is severely impaired, some form of drastic surgical procedure is needed. Fusion of the metacarpophalangeal joints can be done and will correct the fingers in relation to their metacarpals. The functional penalty is high unless the interphalangeal joints are normal. Most surgeons prefer to try to maintain motion by using some form of excisional arthroplasty to align the fingers correctly. Resistance to the original deforming forces must be supplied in some manner. When arthroplasty alone is performed, this resistance must come from attempts to repair the collateral ligaments and periarticular scarring. Unfortunately there will be a trade-off between scarring and motion: the greater the scarring, the less the motion, and the greater are the functional limitations.

Tsuge and co-workers have tried supplying an active force against the ulnar deviators by using a four-tailed graft inserted into the radial side of the hoods of the joints and activated by the brachioradialis muscle. This is an attractive concept, but I have no personal experience with this operation. The authors reported a satisfactory 3-year follow-up.

Internal splinting by prosthetic replacement would seem to supply the ideal solution. This would be true if we had a perfect prosthetic device that never wore out. As yet we do not. I believe that the devices I have discussed in Chapter 8 represent the best examples of the current state of the art, and I will continue to use some of them for my patients. I have set myself severe limitations on the indications for prosthetic replacements and insist on the presence of a significant, demonstrable loss of function before I will use them. Prostheses should not necessarily be inserted in the metacarpophalangeal joints of all the fingers. They should be used only where the joint destruction is so great that arthroplasty and soft-tissue procedures cannot be expected to give a reasonable result.

Although severe dislocation of the joint may be found in the small finger, this does not necessarily mean that prosthetic replacement is essential. Greater destruction of joint mechanism may be present in a more radial finger.

Ulnar drift arising principally in the radial side of the hand is seen in Fig. 10-21, which shows the left hand of a 68-year-old retired schoolteacher. Eighteen years ago a prosthesis was placed in the index finger. Synovectomies of the other metacarpophalangeal joints with repositioning of all the extrinsic tendons was also done. Two years after surgery the ulnar drift remained corrected and the hand was functioning well. At a later follow-up visit it was observed that considerable motion had been lost in the joint, but the patient remained pleased with the result.

Ulnar drift more commonly arises in the small and ring fingers, as seen in Fig. 10-22. Over 20 years ago prostheses were inserted into the ring and small finger metacarpophalangeal joints. The original indication for surgery was the necessity for this executive to be able to write and shake hands with his business contacts. He is still able to do so with ease, but the range of motion in the small finger joint has steadily reduced until now there is only a jog of voluntary motion. The ring finger shows about 15 degrees of controlled flexion from the neutral position.

If the concept of using a prosthesis as an internal splint is kept in mind, the selection of the fingers suitable for prosthetic replacement is made easier. I have used virtually all combinations of arthroplasty and prosthetic replacement that are possible at the metacarpophalangeal joint. Replacement of all the metacarpophalangeal joints of the fingers is occasionally necessitated by gross dislocation of the joints, combined with the need for exceptionally good stability in these joints. The patient who benefits most from such total replacement is one who needs fine control of finger movements, such as a barber or professional musician.

I have not thought it sensible to try to record a detailed survey of the results of surgical correction for ulnar drift. They are largely the results of individual operations discussed elsewhere in this book. The short-term results of any well-conceived and well-performed operation will usually be pleasing, but if surgical correction has been confined to the area of the metacarpophalangeal joints, the unrestrained forces in the flexor tendons and malalignment of the wrist will inevitably influence the long-term results.

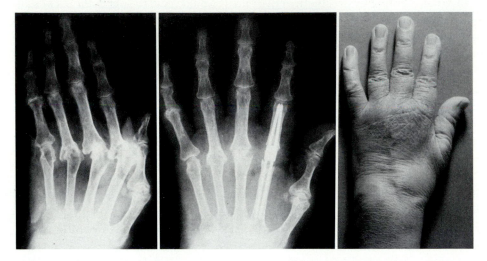

Fig. 10-21. Radially induced ulnar drift. Imbalance of forces created by selective disease of the index and long finger metacarpophalangeal joints has been corrected by the use of a prosthesis as an internal splint. Note that restoration of balance by internal splinting allowed a proper reorientation of the less affected fingers.

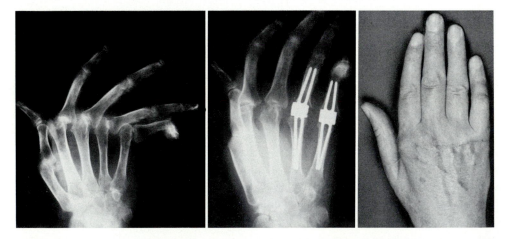

Fig. 10-22. Ulnar-side induced ulnar drift. In this patient the unbalanced pull of the hypothenar muscles was corrected by internal splinting with two prostheses. Note that restoration of balance by internal splinting allowed a proper reorientation of the less affected fingers.

This book started with a quotation from a well-known surgeon, and I end it with a quotation from another surgeon whom I greatly admire.

Good clinical investigation is the touchstone of good surgical research now, just as it was with Lister and Halsted. The surgical investigator must be a bridgetender, channeling knowledge from biologic science to the patient's bedside and back again. He traces his origin from both ends of the bridge. He is thus a bastard, and is called this by everybody. Those at one end of the bridge say he is not a very good scientist, and those at the other say he does not spend enough time in the operating room.

F.D. MOORE*

It is this quotation that continues to give me courage as I try to remain both a scientist and a clinician studying and treating the fascinating biomechanical disturbances created by rheumatoid disease.

This edition is this bastard's view of this problem at this time; I have no doubt I will continue to change my views in years to come.

---

*From Moore, F.D.: The university in American surgery, Surgery **44**:1, 1958.

An outline for examination of the arthritic hand

This plan is not exhaustive but it should be helpful in developing a complete system of examination. The figures referred to illustrate either pathological states or appropriate tests.

Invite your patient to demonstrate painful or tender areas. Avoid these areas until the end of the examination.

INSPECTION
   Posture of elbow, wrist, hand, thumb, and fingers at rest
   Skin
      Thinness and texture
      Pressure nodules
      Ecchymoses or petechial hemorrhages
   Nails
      Psoriasis
      Petechial hemorrhages
   Synovial swellings
      Joints
      Around tendons
   Muscular wasting
      Forearm
      Intrinsic muscles
ACTIVE MOTION
   Demonstrate the motions for your patient to copy.
   Elbow
      Flexion/extension
      Pronation/supination
   Wrist
      Forearm pronated and fingers relaxed
      Palmar/dorsiflexion
      Radial/ulnar deviation
   Fingers
      1. **Wrist neutral—forearm pronated**
         Open hand: extensors all working? (Fig. 6-12, p. 128)
         Fist making: extensors dislocate? (Fig. 10-5, p. 260)
         Abduction and adduction of fingers

284

2. **Wrist neutral—forearm supinated**

Fist making: flexors (superficialis and profundus) working?

Open hands: triggering present? (Fig. 5-14, p. 108)

Thumb

Flexion/extension

Abduction/adduction

Opposes to small finger?

POSTURE AND MOTION

Can your patient make power grasp and precision motion postures? (Fig. 2-10, p. 28)

Select specific areas and joints for further examination.

PALPATION AND PASSIVE MOTION

Elbow

Synovial swelling?

Radial head motion: crepitations?

Dorsum and palm

Extensor tendon synovitis (Fig. 6-2, p. 113)

Extensor tendon nodules (Fig. 5-15, p. 108)

Flexor tendon synovitis (Fig. 6-5, p. 118)

Flexor tendon nodules (Fig. 5-13, p. 107)

Thumb

Posture at rest

Intrinsic + ve/extrinsic − ve (Fig. 9-2, p. 229)

90-90 degree deformity (Fig. 9-5, p. 232)

Joints

1. CMC **joint**

Synovitis?

Capsule lax to passive testing?

Grinding test positive?

2. MP **joint**

Synovitis? (Fig. 7-7, p. 163)

Passive subluxation/dislocation possible?

Collateral ligaments intact? (Fig. 9-8, p. 234)

3. IP **joint**

Synovitis?

Passive subluxation/dislocation possible?

Collateral ligaments intact?

Extensor action

Extensor pollicis longus acting? (Fig. 5-9, p. 103)

Extensor pollicis brevis acting?

Flexor action

Flexor pollicis longus intact and acting?

Flexor pollicis longus triggering?

Intrinsic tightness? (Figs. 9-6 and 9-12, pp. 233 and 244)

Fingers

Flexor sheath synovial swelling (Fig. 6-7, p. 121)

Shifting flexor tendon (Fig. 10-17, p. 275)

Triggering (Fig. 5-14, p. 108)

Finger joints

1. DIP Joint

Posture at rest: mallet or hyperextension

Synovial swelling

Heberden's nodes?

Mucous cyst?

Integrity of joint ligaments: dorsopalmar (Fig. 7-3, p. 155)

Integrity of joint ligaments: lateral

2. PIP joint

Posture at rest

Swan-neck deformity (Fig. 5-2, p. 93)

Swan-neck testing (Fig. 5-3, p. 94)

Boutonniere deformity (Fig. 5-11, p. 104)

Synovial swelling: herniations (Fig. 8-1, p. 180)

Intrinsic tightness: one/both sides (Fig. 6-17, p. 137)

Dislocation of lateral bands (Fig. 5-12, p. 105)

Integrity of joint ligaments: dorsopalmar

Integrity of joint ligaments: lateral

Subluxation or dislocation of joint (Fig. 6-24, p. 148)

3. MP joint in flexion

Integrity of collateral ligaments in 90-degree flexion (Fig. 7-5, p. 157)

4. MP joint in extension

Posture at rest

Synovial swelling; use 3 digits (Fig. 7-7, p. 163)

Subluxation or dislocation of joint (Fig. 5-6, p. 97)

Intrinsic tightness in ulnar/radial deviation (Fig. 6-17, p. 137)

PERIPHERAL NERVES

Are there symptoms or signs compatible with neuropathy or entrapment syndromes?

Radial

Lack of digital extension due to entrapment at elbow?

Lack of digital extension due to tendon rupture?

Ulnar

Sensory or motor loss due to entrapment at elbow

Sensory or motor loss due to entrapment in Guyon's canal

Median

Sensory or motor loss due to carpal tunnel compression—test with both wrists in flexion (Fig. 5-1, p. 90)

References

This list of articles on the rheumatoid hand is not meant to be complete; there are many others that could be included. Some have been deliberately excluded; others, no doubt, have been omitted through ignorance.

The articles quoted have been useful to my work, and I am grateful to the authors for the help they have given to me. Under each chapter I have included papers that are either directly cited or whose contents merit their inclusion in the context of the chapter.

CHAPTER 1

Bleifield, C.J., and Inglis, A.E.: The hand in systemic lupus erythematosus, J. Bone Joint Surg. **56-A:**1207-1215, 1974.

Brown, P.W.: Hand surgery in rheumatoid arthritis, Semin. Arthritis Rheum. **5:**327-363, 1976.

Cats, A., and Pit, A.A.: Clinical significance of rheumatoid vasculitis and the incidence of digital vascular lesions, Folia Med. Neerl. **12**(5-6):159-165, 1969.

Conaty, J.P., and Nickel, V.L.: Functional incapacitation in rheumatoid arthritis; a rehabilitation challenge, J. Bone Joint Surg. **53-A:**624-637, 1971.

Copeman, W.S.C.: Some thoughts on the surgical treatment of rheumatic diseases, Ann. R. Coll. Surg. Engl. **43:**274-286, 1968.

Garner, R.W., Mowat, A.G., and Hazleman, B.L.: Wound healing after operations on patients with rheumatoid arthritis, J. Bone Joint Surg. **55-B:**134-144, 1973.

Granberry, W.M., and Mangum, G.L.: The hand in the child with juvenile rheumatoid arthritis, J. Hand Surg. **5:**105-113, 1980.

Hart, F.D.: Rheumatoid arthritis; extra-articular manifestations, Br. Med. J. **3:**130-136, 1969.

Hart, F.D.: Rheumatoid arthritis; extra-articular manifestations, II, Br. Med. J. **2:**747-752, 1970.

Jacoby, R.K., Jayson, M.I.V., and Cosh, J.A.: Onset, early stages, and prognosis of rheumatoid arthritis, Br. Med. J. **2:**96-100, 1973.

Jensen, P.S.: Hemochromatosis, a disease often silent but not invisible, AJR **126:**343-351, 1976.

Kinnealey, M.: The relationship between self-concept and hand deformity in rheumatoid arthritis, Am. J. Occup. Ther. **24**(4):294-297, 1970.

Lewis, R.A., Adams, J.P., Gerber, N.L., Decker, J.L., and Parsons, B.: The hand in mixed connective tissue disease, J. Hand Surg. **3:**217-222, 1978.

Lipscomb, P.R.: Surgery of the arthritic hand, Sterling Bunnell Memorial Lecture, Mayo Clin. Proc. **40:**132-164, 1965.

Martel, W., Stuck, K.J., Dworin, A.M., and Hylland, R.G.: Erosive osteoarthritis and psoriatic arthritis, a radiologic comparison, AJR **134:**125-135, 1980.

Millender, L.H.: Surgery of the hand in osteoarthritis, Orthop. Review **9:**73-81, 1980.

Moberg, E.: Cartilage lesions. In Hijmans, W., Paul, W.D., and Herschel, H., editors: Early synovectomy in rheumatoid arthritis, Amsterdam, 1969, Excerpta Medica Foundation, pp. 173-177.

Moberg, E., Wassen, E., Kjellberg, S.R., Zettergren, L., Scheller, S., and Aschan, W.: The early pathological changes in rheumatoid arthritis, Acta Chir. Scand. **357**(supp.):142-147, 1966.

Nalebuff, E.A.: Discussion of Preston, R.L.: Early synovectomy in rheumatoid arthritis, introductory paper on the orthopaedic aspects. In Hijmans, W., Paul, W.D., and Herschel, H., editors: Early synovectomy in rheumatoid arthritis, Amsterdam, 1969, Excerpta Medica Foundation, p. 48.

Schlenker, J.D., Clark, D.D., and Weckersen, E.C.: Calcinosis circumscripta of the hand in scleroderma, J. Bone Joint Surg. **55-A:**1051-1056, 1973.

Smyth, C.J.: Optimum therapeutic program in seropositive nodular rheumatoid arthritis, Med. Clin. North Am. **52:**687-698, 1968.

Sones, D.A.: The medical management of rheumatoid arthritis and the relationship between the rheumatologist and the orthopedic surgeon, Orthop. Clin. North Am. **2**:613-621, 1971.

Stern, H.S., and Lloyd, G.L.: Metacarpal shortening, Hand **10**:202-204, 1978.

Straub, L.R., Smith, J.W., Carpenter, G.K., and Dietz, G.H.: Surgery of gout in the upper extremity, J. Bone Joint Surg. **43-A**:731-752, 1961.

Swezey, R.L.: Dynamic factors in deformity of the rheumatoid arthritic hand, Bull. Rheum. Dis. **22**:649-656, 1971-1972.

Wright, V., Longfield, M.D., and Dowson, D.: Joint stiffness; its characterization and significance, Biomed. Eng. **4(1)**:8-14, 1969.

CHAPTER 2

Backhouse, K.M.: The mechanics of normal digital control in the hand and an analysis of the ulnar drift of rheumatoid arthritis, Ann. R. Coll. Surg. Engl. **43**:154-173, 1968.

Backhouse, K.M.: Extensor expansion of the rheumatoid hand, Ann. Rheum. Dis. **31**:112-117, 1972.

Capener, N.: The hand in surgery, J. Bone Joint Surg. **38-B**:128-151, 1956.

Flatt, A.E.: Kinesiology of the hand. In the American Academy of Orthopaedic Surgeons: Instructional course lectures, vol. 18, St. Louis, 1961, The C.V. Mosby Co., pp. 266-281.

Hakstian, R.W., and Tubiana, R.: Ulnar deviation of the fingers: the role of joint structure and function, J. Bone Joint Surg. **49-A**:299-316, 1967.

Keller, A.D., Taylor, C.L., and Zahn, V.: Studies to determine the functional requirements for hand and arm prosthesis, Department of Engineering, University of California at Los Angeles, 1947.

Landsmeer, J.M.F.: Studies in the anatomy of articulation. II. Patterns of movements of biomuscular biarticular systems, Acta Morphol. Neerl. Scand. **3**:304-321, 1961.

Landsmeer, J.M.F.: Power grip and precision handling, Ann. Rheum. Dis. **21**:164-170, 1962.

Linscheid, R.L., and Dobyns, J.H.: Rheumatoid arthritis of the wrist, Orthop. Clin. North Am. **2**:649-665, 1971.

Littler, J.W.: On the adaptability of man's hand, The Hand **5**:187-191, 1973.

Marmor, L.: Hand surgery in rheumatoid arthritis, Arthritis Rheum. **5**:419-424, 1962.

McMurtry, R.Y., Youm, Y., Flatt, A.E., and Gillespie, T.E.: Kinematics of the wrist II, J. Bone Joint Surg. **60-A**:955-961, 1978.

Napier, J.R.: The prehensile movements of the human hand, J. Bone Joint Surg. **38-B**:902-913, 1956.

Smith, E.M., Juvinall, R.C., Bender, L.F., and Pearson, J.R.: Flexor forces and rheumatoid metacarpophalangeal deformity, J.A.M.A. **198**:130-134, 1966.

Stetson, R.H., and McDill, J.A.: Mechanism of different types of movements, Psychol. Monogr. **32(3)**:18, 1923.

Swanson, A.B., deGroot, G.A., Hehl, R.W., Waller, T.J., and Boeve, N.R.: Pathogenesis of rheumatoid deformities in the hand. In Cruess, R., and Mitchell, N., editors: Surgery of rheumatoid arthritis, Philadelphia, 1971, J.B. Lippincott Co.

Taylor, C., and Schwartz, R.J.: The anatomy and mechanics of the human hand, Artif. Limbs **2**:22-35, 1955.

Van der Meulen, J.C.: Causes of prolapse and collapse of the proximal interphalangeal joint, The Hand **4**:147-153, 1972.

Youm, Y., McMurtry, R.Y., Flatt, A.E., and Gillespie, T.E.: Kinematics of the Wrist, I, J. Bone Joint Surg. **60-A**:423-431, 1978.

CHAPTER 3

Bennett, R.L.: Orthotic devices to prevent deformities of the hand in rheumatoid arthritis, Arthritis Rheum. **8**:1006-1018, 1965.

Convery, F.R., Conaty, J.P., and Nickel, V.L.: Dynamic splinting of the rheumatoid hand, Orthot. Prosthet. **21**:249-254, 1967.

Cordery, J.C.: Joint protection, Am. J. Occup. Ther. **19**:285-293, 1965.

Ehrlich, G.E., and DiPiero, A.M.: Stretch gloves; noctural use to ameliorate morning stiffness in arthritic hands, Arch. Phys. Med. Rehabil. **51**:479-480, 1971.

Fess, E.E., Gettle, K.S., and Strickland, J.W.: Hand splinting, St. Louis, 1981, The C.V. Mosby Co.

Kelly, M.: The correction and prevention of deformity in rheumatoid arthritis; active immobilization, Can. Med. Assoc. J. **81**:827-831, 1959.

Landsmeer, J.M.F.: A report on the coordination of the interphalangeal joints of the human finger and its disturbances, Acta Morphol. Neerl. Scand. **2**:59-84, 1959.

Madden, J.W., De Vore, G., and Arem, A.: A rational postoperative management program for metacarpophalangeal joint implant arthroplasty, J. Hand Surg. **2**:358-366, 1977.

Melvin, J.L.: Rheumatic disease: occupational therapy and rehabilitation, Philadelphia, 1977, F.A. Davis Co.

Mongan, E.S., Boger, W.M., Gilliland, B.C., and Meyerowitz, S.: Synovectomy in rheumatoid arthritis, Arthritis Rheum. **13**:761-768, 1970.

Quest, I.M., and Cordery, J.C.: A functional ulnar deviation cuff for the rheumatoid deformity, Am. J. Occup. Ther. **25:**32-40, 1971.

Rembe, E.C.: Use of cryotherapy on the postsurgical rheumatoid hand, J. Am. Phys. Ther. Assoc. **50:**19-23, 1970.

Rhinelander, F.W.: The effectiveness of splinting and bracing on rheumatoid arthritis, Arthritis Rheum. **2:**270-277, 1959.

Rose, D.L., and Kendell, H.W.: Rehabilitation of hand function in rheumatoid arthritis, J.A.M.A. **148:**1408-1413, 1952.

Rose, D.L., and Wallace, L.I.: A remedial occupational therapy program for the residuals of rheumatoid arthritis of the hand, Am. J. Phys. Med. **31:**5-13, 1952.

Rotstein, J.: Simple splinting, Philadelphia, 1965, W.B. Saunders Co.

Savill, D.L.: The use of splints in management of the rheumatoid hand. In La main rheumatismale, Paris, 1966, L'Expansion Scientifique Française, pp. 55-56.

Savill, D.L.: The use of splints in the management of the rheumatoid hand. In Tubiana, R., editor: Le main rheumatoide, Groupe d'Etude de la Main, monograph no. 3, Paris, 1969, L'Expansion Scientifique Française, pp. 219-228.

Souter, W.A.: Splintage in the rheumatoid hand, The Hand **3:**144-151, 1971.

Swanson, A.B.: Silicone rubber implants for replacement of arthritic or destroyed joints in the hand, Surg. Clin. North Am. **48:**1113-1127, 1968.

Swanson, A.B.: A dynamic brace for finger-joint reconstruction in arthritis. In Cruess, R., and Mitchell, N., editors: Surgery of rheumatoid arthritis, Philadelphia, 1971, J.B. Lippincott Co., pp. 199-203.

Wozny, W., and Long, C.: Electromyographic kinesiology of the rheumatoid hand, Arch. Phys. Med. Rehabil. **47:**699-704, 1966.

CHAPTER 4

Albright, J.A., and Chase, R.A.: Palmarshelf arthroplasty of the wrist in rheumatoid arthritis, J. Bone Joint Surg. **52-A:**896-906, 1970.

Arkless, R.: Rheumatoid wrists, Radiology **88:**534-549, 1967.

Bäckdahl, M.J.: The caput ulnae syndrome in rheumatoid arthritis, Acta Rheumatol. Scand. **5**(supp.):1-75, 1963.

Backhouse, K.M., and Kay, A.: The hand in rheumatoid arthritis, Hosp. Med., pp. 329-334, Jan., 1967.

Campbell, R.D., Jr., and Straub, L.R.: Surgical considerations for rheumatoid disease in the forearm and wrist, Am. J. Surg. **109:**361-367, 1965.

Carroll, R.E., and Dick, H.M.: Arthrodesis of the wrist for rheumatoid arthritis, J. Bone Joint Surg. **53-A:**1365-1369, 1971.

Clayton, M.L.: Surgical treatment at the wrist in rheumatoid arthritis, a review of thirty-seven patients, J. Bone Joint Surg. **47-A:**741-750, 1965.

Cracchiolo, A., III, and Marmor, L.: Resection of the distal ulna in rheumatoid arthritis, Arthritis Rheum. **12:**415-422, 1969.

Dee, R.: Total replacement of the elbow joint, Orthop. Clin. North Am. **4**(2):415-433, 1973.

DeLeeuw, B.: The stratigraphy of the dorsal wrist region, Thesis, University of Leiden, Holland, 1962.

Dickson, R.A., Stein, H., and Bentley, G.: Excision arthroplasty of the elbow in rheumatoid disease, J. Bone Joint Surg. **58-B:**227-229, 1976.

Fernandez-Palazzi, F., and Vainio, K.: Synovectomy of carpal joints in rheumatoid arthritis. A report of 47 cases, Arch. Inter-Am. Rheum. **8:**238-258, 1965.

Fisk, G.R.: Carpal instability and the fractured scaphoid, Ann. R. Coll. Surg. Engl. **46:**63-76, 1970.

Green, D.P.: Pisotriquetral arthritis, J. Hand Surg. **4:**465-467, 1979.

Harrison, M.O., Freiberger, R.H., and Ranawat, C.S.: Arthrography of the rheumatoid wrist joint, Am. J. Roentgenol. Radium Ther. Nucl. Med. **112**(3):480-486, 1971.

Inglis, A.E., Ranawat, C.S., and Straub, L.R.: Synovectomy and debridement of the elbow in rheumatoid arthritis, J. Bone Joint Surg. **53-A:**652-662, 1971.

Kessler, I., Raunio, P., and Vainio, K.: The rheumatoid hand; a comparative study of affected sites, Acta Rheumatol. Scand. **11:**241-246, 1965.

Kirk Watson, H., and Hempton, R.F.: Limited wrist arthrodeses, triscaphoid joint, I, J. Hand Surg. **5:**320-327, 1980.

Linscheid, R.L., and Dobyns, J.H.: Rheumatoid arthritis of the wrist, Orthop. Clin. North Am. **2:**649-665, 1971.

Linscheid, R.L., Dobyns, J.H., Beabout, J.W., and Bryan, R.S.: Traumatic instability of the wrist, diagnosis, classification, and pathomechanics, J. Bone Joint Surg. **54-A:**1612-1632, 1972.

Lipscomb, P.R.: Synovectomy of the wrist for rheumatoid arthritis, J.A.M.A. **194:**655-659, 1965.

Mannerfelt, L., and Malmsten, M.: Arthrodesis of the wrist in rheumatoid arthritis; a technique without external fixation, Scand. J. Plast. Reconstr. Surg. **5:**124-130, 1971.

Marmor, L.: Surgery of the rheumatoid elbow, J. Bone Joint Surg. **54-A:**573-578, 1972.

Mikkelsen, O.A.: Arthrodesis of the wrist in rheumatoid arthritis, The Hand **12:**149-153, 1980.

Nalebuff, E.A., and Millender, L.H.: Arthrodesis of the rheumatoid wrist, Orthop. Rev. **1:**13-18, 1972.

Pahle, J.A., and Raunio, P.: The influence of wrist position on finger deviation in the rheumatoid hand, J. Bone Joint Surg. **51-B:**664-676, 1969.

Peacock, E.E., Jr., and Holbrook, J.P.: Early radical synovectomy of the arthritic wrist, Hosp. Pract., Feb., 1973, p. 143.

Peterson, L.F.A., and Janes, J.M.: Surgery of the rheumatoid elbow, Orthop. Clin. North Am. **2:**667-677, 1971.

Porter, B.B., Richardson, C., and Vainie, K.: Rheumatoid arthritis of the elbow: the results of synovectomy, J. Bone Joint Surg. **56-B:**427-437, 1974.

Rana, N.A., and Taylor, A.R.: Excision of the distal end of the ulna in rheumatoid arthritis, J. Bone Joint Surg. **55-B:**96-105, 1973.

Savill, D.L.: Some aspects of rheumatoid hand surgery. In La main rheumatismale, Paris, 1966, L'Expansion Scientifique Francaise, pp. 27-29.

Shapiro, J.S.: A new factor in the etiology of ulnar drift, Clin. Orthop. **68:**32-43, 1970.

Smith-Petersen, M.N., Aufranc, O.E., and Larson, C.B.: Useful surgical procedures for rheumatoid arthritis involving joints of the upper extremity, Arch. Surg. **46:**764-770, 1943.

Souter, W.A.: Arthroplasty of the elbow, Orthop. Clin. North Am. **4:**395-413, 1973.

Stack, H.G., and Vaughan-Jackson, O.J.: The zigzag deformity in the rheumatoid hand, The Hand **3:**62-67, 1971.

Stillman, K.: Resection arthroplasty of the wrist in rheumatoid arthritis, Proceedings of the International Symposium on Surgery of the Hand, Rotterdam, Netherlands, 1981.

Straub, L.R., and Ranawat, C.S.: The wrist in rheumatoid arthritis, J. Bone Joint Surg. **51-A:**1-20, 1969.

Swezey, R.L., and Alexander, S.J.: Notching of the carpal navicular, Ann. Rheum. Dis. **28(1):**45-48, 1969.

Taleisnik, J.: Rheumatoid synovitis of the volar compartment of the wrist joint, J. Hand Surg. **4:**526-535, 1979.

Wilson, D.W., Arden, G.P., and Ansell, B.M.: Synovectomy of the elbow in rheumatoid arthritis, J. Bone Joint Surg. **55-B:**106-111, 1973.

CHAPTER 5

Addison, N.V.: Spontaneous rupture of extensor tendons of wrist joint, Br. J. Surg. **41:**511-514, 1953-1954.

Backhouse, K.M., Kay, A.G.L., Coomes, E.N., and Kates, A.: Tendon involvement in the rheumatoid hand, Ann. Rheum. Dis. **30:**236-242, 1971.

Barnes, C.G., and Currey, H.L.F.: Carpal tunnel syndrome in rheumatoid arthritis, Ann. Rheum. Dis. **26:**226-233, 1967.

Boyes, J.H.: The rheumatoid hand; its treatment, University of Minnesota Continuation Course (private circulation), 1961.

Boyes, J.H.: The role of the intrinsic muscles in rheumatoid deformities. In Tubiana, R., editor: La main rhumatoide, Groupe d'Etude de la Main, monograph no. 3, Paris, 1969, L'Expansion Scientifique Française, pp. 63-64.

Brewerton, D.A.: The rheumatoid hand, Proc. R. Soc. Med. **59:**225-228, 1966.

Chamberlain, M.A., and Bruckner, F.E.: Rheumatoid neuropathy; clinical and electrophysiological features, Ann. Rheum. Dis. **29:**609-616, 1970.

Chang, L.W., Gowans, J.D.C., Granger, C.V., and Millender, L.H.: Entrapment neuropathy of the posterior interosseous nerve, Arthritis Rheum. **15:**350-352, 1972.

Davalbhakta, V.V., and Bailey, B.N.: Trigger wrist; report of two cases, Br. J. Plast. Surg. **25:**376-379, 1972.

Davies, D.V.: Blood supply to the tendon of extensor pollicis longus, Br. Med. J. **2:**56, 1951.

Dobyns, J.H., and Linscheid, R.L.: Rheumatoid hand repairs, Orthop. Clin. North Am. **2:**629-647, 1971.

Ferlic, D.C., and Clayton, M.L.: Flexor tenosynovectomy in the rheumatoid finger, J. Hand Surg. **3:**364-367, 1978.

Howard, L.D., Jr.: Surgical treatment of rheumatic tenosynovitis, Am. J. Surg. **89:**1163-1168, 1955.

Ishikawa, K., Patiala, H., Raunio, P., and Vainio, K.: Carpal tunnel syndrome in juvenile rheumatoid arthritis, Arch. Orthop. Unfall-Chir **82:**85-91, 1975.

Kellgren, J.H., and Ball, J.: Tendon lesions in rheumatoid arthritis, Ann. Rheum. Dis. **9:**48-65, 1950.

Kestler, O.C.: Histopathology of the intrinsic muscles of the hand in rheumatoid arthritis, Ann. Rheum. Dis. **8:**42-58, 1949.

Laine, V.A.I., Sairanen, E., and Vainio, K.: Finger deformities caused by rheumatoid arthritis, J. Bone Joint Surg. **39-A:**527-533, 1957.

Mannerfelt, L., and Norman, O.: Attrition ruptures of flexor tendons in rheumatoid arthritis caused by bony spurs in the carpal tunnel, J. Bone Joint Surg. **51-B:**270-277, 1969.

Marmor, L., Lawrence, J.F., and Dubois, E.L.: Posterior interosseous nerve palsy due to rheumatoid arthritis, J. Bone Joint Surg. **49-A**:381-382, 1967.

Millender, L.H., Nalebuff, E.A., and Holdsworth, D.E.: Posterior interosseous-nerve syndrome secondary to rheumatoid synovitis, J. Bone Joint Surg. **55-A**:753-757, 1973.

Millender, L.H., and Nalebuff, E.A.: Preventative surgery—tenosynovectomy and synovectomy, Orthop. Clin. North Am. **6**:765-792, 1975.

Pallis, C.A., and Scott, J.T.: Peripheral neuropathy in rheumatoid arthritis, Br. Med. J. **1**:1141-1147, 1965.

Paul, W.D.: Systemic manisfestations of rheumatoid arthritis (rheumatoid disease) accentuated by steroid therapy. J. Iowa Med. Soc. **51**:205-216, 1961.

Paul, W.D., Hodges, R.E., Bean, W.B., Routh, J.I., and Daum, K.: Effects of nitrogen mustard therapy in patients with rheumatoid arthritis, Arch. Phys. Med. Rehabil. **35**:371-380, 1954.

Polley, H.F., and Lipscomb, P.R.: Les affections rhumatismales et le syndrome du canal carpieh, Med. Hyg. **24**:408-409, 1966.

Popelka, S., and Vainio, K.: Compression of the deep branch of the radial nerve in patients with rheumatoid arthritis, Clin. Orthop. Traum. Chech. **38**:195-199, 1971.

Riddell, D.M.: Spontaneous rupture of the extensor pollicis longus, J. Bone Joint Surg. **45-B**:506-510, 1963.

Riley, M., and Harrison, S.H.: Interosseous muscle biopsy during hand surgery for rheumatoid arthritis, Br. J. Plast. Surg. **21**:342-346, 1968.

Smith, F.M.: Late rupture of extensor pollicis longus tendon following Colles' fracture, J. Bone Joint Surg. **28**:49-59, 1946.

Sokoloff, L., Wilens, S.L., Bunim, J.J., and McEwen, C.: Diagnostic value of histologic lesions of striated muscle in rheumatoid arthritis, Am. J. Med. Sci. **219**:174-182, 1950.

Steiner, G., Freund, H., Leichtentriff, B., and Maun, M.: Lesions of skeletal muscles in rheumatoid arthritis nodular polymyositis, Am. J. Pathol. **22**:103-145, 1946.

Strandberg, B.: The frequency of myopathy in patients with rheumatoid arthritis treated with triamcinolone, Acta Rheumatol. Scand. **8**:31-44, 1962.

Straub, L.R.: The etiology of finger deformities in the hand affected by rheumatoid arthritis, Bull. Hosp. Joint Dis. **21**:322-329, 1960.

Straub, L.R., and Wilson, E.H.: Spontaneous rupture of extensor tendons in the hand associated with rheumatoid arthritis, J. Bone Joint Surg. **38A**:1208-1217, 1956.

Swezey, R.L., and Fiegenberg, D.S.: Inappropriate intrinsic muscle action in the rheumatoid hand, Ann. Rheum. Dis. **30**:619-625, 1971.

Swezey, R.L.: Dynamic factors in deformity of the rheumatoid arthritis hand, Bull. Rheum. Dis. **22**:649-656, 1971-1972.

Trevor, D.: Rupture of extensor pollicis longus tendon after Colles' fracture, J. Bone Joint Surg. **32-B**:370-375, 1950.

Vainio, K.: Carpal canal syndrome caused by tenosynovitis, Acta Rheumatol. Scand. **4**:22-27, 1957.

Vainio, K.: Synovectomies of the hand and wrist in rheumatoid arthritis. In La Main Rhumatismale, Paris, 1966, Expansion Scientifique Française, pp. 22-24.

Vainio, K.: Rheumatoid changes in the metacarpophalangeal region as a cause of Bunnell's sign, Ann. Rheum. Dis. **26**:328, 1967.

Vaughan-Jackson, O.J.: Rupture of extensor tendons by attrition at the inferior radioulnar joint; report of two cases, J. Bone Joint Surg. **30-B**:528-530, 1948.

Vaughan-Jackson, O.J.: Attrition ruptures of tendons as a factor in the production of deformities in the rheumatoid hand, Proc. R. Soc. Med. **52**:132-134, 1959.

Welsh, R.P., and Hastings, D.E.: Swan-neck deformity in rheumatoid arthritis of the hand, Hand **9**:109-116, 1977.

Wissinger, H.: Digital flexor lag in rheumatoid arthritis, Plast. Reconstr. Surg. **47**:465-468, 1971.

CHAPTER 6

Abernathy, P.J., and Dennyson, W.G.: Decompression of the extensor tendons at the wrist in rheumatoid arthritis, J. Bone Joint Surg. **61-B**:64-68, 1979.

Ellison, M.R., Flatt, A.E., and Kelly, K.J.: Ulnar drift of the fingers in rheumatoid disease, J. Bone Joint Surg. **53-A**:1061-1082, 1971.

Ferlic, D.C., and Clayton, M.L.: Flexor tenosynovectomy in the rheumatoid finger, J. Hand Surg. **3**:364-367, 1978.

Fowler, S.B., and Riordan, D.C.: Surgical treatment of rheumatoid deformities of the hand, J. Bone Joint Surg. **40-A**:1431-1432, 1958.

Gray, R.G., Kiem, I.M., and Gottlieb, N.L.: Intratendon sheath corticosteroid treatment of rheumatoid arthritis—associated and idiopathic hand flexor tenosynovitis, Arthritis Rheum. **21**:92-96, 1978.

Harrison, S.H., Swannell, A.J., and Ansell, B.M.: Repair of extensor pollicis longus using extensor pollicis brevis in rheumatoid arthritis, Ann. Rheum. Dis. **31**:490-492, 1972.

Harrison, S.H., Ansell, B., and Hall, M.A.: Flexor synovectomy in the rheumatoid hand, Hand **8**:13-16, 1976.

Jackson, I. T., and Paton, K. C.: The extended approach to flexor tendon synovitis in rheumatoid arthritis, Br. J. Plast. Surg. **26**:122-131, 1973.

Kaplan, E.: Anatomy, injuries and treatment of the extensor apparatus, Clin. Orthop. **13**:24-41, 1959.

Littler, J.W.: Referred to in Riordan, D.C., and Harris, C.: Intrinsic contracture in the hand and its surgical treatment, J. Bone Joint Surg. **36-A**:10-20, 1954.

Littler, J.W.: Restoration of the oblique retinacular ligament for correcting hyperextension deformity of the proximal interphalangeal joint. In La main rhumatismale, Paris, 1966, L'Expansion Scientifique Française, pp. 39-41.

Nalebuff, E.A., and Millender, L.H.: Surgical treatment of the boutonniere deformity in rheumatoid arthritis, Orthop. Clin. North Am. **6**:753-763, 1975.

Ranawat, C.S., and Straub, L.R.: Volar tenosynovitis of wrist in rheumatoid arthritis, Arthritis Rheum. **13**:112-117, 1970.

Straub, L.R.: The intrinsic muscles in disease with particular reference to the rheumatoid hand. In Dixiéme Congrés International de Chirurgie Orthopédique et de Traumatologie, Paris, 4-9 Sept., 1966. Bruxelles, 1967, Les Publications "Acta Medica Belgica," pp. 863-872.

Zancolli, E.: Structural and dynamic bases of hand surgery, Philadelphia, 1968, J.B. Lippincott Co., p. 139.

CHAPTER 7

Berglöf, F.E.: Osmic acid in arthritis therapy, Acta Rheumatol. Scand. **5**:70-74, 1959.

Brewerton, D.A.: The tangential radiographic projection for demonstrating involvement of metacarpal heads in rheumatoid arthritis, Br. J. Radiol. **40**:233-234, 1967.

Brooks, A.: Personal communication, 1973.

Currey, H.L.F.: Intra-articular Thiotepa in rheumatoid arthritis, Ann. Rheum. Dis. **24**:382, 1965.

Ellison, M.R., and Flatt, A.E.: Arthritis Rheum. **14**:216-222, 1971.

Fearnley, M.E.: Intra-articular Thiotepa therapy in rheumatoid arthritis, Ann. Phys. Med. **7**:294-298, 1964.

Flatt, A.E.: Restoration of rheumatoid finger joint function; interim report on trial of prosthetic replacement, J. Bone Joint Surg. **43-A**:753-774, 1961.

Flatt, A.E.: Intra-articular Thio-tepa in rheumatoid disease of the hands, Rheumatism **18**:70-73, 1962.

Flatt, A.E.: Restoration of rheumatoid finger joint function, III, J. Bone Joint Surg. **54-A**:1317-1322, 1972.

Flatt, A.E., and Fischer, G.W.: Biomechanical factors in the replacement of rheumatoid finger joints, Ann. Rheum. Dis. **28**(supp.):36-41, 1969.

Gatter, R.A., and McCarthy, D.J., Jr.: A study of distal interphalangeal joint tenderness in rheumatoid arthritis, Arthritis Rheum. **9**:325-326, 1966.

Gillespie, T.E., Flatt, A.E., Youm, Y., and Sprague, B.L.: Biomechanical evaluation of metacarpophalangeal joint prosthesis designs, J. Hand Surg. **4**:508-521, 1979.

Gristina, A.G., Pace, N.A., Kantor, T.G., and Thompson, W.A.: Intra-articular Thio-tepa compared with Depo-medrol and procaine in the treatment of arthritis, J. Bone Joint Surg. **52-A**:1603-1610, 1970.

Jimenez, D.C.: Treatment of dysreaction diseases with nitrogen mustards, Ann. Rheum. Dis. **10**:144-151, 1951.

Kay, G.L.: Natural history of synovial hypertrophy in the rheumatoid hand, Ann. Rheum. Dis. **30**:98-102, 1971.

Kidd, K.L., and Peter, J.B.: Erosive osteoarthritis, Radiology **86**:640-647, 1966.

Linscheid, R.L., and Chao, E.Y.S.: Biomechanical assessment of finger function in prosthetic joint design, Orthop. Clin. North Am. **4**:317-330, 1973.

Lipscomb, P.R.: Surgery of the Arthritic hand, Sterling Bunnell Memorial Lecture, Mayo Clin. Proc. **40**:132-164, 1965.

Mason, R.M.: Early synovectomy in rheumatoid arthritis. In Hijmans, W., Paul, W.D., and Herschel, H., editors: Early synovectomy in rheumatoid arthritis, Amsterdam, 1969, Excerpta Medica Foundation, pp. 50-60.

McCarty, D.J., Jr., and Gatter, R.A.: A study of distal interphalangeal joint tenderness and rheumatoid arthritis, Arthritis Rheum. **9**:325-336, 1966.

McMaster, M.: The natural history of the rheumatoid metacarpophalangeal joint, J. Bone Joint Surg. **54-B**:687-697, 1972.

Menkes, C.J., Tubiana, R., Galmiche, B., and Del Barre, F.: Intra-articular injection of radioisotopic beta emitters, Orthop. Clin. North Am. **4**:1113-1125, 1973.

Mickelson, M., and Cooper R.R.: Ligament ultrastructural changes in rheumatoid arthritis, I and II, Iowa Chapter, Arthritis Foundation Med. Info. Bull. **12**(3-4):13-16 and **12**(5-6):9-11, 1971.

Mondragón Kalb, M.: Thiotepa en el tratamiento de la arthritis rheumatoide, Medecina (Mex.) **15**(4):82-84, 1965.

Niebauer, J.J., Shawn, J.L., and Doren, W.W.: Silicone-Dacron hinge prosthesis, design, evaluation and application, Ann. Rheum. Dis. **28**(supp.):56-58, 1969.

Peter, J.B., Pearson, C.M., and Maiuror, L.: Erosive osteoarthritis of the hands, Arthritis Rheum. **9**:365-388, 1966.

Scherbel, A.L., Schucher, S.L., and Weyman, J.S.: Intra-articular administration of nitrogen mustard alone and combined with corticosteroid for rheumatoid arthritis, Cleve. Clin. Q. **24**:78-89, 1957.

Smith, R.J., and Kaplan, E.F.: Rheumatoid deformities at the metacarpophalangeal joints of the fingers, J. Bone Joint Surg. **49-A**:31-47, 1967.

Steindler, A.: Arthritic deformities of the wrist and finger, J. Bone Joint Surg. **33-A**:849-862, 1951.

Swanson, A.B.: Finger joint replacement by silicone rubber implants and the concept of implant fixation by encapsulation, Ann. Rheum. Dis. **28**(5)(supp., Artificial finger joints): 47-55, 1969.

Vainio, K., and Julkunen, H.: Intra-articular nitrogen mustard treatment of rheumatoid arthritis, Acta Rheumatol. Scand. **6**(fasc. 1):25-30, 1960.

Wenley, W.G., and Glick, E.N.: Medical synovectomy with Thiotepa, Ann. Phys. Med. **7**:287-293, 1964.

Young, A.C.: Early radiographic signs of rheumatic disease, Proc. R. Soc. Med. **52**:208-210, 1960.

Zuckner, J., et al.: Evaluating intra-articular Thiotepa in rheumatoid arthritis, Ann. Rheum. Dis. **25**:178-183, 1966.

CHAPTER 8

Ansell, B.M., Harrison, S.H., Little, H., and Thouas, B.: Synovectomy of proximal interphalangeal joints, Br. J. Plast. Surg. **23**:380-385, 1970.

Aptekar, R.G., and Duff, I.F.: Metacarpophalangeal joint surgery in rheumatoid arthritis, Clin. Orthop. **83**:123-127, 1972.

Ashbell, T.S.: The scalloped dorsal metacarpophalangeal skin incision, J. Bone Joint Surg. **51-A**:787-788, 1969.

Bailey, B.N.: Dermal arthroplasty, The Hand, **3**:135-137, 1971.

Beckenbaugh, R.D., Dobyus, J.H., Linscheid, R.L., and Bryan, R.S.: Review and analysis of silicone rubber metacarpophalangeal implants, J. Bone Joint Surg. **58-A**:483-487, 1976.

Biddulph, S.L.: Extensor indicis proprius transfer to supplement replacement arthroplasty for the rheumatoid hand, Orthopaedia **3**:9-11, 1975.

Branemark, P.I., Ekholm, R., and Goldie, I.: Physiologic aspects on the timing of synovectomy in rheumatoid arthritis. In Hijmans, W., Paul, W.D., and Herschel, H., editors: Early synovectomy in rheumatoid arthritis, Amsterdam, 1969, Excerpta Medica Foundation, pp. 11-19.

Carroll, R.E., and Hill, N.A.: Small joint arthrodesis in hand reconstruction, J. Bone Joint Surg. **51-A**:1219-1221, 1969.

Carroll, R.E., and Taber, T.H.: Digital arthroplasty of the proximal interphalangeal joint, J. Bone Joint Surg. **36-A**:912-920, 1954.

Christie, A.J., Weinberger, K.A., and Dietrich, M.: Silicone lymphadenopathy and synovitis, J.A.M.A. **237**:1463-1464, 1977.

Crawford, G.P.: Dual curved incisions for trans-metacarpophalangeal surgery, Plast. Reconstr. Surg. **61**:616-618, 1978.

Currey, H.L.F.: Intra-articular Thiotepa in rheumatoid arthritis, Ann. Rheum. Dis. **24**:382-388, 1965.

Curtis, R.M.: Capsulectomy of the interphalangeal joints of the fingers, J. Bone Joint Surg. **36-A**:1219-1232, 1954.

Ellison, M.R., and Flatt, A.E.: Intra-articular Thiotepa in rheumatoid disease, Arthritis Rheum. **14**:216-222, 1971.

Ellison, M.R., Kelly, K.J., and Flatt, A.E.: The results of surgical synovectomy of the digital joints in rheumatoid disease, J. Bone Joint Surg. **53-A**:1041-1060, 1971.

Flatt, A.E.: The considered use of digital joint prostheses. In Transactions of the Fifth International Congress of Plastic and Reconstructive Surgery, 1971, Butterworths, Australia, pp. 638-648.

Flatt, A.E., and Ellison, M.R.: Restoration of rheumatoid finger joint function, III, J. Bone Joint Surg. **54-A**:1317-1322, 1972.

Froimson, A.I.: Hand reconstruction in arthritis mutilans, J. Bone Joint Surg. **53-A**:1377-1382, 1971.

Girzadas, D.V., and Clayton, M.L.: Limitations of the use of metallic prosthesis in the rheumatoid hand, Clin. Orthop. **67**:127-132, 1969.

Goldie, I., and Wellisch, M.: The presence of nerves in original and regenerated synovial tissue in patients synovectomised for rheumatoid arthritis, Acta Orthop. Scand. **40**:143-152, 1969.

Goldner, J., and Urbaniak, J.R.: The clinical experience with silicone-Dacron metacarpophalangeal and interphalangeal joint prostheses. Presented at Biomaterials Conference, Clemson University, April 4, 1972.

Granowitz, S., and Vainio, K.: Proximal interphalangeal joint arthrodesis in rheumatoid arthritis, Acta Orthop. Scand. **37**:301-310, 1966.

Harrison, H.: Excision arthroplasty of the metacarpophalangeal joints. In Tubiana, R., editor: La main rheumatoide, Groupe d'Etude de la Main, monograph no. 3, Paris, 1969, L'Expansion Scientifique Francaise, pp. 159-164.

Harrison, S.H.: Reconstructive arthroplasty of the metacarpophalangeal joint using the extensor loop operation, Br. J. Plast. Surg. 24:307-309, 1971.

Hellum, C., and Vainio, K.: Arthroplasty of the metacarpophalangeal joints in rheumatoid arthritis with transposition of the interosseus muscles, Scand. J. Plast. Reconstr. Surg. 2:139-143, 1968.

Jackson, I.T.: Surgical treatment of the hand in rheumatoid arthritis, Gazzetta Sanitaria, 19:84-91, 1970.

Lipscomb, P.R.: Surgery for rheumatoid arthritis— timing and techniques: summary, J. Bone Joint Surg. 50-A:614-617, 1968.

Lipscomb, P.R.: Is early synovectomy of the small joints of the hand worthwhile? In Cramer, L.M., and Chase, R.A., editors: Symposium on the hand, vol. 3, St. Louis, 1971, The C.V. Mosby Co., pp. 29-32.

Madden, J.W., De Vore, G., and Arem, A.J.: A rational post-operative management program for metacarpophalangeal joint implant arthroplasty, J. Hand Surg. 2:358-366, 1977.

Moberg, E.: Arthrodesis of finger joints, Surg. Clin. North Am. 40:465-470, 1960.

Newmeyer, W.L., Kilore, E.S., Jr., and Graham, W.P., III: Mucous cysts: the dorsal distal interphalangeal joint ganglion, Plast. Reconstr. Surg. 53:313-315, 1974.

Nicolle, F.V., Holt, P.J.L., and Calnan, J.S.: Prophylactic synovectomy of the joints of the rheumatoid hand, Ann. Rheum. Dis. 30:476-480, 1971.

Niebauer, J.J.: Dacron-silicone prosthesis for the metacarpophalangeal and interphalangeal joints. In Cramer, L.M., and Chase, R.A., editors: Symposium on the hand, vol. 3, St. Louis, 1971, The C.V. Mosby Co., pp. 96-105.

Preston, R.L.: Early synovectomy in rheumatoid arthritis: introductory paper on the orthopaedic aspects. In Hijmans, W., Paul, W.D., and Herschel, H., editors: Early synovectomy in rheumatoid arthritis, Amsterdam, 1969, Excerpta Medica Foundation, pp. 44-49.

Raunio, P.: Prophylactic value of synovectomy of the proximal interphalangeal joint in rheumatoid arthritis, Scand. J. Rheumatol. 6(supp. 19): 1-88, 1977.

Rhodes, K., Jeffs, J.V., and Scott, J.T.: Experience with Silastic prostheses in rheumatoid hands, Ann. Rheum. Dis. 31:103-108, 1972.

Solomon, W.M., and Stecher, R.M.: Chronic absorptive arthritis and opera glass hand, Ann. Rheum. Dis. 9:209-220, 1950.

Strang, R.F.A., and Hueston, J.T.: Healing of bony rheumatoid lesions after synovectomy of metacarpophalangeal joints, Med. J. Austr. 1:809, 1968.

Steffee, A.D., Beckenbaugh, R.D., Linscheid, R.L., and Dobyns, J.H.: The development, technique and early clinical results of total joint replacement for the metacarpophalangeal joints of the fingers. Orthopedics 4:175-180, 1981.

Swanson, A.B.: Complications of silicone elastomer prostheses, J.A.M.A. 238:939, 1977.

Swanson, A.B.: Flexible implant arthroplasty for arthritic finger joints, J. Bone Joint Surg. 54-A:435-455, 1972.

Thompson, M., Douglas, G., and Davidson, E.P.: Evaluation of synovectomy in rheumatoid arthritis, Proc. R. Soc. Med. 66:197-199, 1973.

Tupper, J.W.: The volar plate arthroplasty for rheumatoid arthritis. Proceedings of the fifteenth annual meeting of the Japanese Society for Surgery of the Hand, Niigota, Japan, 1972, p. 24.

Vainio, K.: Arthrodeses and arthroplasties in the treatment of the rheumatoid hand. In La main rhumatismale, Paris, 1966, Expansion Scientifique Française, pp. 30-35.

Vainio, K., Reiman, I., and Pulkki, T.: Results of arthroplasty of the metacarpophalangeal joints in rheumatoid arthritis, Reconstr. Surg. Traumatol. 9:1-7, 1967.

Vaughan-Jackson, O.J.: Long-term evaluation of the results of surgery of the rheumatoid hand. In Tubiana, R., editor: La main rhumatoide, Groupe d'Etude de la Main monograph no. 3, Paris, 1969, L'Expansion Scientifique Française, p. 103.

Weilby, A.: Resection arthroplasty of the metacarpophalangeal joint a.m. Tupper using interposition of the volar plate, Scand. J. Plast. Reconstr. Surg. ll:239-242, 1977.

Wilde, A.H.: Synovectomy of the proximal interphalangeal joint of the finger in rheumatoid arthritis, J. Bone Joint Surg. 56-A:71-78, 1974.

Wilde, A.H., and Sawmiller, S.R.: Synovectomy of the proximal interphalangeal joint of the finger in rheumatoid arthritis, Cleve. Clin. Q. 36:155-161, 1969.

Zachariae, L.: Experience of Flatt finger joint prostheses, Acta Orthop. Scand. 38:329-340, 1967.

CHAPTER 9

Amadio, P., Millender, L.H., and Smith: Silicone spacer or tendon spacer for trapezium resection arthroplasty, J. Hand Surg. 7:237-244, 1982.

Ashworth, C.R., Blatt, G., Chuinard, R.G., and Stark, H.H.: Silicone rubber interposition arthroplasty of the carpometacarpal joint of the thumb, J. Hand Surg. 2:345-357, 1977.

Brewerton, D.A.: The rheumatoid hand, Proc. R. Soc. Med. 59:225-228, 1966.

Brumfield, R.H., and Conaty, J.P.: Reconstructive surgery of the thumb in rheumatoid arthritis, Orthopedics 3:529-533, 1980.

Burton, R.I.: Basal joint arthrosis of the thumb, Orthop. Clin. North Am. **4**:331-348, 1973.

Campbell, C.S.: Gamekeeper's thumb, J. Bone Joint Surg. **37-B**:148-149, 1955.

Carroll, R.E., and Hill, N.A.: Arthrodesis of the carpo-metacarpal joint of the thumb, J. Bone Joint Surg. **55-B**:292-294, 1973.

Clayton, M.L.: Surgery of the thumb in rheumatoid arthritis, J. Bone Joint Surg. **44-A**:1376-1386, 1962.

Eaton, R.G.: Replacement of the trapezium for arthritis of the basal articulations, J. Bone Joint Surg. **61-A**:76-82, 1979.

Eaton, R.G., and Littler, W.: Ligament reconstruction for the painful thumb carpometacarpal joint, J. Bone Joint Surg. **55-A**:1655-1666, 1973.

Ferlic, D.C., Serot, D.I., and Clayton, M.L.: The use of the Flatt hinge prosthesis in the rheumatoid thumb, Hand **10**:94-98, 1978.

Gervis, W.H.: A review of excision of the trapezium for osteoarthritis of the trapezio-metacarpal joint after twenty five years, J. Bone Joint Surg. **55-B**:56-57, 1973.

Goldner, J.L., and Clippinger, F.W.: Excision of the greater multangular bone as an adjunct to mobilization of the thumb, J. Bone Joint Surg. **41-A**:609-625, 1959.

Haffajee, D.: Endoprosthetic replacement of the trapezium for arthrosis in the carpometacarpal joint of the thumb, J. Hand Surg. **2**:141-148, 1977.

Inglis, A.E., Hamlin, C., Sengelmann, R.P., and Straub, L.R.: Reconstruction of the metacarpophalangeal joint of the thumb in rheumatoid arthritis, J. Bone Joint Surg. **54-A**:704-712, 1972.

Kaplan, E.B.: Pathology and treatment of gamekeeper's thumb, J. Bone Joint Surg. **43-A**:608, 1961.

Kessler, I.: Aetiology and management of adduction contracture of the thumb in rheumatoid arthritis, The Hand **5**:170-174, 1973.

Kessler, I.: Silicone arthroplasty of the trapeziometacarpal joint, J. Bone Joint Surg. **55-B**:285-291, 1973.

Kessler, I.: A simplified technique to correct hyperextension deformity of the metacarpophalangeal joint of the thumb, J. Bone Joint Surg. **61-A**:903-905, 1979.

Millender, L.H., Nalebuff, E.A., Amadio, P., and Phillips, C.: Interpositional athroplasty for rheumatoid carpometacarpal joint disease, J. Hand Surg. **6**:533-541, 1978.

Nalebuff, E.A.: Diagnosis, classification and management of rheumatoid thumb deformities, Bull. Hosp. Joint Dis. **24**:119-137, 1968.

Nalebuff, E.A.: Personal communication, 1973.

Poppen, N.K., and Niebauer, J.J.: "Tie-in" trapezium prosthesis: long-term results, J. Hand Surg. **5**:445-450, 1978.

Pulkki, T.: Rheumatoid deformities of the hand, Acta Rheum. Scand. **7**:85-88, 1961.

Ratliff, A.H.C.: Deformities of the thumb in rheumatoid arthritis, The Hand **3**:138-143, 1971.

Swanson, A.B.: Disabling arthritis at the base of the thumb, J. Bone Joint Surg. **54-A**:456-471, 1972.

Swanson, A.B., and Herndon, J.H.: Flexible (silicone) implant arthroplasty of the metacarpophalangeal joint of the thumb, J. Bone Joint Surg. **59-A**:362-368, 1977.

Weinman, D.T., and Lipscomb, P.R.: Degenerative arthritis of the trapeziometacarpal joint; arthrodesis or excision? Mayo Clin. Proc. **42**:276-287, 1967.

CHAPTER 10

Backhouse, K.M.: Extensor expansion of the rheumatoid hand, Ann. Rheum. Dis. **31**:112-117, 1972.

Backhouse, K.M.: The mechanics of normal digital control in the hand and an analysis of the ulnar drift of rheumatoid arthritis, Ann. R. Coll. Surg. Engl. **43**:154-173, 1968.

Billich, H.U.: Mitteilungen aus den grenz, Gebieten der Medizin and Chirurgie, **39/40**:638-647, 1926/1928.

Boyce, T., Youm, Y., Sprague, B.L., and Flatt, A.E.: Clinical and experimental studies on the effect of extensor carpi radialis longus transfer in the rheumatoid hand, J. Hand Surg. **3**:390-394, 1978.

Clark, I.P., James, D.F., and Colwill, J.C.: Intraarticular pressure as a factor in initiating ulnar drift, J. Bone Joint Surg. **60-A**:325-327, 1978.

Fearnley, G.R.: Ulnar deviation of fingers, Ann. Rheum. Dis. **10**:126-136, 1951.

Flatt, A.E.: The pathomechanics of ulnar drift, Final Report Social and Rehab. Services Grant No. RD2226M, 1971.

Hakstian, R.W., and Tubiana, R.: Ulnar deviation of the fingers; the role of joint structure and function, J. Bone Joint Surg. **49-A**:299-316, 1967.

Harrison, D.H., Harrison, S.H., and Smith, P.: Realignment procedure for ulnar drift of the metacarpophalangeal joint in rheumatoid arthritis, Hand **11**:163-168, 1979.

Harvey-Kemble, J.V.: Functional disability in the rheumatoid hand, Hand **9**:234-241, 1977.

Hastings, D.E., Evans, J.A., and Hewitson, W.A.: Rheumatoid wrist deformities and their relation to ulnar drift, J. Bone Joint Surg. **54-A**:1797, 1972.

Hueston, J.T.: The role of the intrinsic muscles in the production of metacarpophalangeal subluxation in the rheumatoid hand, Plast. Reconstr. Surg. **52:**342-345, 1973.

Landsmeer, J.M.F.: Anatomical and functional investigations on the articulation of the human fingers, Acta Anat. (Basel) **25**(supp. 24):5-69, 1955.

Landsmeer, J.M.F.: A report on the coordination of the interphalangeal joints of the human finger and its disturbances, Acta Morphol. Neerl. Scand. **2:**59-84, 1953.

Landsmeer, J.M.F.: Studies in the anatomy of articulation, II, Acta Morphol. Neerl. Scand. **3:**304-321, 1961.

Linscheid, R.L., and Dobyns, J.H.: Rheumatoid arthritis of the wrist, Orthop. Clin. North Am. **2:**649-655, 1971.

Lundblom, A.: On congenital ulnar deviation of the fingers of familial occurrence, Acta Orthop. Scand. **3/4:**393-404, 1932-1933.

Nicholle, F.V.: Surgical correction of ulnar drift in the rheumatoid hand, Hand **11:**157-162, 1979.

Pahle, J.A., and Raunio, P.: The influence of wrist position on finger deviation in the rheumatoid hand, J. Bone Joint Surg. **51-B:**664-676, 1969.

Shapiro, J.S., Heijna, W., Nasatir, S., and Ray, R.D.: The relationship of wrist motion to ulnar phalangeal drift in the rheumatoid patient, The Hand **3:**68-75, 1971.

Smith, E.M., Juvinall, R.C., Bender, L.F., and Pearson, J.R.: Flexor forces and rheumatoid metacarpophalangeal deformity, J.A.M.A. **198:**130-134, 1966.

Smith, R.J., and Kaplan, E.B.: Rheumatoid deformities at the metacarpophalangeal joints of the fingers, J. Bone Joint Surg. **49-A:**31-47, 1967.

Snorrason, E.: The problem of ulnar deviation of the fingers in rheumatoid arthritis, Acta Med. Scand. **140**(fasc. V):359-363, 1951.

Straub, L.R.: The etiology of finger deformities in the hand affected by rheumatoid arthritis, Bull. Hosp. Joint Dis. **21:**322-329, 1960.

Straub, L.R.: Surgical rehabilitation of the hand and upper extremity in rheumatoid arthritis, Bull. Rheum. Dis. **12:**5, 265-268, 1962.

Taleisnik, J.: Rheumatoid synovitis of the volar compartment of the wrist joint, J. Hand Surg. **4:**526-534, 1979.

Tsuge, K., Sanada, Y., and Nagayama, Y.: Surgical treatment of rheumatoid hand, Hiroshima J. Med. Sci. **15:**103-120, 1966.

Vainio, K., and Oka, M.: Ulnar deviation of the fingers, Ann. Rheum. Dis. **12:**122-124, 1953.

Vainio, K.: Personal communication, 1969.

Wise, K.S.: Anatomy of the metacarpophalangeal joints with observations of the aetiology of ulnar drift, J. Bone Joint Surg. **57-B:**485-490, 1975.

Zancolli, E.: Structural and dynamic bases of hand surgery, Philadelphia, 1968, J.B. Lippincott Co.

Author index

Subject index*

---

*Numerals in italics refer to pages on which
illustrations appear.